KU-051-931

The DRCOG Revision Guide

BRITISH MEDICAL ASSOCIATION

1000803

The DRCOG Revision Guide
Examination Preparation and Practice Questions

SECOND EDITION

SUSAN WARD
King's Mill Hospital, Sherwood Forest Hospitals Trust, Mansfield

LISA JOELS
Royal Devon and Exeter NHS Foundation Trust

ELAINE MELROSE
Retired Consultant Obstetrician and Gynaecologist, Ayrshire, Scotland

SRINIVAS VINDLA
King's Mill Hospital, Sherwood Forest Hospitals Trust, Mansfield

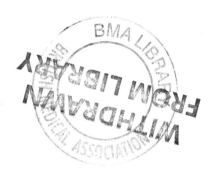

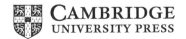
CAMBRIDGE
UNIVERSITY PRESS

CAMBRIDGE
UNIVERSITY PRESS

University Printing House, Cambridge CB2 8BS, United Kingdom

One Liberty Plaza, 20th Floor, New York, NY 10006, USA

477 Williamstown Road, Port Melbourne, VIC 3207, Australia

4843/24, 2nd Floor, Ansari Road, Daryaganj, Delhi – 110002, India

79 Anson Road, #06-04/06, Singapore 079906

Cambridge University Press is part of the University of Cambridge.

It furthers the University's mission by disseminating knowledge in the pursuit of education, learning, and research at the highest international levels of excellence.

www.cambridge.org
Information on this title: www.cambridge.org/9781316638620
DOI: 10.1017/9781316986745

© Susan Ward, Lisa Joels, Elaine Melrose, and Srinivas Vindla 2014, 2017

This publication is in copyright. Subject to statutory exception and to the provisions of relevant collective licensing agreements, no reproduction of any part may take place without the written permission of Cambridge University Press.

First published 2014
Second edition 2017

Printed in the United Kingdom by Clays, St Ives plc

A catalogue record for this publication is available from the British Library.

Library of Congress Cataloging-in-Publication Data
Names: Ward, Susan, 1957– | Joels, Lisa. | Melrose, Elaine | Vindla, Srinivas. |
Royal College of Obstetricians and Gynaecologists (Great Britain)
Title: The DRCOG revision guide: examination preparation and practice questions /
Susan Ward, King's Mill Hospital, Mansfield ; Lisa Joels, Elaine Melrose, Srinivas Vindla.
Other titles: Diploma of the Royal College of Obstetricians and Gynaecologists
revision guide
Description: Second edition. | Cambridge: Cambridge University Press, 2017. |
"The Diploma of the Royal College of Obstetricians and Gynaecologists" –
Introduction. | Includes bibliographical references and index.
Identifiers: LCCN 2016059495 | ISBN 9781316638620 (hard back)
Subjects: LCSH: Gynecology – Examinations, questions, etc. | Obstetrics – Examinations,
questions, etc. | Gynecology – Great Britain – Examinations,
questions, etc. | Obstetrics – Great Britain – Examinations, questions, etc.
Classification: LCC RG111.W37 2017 | DDC 618.10076–dc23
LC record available at https://lccn.loc.gov/2016059495

ISBN 978-1-316-63862-0 Paperback

Cambridge University Press has no responsibility for the persistence or accuracy of URLs for external or third-party Internet Web sites referred to in this publication and does not guarantee that any content on such Web sites is, or will remain, accurate or appropriate.

....

Every effort has been made in preparing this book to provide accurate and up-to-date information that is in accord with accepted standards and practice at the time of publication. Although case histories are drawn from actual cases, every effort has been made to disguise the identities of the individuals involved. Nevertheless, the authors, editors, and publishers can make no warranties that the information contained herein is totally free from error, not least because clinical standards are constantly changing through research and regulation. The authors, editors, and publishers therefore disclaim all liability for direct or consequential damages resulting from the use of material contained in this book. Readers are strongly advised to pay careful attention to information provided by the manufacturer of any drugs or equipment that they plan to use.

Contents

Foreword

This up-to-date revision text for the DRCOG examination fills a well-recognised gap in the market for potential candidates. The authors have taken a structured approach to the layout with an initial short section providing guidance on how to answer the different types of question found in the examination. For each of the seven modules in the women's health syllabus, a bank of questions has been written as single best answers (SBAs) and extended matching questions (EMQs) to ensure that the candidate is tested on relevant knowledge, whilst becoming familiar with the question styles. The rationale for the correct answer is then concisely explained in the answer section.

In addition, there are two complete mock examination papers in the same format as the actual examination to enable candidates to test their time management. All four authors have been members of the DRCOG subcommittee, so that the questions have been produced in the same way as questions in the actual examination – by a committee – which is a unique selling point when compared to other books on the market. The questions have been tested with real candidates sitting the DRCOG examination recently to check that the level of difficulty is appropriate.

I am delighted that this book has been produced, and I am sure that it will become the required reading for all DRCOG candidates.

Corinne Hargreaves, MRCOG
Consultant in Obstetrics and Gynaecology
Chair of the DRCOG Subcommittee 2011–2014

Abbreviations

A&E	Accident and Emergency
ABC	Airway, breathing, circulation
AFP	Alpha fetoprotein
AIDS	Acquired Immunodeficiency Syndrome
APH	Antepartum haemorrhage
BMI	Body Mass Index
BP	Blood Pressure
BV	Bacterial vaginosis
CBT	Cognitive Behavioural Therapy
CIN	Cervical intra-epithelial neoplasia
CNST	Clinical Negligence Scheme for Trusts
COC	Combined Oral Contraceptive Pill
CSF	Cerebrospinal fluid
CT	Computerized Tomography
CTG	Cardiotocograph
CTPA	Computed tomography pulmonary angiogram
CVS	Chorionic villus sampling
DNA	Deoxyribonucleic acid
DRCOG	Diploma of the Royal College of Obstetricians and Gynaecologists
DVT	Deep Vein Thrombosis
EC	Emergency contraception
ECG	Electrocardiogram
ECV	External cephalic version
EMQ	Extended Matching Question
FBC	Full blood count
FBS	Fetal blood sampling
FGM	Female Genital Mutilation
FSH	Follicle Stimulating Hormone
FSRH	Faculty of Sexual and Reproductive Health
GA	General Anaesthetic
GBS	Group B streptococcus
GI	Gastro-intestinal
GMC	General Medical Council
GnRH	Gonadotrophin Releasing Hormone
GP	General practitioner
GTT	Glucose tolerance test
GUM	Genitourinary Medicine
HAART	Highly active antiretroviral therapy
hCG	Human Chorionic Gonadotrophin
HIV	Human Immunodeficiency Virus
HPV	Human Papilloma Virus
HRT	Hormone Replacement Therapy
HSG	Hysterosalpingogram

HVS	High vaginal swab
HyCoSy	Hystero-salpingo contrast sonography
IM	Intramuscular
INR	International normalized ratio
IUCD	Intrauterine Contraceptive Device
IUD	Intrauterine Device
IUFD	Intra-uterine fetal death
IUGR	Intrauterine Growth Restriction
IUS	Intrauterine System
IV	Intravenous
IVF	In Vitro Fertilization
IVP	Intravenous Pyelogram
IVU	Intravenous Urogram
KUB	Kidney, Ureter, and Bladder (x-ray)
LARC	Long-acting reversible contraceptive
LFT	Liver Function Test
LH	Luteinizing Hormone
LHRH	Luteinizing Hormone Releasing Hormone
LLETZ	Large Loop Excision of the Transformation Zone (of the Cervix)
LMP	Last Menstrual Period
LMWH	Low molecular weight heparin
MCQ	Multiple Choice Question
MDT	Multidisciplinary Team
MRI	Magnetic Resonance Imaging
MSU	Midstream Specimen of Urine
MSV	Mauriceau-Smellie Veit manoeuvre
NHS	National Health Service
NICE	National Institute for health and care excellence
NG	Nasogastric
OA	Occipito-Anterior
O&G	Obstetrics and Gynaecology
OP	Occipito-Posterior
OSCE	Objective Structured Clinical Examination
PCB	Postcoital bleeding
PCO	Polycystic Ovary
PCOS	Polycystic ovarian syndrome
PCR	Polymerase Chain Reaction
PE	Pulmonary embolus
PID	Pelvic inflammatory disease
POP	Progesterone-only pill
PPH	Post partum haemorrhage
PROM	Premature rupture of the membranes
RCOG	Royal College of Obstetricians and Gynaecologists
RMI	Risk of Malignancy Index
SARC	Sexual Assault Referral Centre
SBA	Single Best Answer
SCBU	Special Care Baby Unit
SSRI	Selective Serotonin Reuptake Inhibitor
STI	Sexually Transmitted Infection
TB	Tuberculosis
TED	Thromboembolic disease prevention compression stockings
TOP	Termination of Pregnancy
TSH	Thyroid stimulating hormone
TVS	Transvaginal Scan

TVT	Tension-Free Vaginal Tape
U&E	Urea and Electrolytes
USS	Ultrasound Scan
UTI	Urinary tract infection
VBAC	Vaginal Birth after Caesarean Section
VIN	Vulval intra-epithelial neoplasia
VTE	Venous thromboembolism
VZIG	Varicella Zoster Immunoglobulin
WHO	World Health Organisation

Introduction

This volume is not a textbook; it is intended as a guide focussing on question practice for candidates studying for the Diploma of the Royal College of Obstetricians and Gynaecologists (DRCOG) examination. It is set out in a format aligned to the DRCOG syllabus with each chapter relating to one of the seven modules, containing examples of the type of questions that could be asked about that particular subject. As well as becoming more familiar with the style of the examination, candidates can use the specimen questions to assess their knowledge about that section of the syllabus and identify where best to concentrate their revision efforts.

The DRCOG is a clinically orientated examination. Any doctor who has spent a few months in a busy obstetric and gynaecology post will have a good chance of passing after spending some time studying. When choosing which books to use for revision it is important to realise that the examination is intended to be relevant to doctors working in general practice in the United Kingdom, where women's health issues represent a large proportion of the workload. There are many books on the market aimed at candidates revising for the DRCOG and also many written for general practitioners (GPs) with an interest in women's health.

The questions in this book have been written by four consultants, all of whom have been on the DRCOG Examination Subcommittee and who have written questions for the actual examination. As well as making suggestions regarding strategy and technique for answering the questions, we have included many examples of both types of question for each section of the syllabus to give you some idea of the form, content, and level of difficulty of the questions you might encounter in the examination.

The chapters represent each of the seven sections of the syllabus. Each chapter contains twenty SBA questions and six EMQs with five parts to each question – a total of 140 SBAs and 210 EMQs within the main part of the book. This should give you plenty of practice!

In addition, there is a separate mock exam in the two-part format currently used for the DRCOG examination that you could use to practise time management.

As each of the authors has participated in the setting of the actual examination over the last few years, we have tried to give you some idea of the thought processes behind the answers provided. These comments are representative of the discussions around the table at the DRCOG Examination Subcommittee meetings where the examination is constructed. The committee consists of a group of obstetricians and gynaecologists with different special interests and GPs. Every time a new question is added to the question bank, the GPs are asked to assess whether the content is 'reasonable knowledge that could be expected of a GP with an interest in women's health in the UK' as the committee is keen to avoid setting questions that test membership examination–level knowledge.

Each paper is standard-set by a group of GPs whose work is very valuable to the college, as they are aware of the level of knowledge expected from candidates sitting the examination. Their input ensures that different diets of the examination are comparable and that it is a fair assessment.

We have tried to give you some suggestions as to where to find the knowledge being tested in the examination. During the meetings where the questions are set, the committee has at its disposal a wide range of textbooks and resources such as the British National Formulary, along with the National Institute for Health and Care Excellence guidelines and the 'Green-top' guidelines produced by the college. These guidelines can be accessed from the Royal College of Obstetricians and Gynaecologists (RCOG) website and are now collected into a compendium available as a book, data stick, or app for your mobile telephone/computer tablet. The guidelines would be a good starting point for your revision because some of the questions are set directly from there. It is also worth familiarising yourself with the report on *Confidential Enquiries into Maternal Deaths in the United Kingdom*; the most recent edition before this book was written was produced in December 2015 covering the maternal deaths between 2009 and 2012 (called the MBRRACE-UK report accessible from the RCOG website). In addition, we have provided a list of other websites where you can find useful information to guide your revision.

We hope you enjoy studying for this examination: your patients will certainly benefit from the knowledge you acquire. Good luck!

The DRCOG Exam

In this chapter we explain the format of the exam and discuss the two different styles of question as a foundation for giving you hints and tips about how to approach the questions and apply your knowledge logically in order to answer correctly. This will be consolidated in subsequent chapters as we explain each of the examples.

The Exam Format and a Bit of History

The format of the examination was changed from a written exam and an Objective Structured Clinical Examination (OSCE) to just a written exam a few years ago with the first new-style paper appearing in April 2007. The new exam comprised two written papers; the first paper consisted of ten EMQs with three parts to each question and eighteen SBA questions. The second was a multiple choice question (MCQ) paper consisting of forty questions each with five parts (200 questions in total).

The format will be changed again from 2017 onwards because it is widely acknowledged that the MCQ true/false style questions are less effective at testing applied clinical knowledge. They do not discriminate as effectively between candidates, and they are not really suitable for assessing medics as they rely on 'absolutes', which seldom exist in medicine.

Now that the MCQs have been removed, the exam you are currently studying for will still be two papers, but paper 1 will have forty EMQs and paper 2 will have sixty SBA questions. Each paper will last ninety minutes and you will get two time warnings: thirty minutes and then ten minutes before the end of the examination.

The questions are weighted differently. The EMQs score 3 for each correct answer and represent 50 per cent of your total marks. The SBA questions score 2 each and comprise the other 50 per cent of your marks. The reason for this is that there is thought to be a great deal more reasoning and application of knowledge needed when answering an EMQ so it is worth more.

At the end of this book there is a complete mock examination – paper 1 and paper 2 – which you could use to practise time management under examination conditions, not forgetting that your answers must be transferred to the computer-marked answer paper before leaving the exam hall on the actual examination day.

The rationale for changing the exam was to improve reliability and validity by removing the subjective aspects of assessment in both the written and face-to-face elements of the OSCE. The whole paper is now marked by computer, significantly improving validity by standardisation. The exam is further improved by a standard setting process whereby a 'more difficult' examination paper will have a lower pass mark than an 'easier' paper, ensuring that the pass mark constantly reflects a competent candidate with the necessary knowledge skills and attitudes.

In reality the pass mark is somewhere between 60 and 70 per cent, usually towards the upper part of the range. It differs between exams because of the standard setting, but if you are scoring more than 70 per cent in your revision practice, you are probably doing well enough to pass. The top mark is usually between 85 and 95 per cent and the highest scoring candidate (on their first attempt) is awarded the DRCOG Prize Medal. Could this be you?

Extended Matching Questions

It is likely that you will have previously come across EMQs during your training. It helps to know that, for each list of options the committee may have written quite a few questions for the bank, but only a couple are used in the actual exam. This explains why some of the options might look a bit unusual or irrelevant, but don't be put off by this. The options in both the EMQs and the SBAs will be in alphabetical order, so that the order in which they appear on the list will not give you any clues as to the correct answer.

The format of the EMQs in the DRCOG examination is shown in this example:

OPTION LIST

A	Ask a shop assistant for help
B	Call the police
C	Continue shopping
D	Give the child a bag of crisps
E	Ignore the child until it stops screaming
F	Lie on the floor and scream
G	Pick up the child and walk out
H	Pour water over the child
I	Smack the child
J	Walk out of the shop

INSTRUCTIONS

Each of the following situations relate to parenting skills. For each situation select the single most appropriate course of action. Each answer may be used once, more than once, or not at all.

1. A 29-year-old woman is carrying out her weekly shopping with her 2-year-old child. Halfway around the supermarket the child becomes fractious and asks for a bag of crisps. When the woman says no, the child throws a temper tantrum lying on the floor, screaming and crying. Other shoppers are beginning to point and stare.

Don't worry, parenting skills aren't part of the DRCOG curriculum, but this example can be used to show how knowledge skills and attitudes can be applied to ensure the correct answer is selected.

How to tackle this question:

The best way of tackling the EMQs is to read very briefly down the list of options but then cover up the options and use your knowledge, skills, and attitudes to work out the answer as if you were answering the questions verbally.

If the first answer that comes in to your head is on the list of options, it is very likely that this is the correct option. Now read the whole option list very carefully and double check that your chosen option is the 'single correct answer'.

You should be aware that there is usually at least one 'distracter' on each list: that is, an option that is nearly correct, but good candidates will know why the distracter is not the correct option. The clinical details given in the stem usually contain the information that you need to separate the correct option from the distracter(s).

Double check the question again to make sure you haven't missed a subtle fact and that you've interpreted the situation correctly.

So how should you answer this question? Use your experience; if you have looked after a toddler (i.e., for a clinical question you will be using your experience of working in obstetrics and gynaecology) this will be a familiar situation. You will need some knowledge of the psychology of parenting (clinical knowledge gained from reading textbooks) and you will need to be aware of child protection issues and safety concerns (ethics and law). Applying your skills/experience, knowledge, and attitudes you can correctly select the answer E – ignore the child until it stops screaming – which will ensure that you finish your shopping and avoid child protection services.

EMQs are specifically designed to test interpretation of a scenario and demonstrate application of knowledge, skills, and attitudes and therefore are unlikely to be found as a paragraph in a textbook. We have deliberately constructed the questions to reflect potential clinical scenarios that could be encountered by a GP or GP trainee.

Two or three questions follow each option list. Each option may be used more than once or not at all, that is, it is possible that one of the options could be the correct answer for two of the questions. If the list of options looks a bit unusual, the reason for this is that the committee writes many more questions to go with each option list so that there is a large bank of questions available looking at various aspects of a clinical scenario. An unusual option may belong to another question on the bank, so don't fall into the trap of assuming that because it's an unusual option that you hadn't thought of, then it must be the correct answer.

Single Best Answer Questions

SBA questions – used to be called 'best of fives' – are similar to EMQs in requiring application of knowledge as opposed to direct recall of facts. The majority of SBAs are also based on a clinical scenario that requires interpretation of facts in order to select the single best answer, but this can be either the most appropriate or the least appropriate answer depending on how the question is phrased. For example, an SBA based on a similar scenario to that in the preceding text might be:

A 29-year-old woman is trying to cope with her 2-year-old child who is having a temper tantrum in the middle of a supermarket. Which of the following is the most appropriate course of action?

A. Distract the child with something interesting to look at

B. Ignore the child until it calms down

C.   Leave the store and go home
D.   Pacify the child with sweets
E.   Remove the child to a safe place

These options initially all look plausible and very similar, however if you reflect on your reading of parenting manuals (textbooks) you will recall that bribing with sweets will set up a vicious cycle resulting in worsening behaviour, and your experience tells you that a toddler in a full-blown tantrum is not distractible. Leaving the store rewards bad behaviour, and if you review carefully the scenario it's hard to imagine a supermarket as being a particularly dangerous place (experience) unless you 'overthink' the question and imagine the child to be next to an unstable display of baked bean cans or something similar. Again the answer is B – ignore the child until it calms down.

The message here is: carefully assess the information given but don't read complexity into the scenario where there is none.

In the actual examination, you can use the question booklet to write on and make notes (as it is not read when it is returned to the College), but you must transfer your answers to the computer-marked sheet before the examination finishes. The risk of leaving gaps on the answer sheet as you progress through the examination is that you might incorrectly transcribe your answers and lose marks when your answers were originally correct. You are supplied with an eraser to make corrections, and you must be very careful when you've finally chosen your answers to make sure that you complete the answer sheet correctly.

The examiners try hard to avoid predictable patterns when selecting the questions. Great care is also taken to avoid questions that have 'always' or 'never' as these are obviously incorrect given the nature of clinical medicine. If a question looks like an 'always or never' scenario, re-read it as you may have missed a crucial part of the question.

Revising for the Exam

The DRCOG exam strives to be relevant to general practice and therefore focuses on core knowledge rather than rarities and minutiae; however, facts such as maternal mortality rate, prevalence, and incidence are considered core knowledge and may feature in the exam. These facts are unlikely to be the topic of your ward rounds, handovers, or reflective practice sessions so it really does pay to revise.

Each examination diet is blueprinted to ensure that all areas of the syllabus are covered, so the best advice is to ensure that you have covered the whole syllabus in your reading and revision, rather than trying to 'spot' questions.

In addition to the textbooks you used as an undergraduate, there are several books on the market covering issues relevant to women's health in general practice, and we suggest that you also access specific texts on contraception and genitourinary medicine. We have provided a list of websites where you will find helpful information about some topics that could come up in the examination, and although this list is not exhaustive, we think you will find that the websites contain interesting revision material.

Doing exam questions is a very good way to revise, and it is highly recommended that you re-read a topic where your score is disappointing – you will be even more disappointed if it comes up in the examination and you have neglected to revisit that topic and top up your knowledge.

Whilst you are revising, don't forget to eat, sleep, and relax too – all these things will improve your performance!

Conclusions

The DRCOG uses two different question formats to test objectively the applied knowledge, skills, and attitudes of all areas of the syllabus to the standard of a GP practising in the United Kingdom. To pass the exam reading and revision is required, but understanding the style of questions and practising questions will improve your chance of success.

Curriculum Module 1

Basic Clinical Skills

Syllabus

▦ You will be expected to understand the patterns of symptoms in patients presenting with obstetric problems, gynaecological problems, and sexually transmitted infections, and in patients in a family planning setting.

▦ You will be expected to demonstrate an understanding of the pathophysiological basis of physical signs and understand the indications, risks, benefits, and effectiveness of investigations in a clinical setting.

▦ You will be required to demonstrate an understanding of the components of effective verbal and nonverbal communication.

▦ You will need to be aware of relevant ethical and legal issues including the implications of the legal status of the unborn child, the legal issues relating to medical certification, and issues related to medical confidentiality.

▦ You will be expected to understand the issues surrounding consent in all clinical situations including postmortem examination and termination of pregnancy.

Learning Outcomes

This module covers history taking; clinical examination and investigation; note keeping; legal issues relating to medical certification; time management and decision making; communication; and ethics and legal issues. It is easy to set clinical questions on history, examination, or investigation, but quite a challenge to set written questions to test the other areas. Previously *viva voce* examinations such as the OSCE were used to test communication skills. The OSCE component of the DRCOG has now been abandoned because nobody ever failed due to poor communication skills.

Although you might imagine that attributes such as 'good time management' could not be tested in a written format, we can test this to some extent – for example whether a candidate can prioritise clinical cases safely – using both EMQ and SBA formats.

We have also tried to look at attitudes and behaviour using written questions concentrating on issues such as consent, domestic violence, and confidentiality. We recommend that you have a look at the General Medical Council (GMC) website (especially 'Duties of a Doctor') to find information about these attitudinal and ethical issues, and of course you should discuss cases with your supervisors in both Obstetrics and Gynaecology (O&G) and general practice.

Single Best Answer Questions

1.1 Pelvic pain is a common problem in women of childbearing age. When taking a history, which of the following symptoms suggests that the diagnosis might be endometriosis?

A. Abdominal distension

B. Dyschezia

C. Pain throughout the menstrual cycle

D. Primary dysmenorrhoea

E. Superficial dyspareunia

Answer [ ]

1.2 Pregnancy is known to provoke episodes of domestic violence, and GPs, midwives, and obstetricians are encouraged to be aware of the possibility. Which of the following might raise the suspicion of domestic abuse?

A. All the family turn up for every antenatal appointment

B. Repeated failure to attend antenatal appointments

C. The woman always brings a female relative to translate for her

D. There is a linear burn across the patient's abdomen that occurred during ironing

E. The woman seems unsure about her request for termination of unwanted pregnancy

Answer [ ]

1.3 Which of these conditions causes primary rather than secondary amenorrhoea?

A. Asherman syndrome

B. Anorexia nervosa

C. Polycystic ovarian syndrome

D. Rokintansky syndrome

E. Sheehan syndrome

Answer [ ]

1.4 A 27-year-old woman attends the surgery for booking in her fourth pregnancy. She has a body mass index (BMI) of 38 and has had three previous caesarean sections, delivering babies of more than 4 kg each time. Which complication is a recognised extra risk factor for her in this pregnancy?

A. Antepartum haemorrhage

B. Placenta accreta

C. Postpartum haemorrhage

D. Intrauterine growth restriction

E. Pre-eclampsia

Answer [ ]

1.5 When a woman presents with an ovarian cyst, the gynaecologist works out the 'risk of malignancy index' (RMI), which helps to evaluate the likelihood of the ovarian cyst being malignant.

Which of the following contributes to the RMI?

A. Solid areas in the cyst on computerized tomography (CT) scan
B. The age of the woman
C. The CA15-3 tumour marker level
D. The menopausal status of the woman
E. A family history of ovarian cancer

Answer   [   ]

1.6 About 15 per cent of pregnant women will be rhesus negative.

When they suffer an early pregnancy complication, which one of these non-sensitised, rhesus negative women does not need anti-D immunoglobulin?

A. Miscarriage less than 12 weeks when the uterus is evacuated surgically or medically
B. Ectopic pregnancy
C. Incomplete miscarriage more than 12 weeks
D. Complete miscarriage less than 12 weeks when bleeding is heavy
E. Threatened miscarriage less than 12 weeks when the fetus is viable

Answer   [   ]

1.7 Maternal deaths in the United Kingdom are reported nationally and the World Health Organisation keeps records of the rates worldwide.

With relation to maternal death, which of these statements is correct?

A. Every maternal death in the United Kingdom is scrutinised to look for substandard care
B. Reducing the number of maternal deaths worldwide by the year 2050 is a 'millennium development goal'
C. The maternal mortality rate is lower in the United States than in the United Kingdom
D. The maternal mortality ratio is defined as the number of maternal deaths per hundred thousand pregnancies
E. There were no maternal deaths from swine flu in the last epidemic

Answer   [   ]

1.8 A nulliparous 22-year-old woman presents with a 3-month history of inter-menstrual bleeding. She is healthy with no other medical problems and is using the withdrawal method for contraception.

Select the most likely diagnosis:

A. Cervical cancer
B. Chlamydia infection
C. Endometrial polyp
D. Nabothian follicle on the cervix
E. Ovarian granulosa cell tumour

Answer   [   ]

1.9 A primigravid woman who is 33 weeks pregnant has just arrived in the United Kingdom from Africa to visit her family. She presents to the surgery feeling ill with joint pains and diarrhoea. She has a temperature and may be infected with the Ebola virus.

Which of the following statements is correct regarding Ebola infection in pregnancy?

A. If she delivers whilst she is ill, she will be able to breast-feed her baby
B. The main Ebola viral load is concentrated in the fetus and placenta
C. The fetus is likely to survive if delivered now because she is in the third trimester
D. The maternal mortality rate is around 10 per cent
E. Viral spread is by inhaled airborne droplets

Answer [ ]

1.10 A 43-year-old smoker attends the emergency department at 35 weeks of gestation complaining of sudden onset of central chest pain. On examination she is pale and sweaty with a tachycardia of 120 bpm. Her temperature and blood pressure are normal.

She has had three normal births in the past. Her BMI is 35 but she is otherwise fit and well, and this pregnancy has been straightforward so far.

Which is the most likely diagnosis?

A. Cardiac ischaemia
B. Chest infection
C. Pneumothorax
D. Pulmonary embolus
E. Reflux oesophagitis

Answer [ ]

1.11 Taking over the gynaecology on-call duties one evening, you are given this list of tasks to be done on the ward.

Select the task that takes priority:

A. Site an intravenous infusion for a severely dehydrated patient with hyperemesis
B. Sign a death certificate as a patient's husband is waiting on the ward for it
C. Review the scan report of a woman with a suspected ectopic pregnancy
D. Review a woman who has just miscarried an 18-week fetus but not delivered the placenta
E. Clerk a new patient that a GP has sent in to hospital with a suspected torted ovarian cyst

Answer [ ]

1.12 You are trying to persuade a postoperative woman with a haemoglobin of 55 g/L that she would not be so breathless if she had a blood transfusion, but she is concerned about the risk of acquiring human immunodeficiency virus (HIV). The chance of acquiring HIV infection as a result of blood transfusion in the United Kingdom is approximately:

A. 1 in 6,000
B. 1 in 60,000
C. 1 in 600,000
D. 1 in 6 million
E. 1 in 60 million

Answer [ ]

1.13 The community midwife doing an antenatal clinic in your GP surgery asks you to see a 37-year-old obese woman who has come for a routine checkup at 32 weeks of gestation in her first pregnancy. Her booking blood pressure in the first trimester was 130/88 mmHg but it is now 160/95 mmHg, and the midwife has checked the blood pressure twice. The woman is asymptomatic. Which is the most appropriate course of action?

A. Urinalysis and prescribe antihypertensives if no proteinuria
B. Send urgent full blood count, urate, and liver function test (LFT)
C. Refer her urgently to hospital for further investigation and treatment
D. Urinalysis and request urgent antenatal appointment if no proteinuria
E. Twenty-four-hour urine collection for protein analysis

Answer [ ]

1.14 A 52-year-old woman presents to your surgery with a very sore vulva. On examination you find thickening of both labia minora with a couple of shallow ulcers on both sides and a split area at the fourchette. What is the most likely diagnosis in her case?

A. Eczema
B. Genital herpes
C. Lichen planus
D. Lichen sclerosus
E. Vulval intra-epithelial neoplasia

Answer [ ]

1.15 The clinical scenarios detailed in the following text describe gynaecological patients admitted as an emergency. Which patient is most likely to have a diagnosis of ectopic pregnancy?

A. Acute onset of central abdominal pain and nausea at 12 weeks of gestation. On examination severe lower abdominal tenderness with generalised guarding and rebound, also foetor oris. White cell count is $18 \times 10^9/l$ and urinalysis is negative.
B. History of 11 weeks' amenorrhea and brown vaginal discharge but no pain. Pelvic examination reveals no tenderness but uterus is small for dates and the cervical os is closed. Serum βhCG is 2,010 IU/ml and scan is awaited.
C. Seven weeks' amenorrhea and vaginal bleeding. Pelvic examination reveals no tenderness. Uterus is soft and slightly enlarged with an open cervical os.

D.   Admitted with bleeding and lower abdominal pain at 8 weeks of gestation. Transvaginal ultrasound scan shows an intrauterine sac with a fetal pole but no heart pulsation detected. Serum βhCG is 150 000 IU/ml.

E.   Patient with lower abdominal and shoulder tip pain who has a copper coil fitted. Last menstrual period was 2 weeks ago and on examination has a tender abdomen with guarding. Urinary hCG test positive in accident and emergency (A&E).

Answer [ ]

1.16 A 46-year-old woman presents to her GP seeking help with her period problems, which date back almost a year. Her cycles are still regular with a cycle of 26 days but the bleeding is now very heavy with clots. She complains of severe secondary dysmenorrhoea but no other pelvic pain. On examination there are no masses palpable in the pelvis. The uterus is enlarged to the size of an orange, smooth, and very tender but mobile with no adnexal tenderness.

Select the most likely gynaecological cause of this clinical picture:

A.   Adenomyosis
B.   Chronic pelvic inflammatory disease
C.   Endometriosis
D.   Endometrial hyperplasia
E.   Fibroids

Answer [ ]

1.17 A 39-year-old woman asks for a hospital referral so that she can be investigated for recurrent miscarriage, having suffered three first trimester pregnancy losses. She believes that her miscarriages are due to stress. She works long hours as a computer programmer and smokes fifteen cigarettes a day. Which of the following factors is the most likely cause of her recurrent miscarriages?

A.   Working with visual display units
B.   Smoking
C.   Advanced maternal age
D.   Natural killer cells
E.   Bacterial vaginosis

Answer [ ]

1.18 In your GP surgery the practice nurse asks you to see a 25-year-old lady who is unable to tolerate speculum examination for her first smear test. The patient tells you that she has experienced severe dyspareunia since her marriage 2 years ago and discloses that she was sexually abused as a child. Which of the following statements about child abuse is untrue?

A.   Abuse in childhood predisposes to depressive illness in later life that does not respond to treatment
B.   Child abuse encompasses neglect as well as physical and sexual abuse
C.   Somatisation as an adult can be a result of child abuse
D.   Women who have been abused as children rarely disclose such a history

E.   Abuse in childhood is known to be associated with illicit drug use as an adult

Answer [ ]

1.19 The mother of a 13-year-old girl attends the surgery for advice. Her daughter has been offered human papilloma virus (HPV) vaccine at school but did not bring an information leaflet home, so she wants to know more about it.

Which one of these statements about the quadrivalent vaccine (Gardasil®) is correct?

A.   She will require three doses of the vaccine over 6 months
B.   The vaccine will reduce the chance of her developing genital warts as well as cervical intraepithelial neoplasia
C.   If she completes the course of vaccinations she will not need cervical smears in the future
D.   The vaccine is not appropriate if she is already sexually active
E.   The vaccine is made from live attenuated HPV

Answer [ ]

1.20 Which one of the following statements is true in relation to women with Turner syndrome?

A.   They have no problems with learning difficulties
B.   Estrogen therapy may result in spontaneous fertility
C.   There is a high prevalence of left-sided congenital heart malformation
D.   Administration of growth hormone at puberty will not produce any extra height
E.   They all have karyotype 46XO

Answer [ ]

Extended Matching Questions

A	CT scan of the pelvis
B	Cystoscopy
C	Diagnostic laparoscopy
D	Dye laparoscopy
E	High vaginal swab for chlamydia
F	Hysterosalpingogram
G	Magnetic resonance imaging (MRI) scan of the pelvis
H	Serum CA125 level
I	Transvaginal ultrasound scan
J	Urodynamic study

Each of these clinical scenarios describes a woman presenting with symptoms of pelvic pain; for each case pick the most appropriate initial investigation given the information that you are presented with.

Each option may be used once, more than once, or not at all.

1.21 Secondary dysmenorrhoea in a 40-year-old nulliparous woman with a BMI of 48. Over the last year her periods have become heavier and she is not currently sexually active.

Answer [ ]

1.22 A 38-year-old woman complains of premenstrual pain, severe secondary dysmenorrhea, and dyschezia

Answer [ ]

1.23 A 24-year-old secretary with noncyclical pain and deep dyspareunia who has been trying to get pregnant for 2 years

Answer [ ]

1.24 A postmenopausal woman with left iliac fossa pain radiating down her leg, whose abdominal ultrasound scan (USS) shows a 9 cm septated cyst adjacent to the uterus on the left side with free fluid around it

Answer [ ]

1.25 A 62-year-old woman with severe urinary frequency for 8 weeks associated with dyspareunia

Answer [ ]

A	Bleeding corpus luteum cyst
B	Ectopic pregnancy
C	Gastroenteritis
D	Heterotopic pregnancy
E	Ovarian hyperstimulation syndrome
F	Ovarian torsion
G	Pelvic sepsis
H	Pulmonary embolism
I	Threatened miscarriage

These women have all undergone assisted conception treatment with in vitro fertilization (IVF) and have developed complications. For each clinical scenario select the most likely diagnosis.

Each option may be used once, more than once, or not at all.

1.26 Following a cycle of IVF, a young woman is pregnant for the first time. She presents to A&E with increasing lower abdominal pain and diarrhoea. She has had brown vaginal loss for a couple of days. On examination she is pale with a tachycardia of 100 bpm but her blood pressure is normal. An urgent ultrasound scan shows an endometrial thickness of 12 mm but no gestation sac seen.

Answer [ ]

1.27 A slightly obese woman with polycystic ovarian syndrome is admitted a week after an IVF cycle during which 12 oocytes were collected. She had an embryo transfer 5 days previously and now has shortness of breath, nausea, and abdominal pain. Her abdomen is distended on examination.

Answer [ ]

1.28 A 27-year-old woman is admitted to the gynaecology ward as an emergency with severe abdominal pain and vomiting. She is unable to lie still and scores her pain 9 out of 10. On examination she is apyrexial, tachycardic, and normotensive. She has a tender mass on the left side of the pelvis. She had a cycle of IVF recently with oocyte recovery 10 days previously, followed by embryo transfer 2 days later.

Answer [ ]

1.29 Three weeks after a cycle of IVF a 34-year-old woman presents to her GP with increasing pain in the lower abdomen and rigors. She only had one embryo replaced in the uterus because only one of the oocytes that were retrieved fertilised.

Answer [ ]

1.30 A pregnant woman is rushed to A&E in the United Kingdom having collapsed at the airport. She had a cycle of IVF in another country 7 weeks ago, during which three embryos were replaced in the uterus. She has a scan picture with her, showing an intrauterine pregnancy with a viable 6-week fetus.

Her blood pressure is 85/45 mmHg, her pulse is 120 bpm, her temperature is 36.5°C and on abdominal examination she has rigidity, rebound tenderness, and guarding. Pelvic examination reveals tenderness in the left adnexa, and she has cervical excitation. Her haemoglobin is 95 g/l and her white cell count is $8 \times 10^9/l$.

Answer [ ]

A	Bacterial vaginosis
B	Beta-haemolytic streptococcus
C	Candida
D	Chlamydia
E	Gonorrhoea
F	Herpes genitalis
G	Primary syphilis
H	Streptococcus A (streptococcus pyogenes)
I	Trichomonas vaginalis

These clinical scenarios relate to women presenting to a hospital clinic or general practice surgery. Select the most likely infecting organism given the clinical information for each woman.

Each option may be used once, more than once, or not at all.

1.31 A 23-year-old woman is admitted 2 days postpartum with severe sepsis. Her temperature is 38°C, pulse 110 bpm; her respiratory rate is raised; and her uterus is enlarged and tender. She has a sore throat with a red pharynx and white spots on her tonsils on examination.

Answer [ ]

1.32 A 55-year-old diabetic woman presents to her GP with a 6-week history of a sore vulva. On examination her vulval skin is red and excoriated.

Answer [ ]

1.33 A 19-year-old presents to the practice nurse with postcoital bleeding and on speculum examination her cervix bleeds on contact.

Answer [ ]

1.34 A primigravid woman is admitted in labour at term. Her uterus is tender and a diagnosis of chorioamnionitis is made. Postnatally the baby develops meningitis.

Answer [ ]

1.35 A 22-year-old woman is admitted to the gynaecology ward with acute retention of urine. On examination she has a sore vulva.

Answer [ ]

A	Colposcopy
B	Colposcopy and cervical biopsy
C	Dilatation and curettage
D	Endometrial biopsy using sampling device
E	Hysteroscopy and endometrial biopsy
F	HPV typing
G	Liquid-based cervical cytology
H	MRI scan of abdomen and pelvis
I	Transvaginal ultrasound scan

The scenarios described in the following text relate to women whose GP suspects that they might have cancer, so they have been referred to a gynaecology clinic with an urgent '2-week wait' appointment. For each patient select the most appropriate investigation given the clinical information described in each case.

Each option may be used once, more than once, or not at all.

1.36 A 48-year-old diabetic woman with a BMI of 48 presents with a history of irregular periods and intermenstrual bleeding. She is nulliparous.

Answer [ ]

1.37 A 26-year-old woman attends for her first smear at the GP's surgery and mentions that she has experienced postcoital bleeding for the last 6 months. Whilst taking the smear, a friable 3 mm diameter red lesion is noted on her cervix, which bleeds profusely.

Answer [ ]

1.38 A 57-year-old woman goes to see her GP complaining of indigestion and abdominal distension. She has had a CA125 blood test done privately and the result is 60 iu/l.

Answer [ ]

1.39 A worried 31-year-old refugee woman presents to the surgery a few weeks after arrival in the country saying that her younger sister has just died of cervical cancer back home. She wishes to be reassured that she does not have it too.

Answer [ ]

1.40 A 32-year-old nulliparous woman presents with lower abdominal pain and severe dysmenorrhoea three years after radiotherapy treatment for cancer of the cervix. On examination her cervix looks normal but atrophic with radiotherapy changes and an ultrasound scan shows that the cavity of the uterus is distended with blood.

Answer [ ]

A	Discuss with on-call consultant
B	Discuss with on-call registrar (Specialty Trainee year 4)
C	Leave for consultant to deal with on his return
D	No action required
E	Phone GP
F	Phone patient
G	Post a prescription to patient
H	Recall urgently to gynaecology clinic next week
I	Refer to gynae-oncology multidisciplinary team (MDT) meeting
J	Routine gynaecology clinic follow up
K	Write to GP
L	Write to patient

The rest of your clinical team are away and your consultant's secretary has asked you to go through some messages and results in his in-tray. For each of the following scenarios select the most appropriate course of action to ensure the best use of National Health Service (NHS) time and resources, as well as considering the safest and most convenient solution for the patient.

Each option may be used once, more than once, or not at all.

1.41 A 28-year-old woman attended the antenatal clinic a few days ago for a growth scan at 28 weeks of gestation and gave a history of an offensive vaginal discharge for the last week. The result of the high vaginal swab is reported as showing clue cells on microscopy and profuse anaerobes on culture.

Answer [ ]

1.42 An 18-year-old woman attended the emergency gynaecology clinic 2 days ago with pelvic pain, discharge, and postcoital bleeding for the preceding fortnight. The endocervical swab result shows chlamydia trachomatis detected by polymerase chain reaction (PCR).

Answer [ ]

1.43 A GP has written a letter about a 30-year-old woman with a 2-year history of pelvic pain. She has been previously seen in the gynaecology clinic by your consultant and was advised to start the combined oral contraceptive pill. She is getting headaches so has discontinued the pill but is still getting pelvic pain.

Answer [ ]

1.44 A 23-year-old woman was seen in the gynaecology clinic 2 weeks ago with a 3-month history of pelvic pain throughout the cycle. Examination showed no abnormality, no tenderness on vaginal examination, and the high vaginal and endocervical swabs were negative. In clinic, you gave her an advice leaflet about irritable bowel syndrome and organised an ultrasound scan. The scan result shows a normal-sized anteverted uterus, both ovaries are clearly seen and are normal. There is no free fluid and there are no adnexal masses.

Answer [ ]

1.45 A 22-year-old woman was admitted as an emergency 1 week ago. She was found to have a torted ovarian cyst and had a laparoscopic oophorectomy. The rest of her pelvis was normal, and she was given that information before discharge. The histology report on the cyst shows a mature cystic teratoma (dermoid cyst).

Answer [ ]

A	Appendicitis
B	Complete mole
C	Ectopic pregnancy
D	Hyperemesis gravidarum
E	Incomplete miscarriage
F	Missed miscarriage
G	Partial hydatidiform mole
H	Threatened miscarriage
I	Urinary tract infection

The following clinical scenarios describe pregnant women presenting with acute problems. In each case select the most likely diagnosis.
Each option may be used once, more than once, or not at all.

1.46 Having had a positive pregnancy test two weeks after her missed period, a 29-year-old primigravid woman is referred to have a scan because of vaginal bleeding. On arrival in the Early Pregnancy Unit the bleeding is noted to be heavy and when you insert a speculum you find that the cervical os is open.

Answer [ ]

1.47 A 28-year-old woman has a transvaginal ultrasound scan on the Early Pregnancy Unit at 8 weeks of gestation because of vaginal bleeding. The uterus is larger than expected with a closed os. The scan shows an abnormal-looking intrauterine sac with a fetal pole but no heart pulsation detected. Her serum βhCG is 150 000 IU/ml.

Answer [ ]

1.48 A 28-year-old woman attends her GP's surgery asking for a pregnancy test after 14 weeks of amenorrhoea. She feels unwell and has been vomiting throughout the day. On examination she is tachycardic, sweaty, and has a tremor. Her uterus is easily palpable and the fundus is just below the umbilicus.

Answer [ ]

1.49 Having reached 11 weeks of gestation, a 22-year-old woman is relieved when her morning sickness disappears. A week later she is devastated when her booking scan shows an irregular sac which is 10 weeks' size. A fetal pole is present but cardiac activity is absent.

Answer [ ]

1.50 A GP refers a pregnant 19-year-old woman at 14 weeks of gestation because she has been vomiting for the last week. She has no diarrhoea but is clinically very dehydrated. Urine dip is positive for ketones, nitrites, and protein.

Answer [ ]

Curriculum Module 2

Basic Surgical Skills

Syllabus

■ You will be expected to demonstrate an understanding of commonly performed obstetric and gynaecological surgical procedures including their complications and the legal issues around consent to surgical procedures.

■ You will need to be aware of commonly encountered infections, including an understanding of the principles of infection control.

■ You will be expected to interpret preoperative investigations and be aware of the principles involved in appropriate preoperative and postoperative care.

Learning Outcomes

Although you might think that this topic is not relevant to GPs with little or no involvement in surgical events happening in secondary care, we feel that some core knowledge is necessary. For example, patients often wish to be able to discuss their proposed treatment with their GP or they may develop a surgical complication after they have left hospital. Increasingly, GPs are taking on postoperative follow-up for patients to move care out of hospital into the community. It is usually the GP who is asked to supply certification for time off work or asked for information about driving, resuming intercourse, and so forth.

Therefore, although you would not be expected to perform the operations yourself, a basic knowledge of the technicalities of gynaecological and obstetric operations is useful in this context, and you may have picked up some of this if you have worked as a junior doctor in obstetrics and gynaecology. Some of the knowledge is transferable from other surgical specialties, and everyone will have some exposure to some sort of surgery during their previous training.

You may need to refer to your undergraduate textbooks, or there may be some guidelines on the RCOG website that you might find useful, for example, 'birth after previous caesarean' and 'blood transfusion in obstetrics'. There are also a set of clinical governance guidelines on the RCOG website (accessible to nonmembers) that cover obtaining consent for many obstetric and gynaecological operations and procedures. These are full of useful information such as the possible complications and are highly recommended source material.

Single Best Answer Questions

2.1 A woman is about to have a caesarean section for placenta praevia and has been counselled about the risk of haemorrhage. She asks if there is a cell saver available for her operation.

Which of these statements is correct regarding the use of intraoperative cell savers in obstetrics?

A. Antibiotics should be given routinely if salvaged blood is transfused.
B. Cell salvage is not recommended for rhesus negative mothers.
C. Cell savers cannot be used in caesarean section because of the risk of amniotic fluid embolism.
D. If the mother is rhesus negative she needs anti-D after reinfusion of salvaged blood.
E. The leucocyte-depletion filter will remove fetal blood cells.

Answer [ ]

2.2 One of the more serious complications of laparoscopy is bowel damage occurring at insertion of the laparoscope. Which of these patient characteristics makes this complication most likely?

A. BMI less than 20
B. BMI more than 40
C. Previous diagnostic laparoscopy
D. Previous caesarean section scar
E. History of endometriosis

Answer [ ]

2.3 If a woman has been delivered by caesarean section in her first pregnancy, it is good practice to read the previous operation notes to see if there were any intraoperative complications.

In which of these indications for caesarean may the surgical details on the operation notes explain an underlying anatomical reason for the caesarean indication?

A. Cord prolapse
B. Breech presentation
C. Failed forceps delivery
D. Fetal distress
E. Placenta praevia

Answer [ ]

2.4 On the labour ward a woman needs an emergency caesarean section for cord prolapse but she cannot sign the consent form as she is illiterate.

Select the best course of action in the absence of her written consent:

A. Ask her husband to sign the consent form
B. Cancel the operation
C. Do the operation without consent in her best interest
D. Get permission through a court order on the telephone
E. Obtain verbal consent

Answer [ ]

2.5 Some elective gynaecological operations are more likely to result in primary haemorrhage, needing transfusion, than others.

Select the operation where cross-matched blood should be available rather than just 'group and save' being requested:

A.   Adhesiolysis
B.   Hysterectomy for dysfunctional uterine bleeding
C.   Myomectomy
D.   Ovarian cystectomy
E.   Posterior vaginal repair

Answer   [   ]

2.6 Elderly women, especially if they have cancer, are more at risk of wound dehiscence. Following a hysterectomy, postoperative dehiscence of an abdominal wound is more likely to occur if:

A.   The urinary catheter is left in too long
B.   The patient is mobilised too early
C.   The patient develops a postoperative ileus
D.   The patient develops a vault haematoma
E.   The wound is transverse rather than vertical

Answer   [   ]

2.7 One of your patients is about to be admitted for a hysterectomy and has been counselled about the 'enhanced recovery pathway' at her pre-op checkup appointment. This care plan has been introduced for patients undergoing major gynaecological surgery to shorten their hospital stay, thereby reducing costs.

Which of these is part of this pathway?

A.   Avoiding dehydration by limiting fluid restriction to 2 hours before surgery
B.   Cooling the patient during surgery
C.   Mechanical bowel preparation helps avoid bowel trauma and enhances recovery
D.   Preloading with a sachet of amino acid solution
E.   Routinely using drains to avoid pelvic haematoma formation

Answer   [   ]

2.8 A patient who is due to have a pelvic floor repair mentions at the preoperative check that she is allergic to latex. Her surgery is scheduled for the middle of the operating list the following morning. Her general health is good and she has no other allergies.

Select the most appropriate action:

A.   Add an 'alert' to the operating list
B.   Cancel the operation
C.   Move her operation to the beginning of the list
D.   Tell the theatre staff at the start of the list during the briefing
E.   Reassure her that nonlatex gloves will be used

Answer   [   ]

2.9 Which procedure requires peri-operative antibiotic prophylaxis?

A. Caesarean section

B. Forceps delivery

C. Laparoscopic removal of ectopic pregnancy

D. Oophorectomy for ovarian cyst

E. Perineal repair of second-degree tear

Answer [ ]

2.10 During an abdominal hysterectomy operation, the risk of ureteric injury is higher if:

A. Ovaries are being conserved

B. Patient is postmenopausal

C. She is immunosuppressed

D. The patient has a duplex kidney

E. There is endometriosis involving the Pouch of Douglas

Answer [ ]

2.11 You are about to sign a consent form with a patient who is having a caesarean section. After you have listed the complications for her, she asks you which is the most common:

A. Wound dehiscence

B. Subsequent subfertility

C. Pseudo-obstruction of the bowel

D. Excess blood loss during surgery

E. Fetal laceration

Answer [ ]

2.12 In the antenatal clinic you see a primigravid woman who has been referred by her community midwife at 37 weeks because the fetus is lying transversely. You organise an USS that shows the reason for the abnormal lie is an 8 cm diameter ovarian cyst filling her pelvis. Your consultant tells you to arrange a caesarean section, and the woman asks you about the management of the cyst. Select the most appropriate advice in this clinical situation:

A. It will be dealt with later as the ovaries are not accessible during a caesarean

B. Spontaneous resolution of the cyst is likely after delivery

C. Removing the cyst at the time of caesarean will require a general anaesthetic

D. Caesarean and removal of the cyst should take place now in case the cyst torts

E. Ovarian cystectomy during a caesarean at 39 weeks is appropriate

Answer [ ]

2.13 You have seen a woman in preoperative assessment clinic who is due to undergo hysterectomy for prolapse in a few weeks' time. Which one of these is the most important factor to warn the anaesthetist about from her case notes?

A. She lives alone and has no postoperative social arrangements for care

B. Her mother had a deep vein thrombosis (DVT) during chemotherapy many years ago

C. She has hypertension, which is adequately treated with bendroflumethiazide

D. She is allergic to penicillin

E. There is a family history of suxamethonium apnoea

Answer [ ]

2.14 You are filling out a thromboprophylaxis risk form in the preoperative assessment clinic, for a woman about to undergo a pelvic floor repair. Which of the following does not contribute to her risk score for venous thromboembolism?

A. The woman has a BMI of 44

B. The woman has inflammatory bowel disease

C. The woman has essential hypertension

D. The woman has protein S deficiency

E. The woman has a history of recent breast cancer

Answer [ ]

2.15 A 45-year-old woman has been put on the waiting list for endometrial ablation to treat her menorrhagia. She visits the GP surgery to ask for further information as she wasn't given adequate time to discuss the procedure in the gynaecology clinic.

Which one of the following statements about endometrial ablation is correct?

A. Endometrial ablation is always done under general anaesthetic

B. Endometrial sampling is not required prior to the procedure

C. It cannot be undertaken in the presence of a caesarean scar

D. She should continue using contraception afterwards

E. The operation has a 90 per cent chance of producing amenorrhoea

Answer [ ]

2.16 A woman attends A&E due to heavy vaginal bleeding a week after having a large loop excision of the transformation zone (LLETZ procedure) for CIN 3. Her pulse and blood pressure are normal and her haemoglobin is 120 g/L.

On speculum examination there is active bleeding from the cervix. What is the most appropriate initial management in this case?

A. Arrange the operating theatre immediately for suturing of the cervix

B. Pack the vagina and give broad spectrum antibiotics

C. Prescribe oral norethisterone and allow home

D. Prescribe tranexamic acid and allow home

E. Take a swab and commence broad spectrum oral antibiotics

Answer [ ]

2.17 You would have concerns about the legitimacy of one of these patients signing their consent form for surgery. Which patient?

A. A girl aged 15 years requesting termination of pregnancy

B. An elderly woman who has had a stroke

C. A woman requesting sterilisation whose husband did not agree

D. A Jehovah's Witness who needs a caesarean for placenta praevia

E. A non-English-speaking woman whose husband is translating for her

Answer [ ]

2.18 An 86-year-old woman presents to the gynaecology outpatient clinic with postmenopausal bleeding. Having examined her, the consultant decides that hysteroscopy and cervical biopsy are necessary, but she is currently taking warfarin because of an artificial heart valve.

Select the most appropriate option regarding her anticoagulation:

A. Change to heparin and omit dose on morning of surgery

B. Continue with current dose of warfarin

C. Omit anticoagulation on morning of surgery

D. Omit warfarin for three days before surgery and check international normalized ratio (INR)

E. Postpone surgery until anticoagulant therapy completed

Answer [ ]

2.19 You are asked to review a woman on the Day Case Unit who had a laparoscopic sterilisation yesterday. She has had four children between the ages of 6 months and 4 years, all delivered by caesarean section using a Pfannenstiel incision. The nurses are concerned because she has abdominal pain and is still not well enough to go home, although your consultant saw her last night after the operating list had finished and discharged her.

When you examine her you notice some watery discharge from her suprapubic incision that is soaking through the dressing.

Which one of the following statements applies to this case?

A. Bowel damage is unlikely because her previous incision was suprapubic

B. She is probably evading being discharged because the children exhaust her

C. She should be sent home because your consultant discharged her

D. There could be a hole in her bladder

E. Unrecognised laparoscopic bowel injury is a likely diagnosis

Answer [ ]

2.20 An asthmatic woman is breathless on return to the Day Case Unit from the operating theatre recovery room and you are asked for advice. She has had an uncomplicated evacuation of uterus performed, but the clinical notes mention that she did have a coughing fit as she was being anaesthetised. Select the most appropriate immediate course of action in this situation:

A. Send her for an urgent chest x-ray
B. Organise a peak flow estimation
C. Prescribe nebulised salbutamol
D. Ask the anaesthetist to review her at the end of the list
E. Check her airway and give her oxygen by face mask

Answer [ ]

Extended Matching Questions

A	CA125 level
B	Chest x-ray
C	Clotting screen
D	CT scan of abdomen and pelvis
E	Electrocardiogram
F	Endocervical chlamydia swab
G	Ferritin
H	Haemoglobin
I	High vaginal swab
J	Plain abdominal x-ray
K	Pregnancy test
L	Thrombophilia screen
M	Ultrasound guided biopsy
N	USS of the pelvis

These clinical scenarios describe women who are on the waiting list for various gynaecological operations. Select the single most appropriate preoperative investigation for each case.

Each option may be used once, more than once, or not at all.

2.21 A 31-year-old woman requesting fertility investigations is to be admitted to the Day Case Unit on day 8 of her next menstrual cycle for a laparoscopy and dye test to check tubal patency because she has a history of pelvic inflammatory disease.

Answer [ ]

2.22 To investigate her severe long-standing menorrhagia a 49-year-old woman is going to undergo hysteroscopy and endometrial biopsy, and she has chosen to have it done under general anaesthetic.

Answer [ ]

2.23 A woman aged 42 years has an USS revealing a left ovarian cyst measuring 9 cm with solid elements in it. The right ovary seems normal on the scan and there is no ascites. Your consultant is trying to decide whether to remove the uterus and other ovary as well as the diseased ovary.

Answer [ ]

2.24 A 32-year-old multiparous woman is admitted as a day case for laparoscopic sterilisation. She has been using a copper coil for contraception but you cannot see the strings, and she thinks it was extruded from the uterus during an unusually heavy period 4 weeks ago.

Answer [ ]

2.25 A 40-year-old woman is going to have a hysterectomy for endometriosis. Scan reveals bilateral chocolate cysts on the ovaries. She has not had any surgery before, but her mother had a DVT following hysterectomy at the same age.

Answer [ ]

A	Chest x-ray
B	CT scan of abdomen and pelvis
C	Electrocardiogram
D	Haemoglobin
E	High vaginal swab
F	Intravenous pyelogram (IVP) x-ray
G	Plain abdominal x-ray
H	Serum calcium
I	USS of kidneys
J	Urea and electrolytes
K	Urine culture

These clinical scenarios describe women developing complications after gynaecological operations. Select the most appropriate investigation for each case.
Each option may be used once, more than once, or not at all.

2.26 Three days after a hysterectomy for endometrial cancer, a 60-year-old woman still has a distended abdomen with no bowel sounds. Which investigation will help you most with planning her management?

Answer [ ]

2.27 An obese 58-year-old woman who normally smokes twenty cigarettes a day develops severe left-sided chest pain two days after a prolapse operation. She is tachycardic and tachypnoeic. On examination you find an inspiratory wheeze but normal air entry all over the chest. Which investigation would you carry out initially?

Answer [ ]

2.28 Having undergone hysteroscopy and insertion of a Levonorgestrel intrauterine system (Mirena®) for menorrhagia under general anaesthetic, a 42-year-old woman was not well enough to be discharged home and has stayed in hospital overnight because of severe lower abdominal pain. The next morning, she is still in pain and has a temperature of 38°C. You cannot locate the coil strings on speculum examination.

Answer [ ]

2.29 On the fourth day following a difficult hysterectomy and bilateral salpingo-oophorectomy operation for endometriosis a 38-year-old woman has a swinging pyrexia and unilateral loin pain. She is still nauseous and seems to have a persistent ileus.

Answer [ ]

2.30 Six days after leaving hospital following a vaginal hysterectomy operation, an anaemic woman is readmitted with further vaginal discharge and pain. She was sent home on iron tablets and analgesics. On readmission she is pyrexial, and bimanual pelvic examination reveals a palpable tender mass at the vault with offensive brown blood in the vagina.

Answer [ ]

A	A guardian with power of attorney should sign the consent form
B	Consent from the patient is valid
C	Defer the operation until a court order can be obtained
D	Defer the operation until an independent interpreter is available
E	Defer the operation until the woman is fully recovered
F	The consent already given is not valid
G	The clinician could go ahead with surgery in the patient's best interests
H	The woman has a right to refuse consent
I	The woman should not be asked to participate in the research
J	Verbal consent from the patient is adequate
K	Written consent could be obtained from the patient's husband

These clinical scenarios describe women in different situations where consent may be an issue. Select the most appropriate advice for each case.

Each option may be used once, more than once, or not at all.

2.31 A 51-year-old woman with severe learning difficulties is brought into A&E as an emergency with prolonged heavy bleeding. On admission her haemoglobin is 93 g/l. She needs a hysteroscopy to investigate the problem but cannot understand what is being proposed.

Answer [ ]

2.32 On the labour ward a primigravid woman has reluctantly had a fetal blood sample done at 4 cm dilatation, and the result shows that the baby is hypoxic. She has a needle phobia and adamantly refuses caesarean section to deliver the baby quickly. Both the obstetric consultant and the paediatrician have explained the possible consequences to her.

Answer [ ]

2.33 A Jehovah's Witness has a hysterectomy operation for endometrial cancer. She specifically states that she will not accept blood transfusion and signs a disclaimer form preoperatively. In the recovery room it becomes apparent that she has internal bleeding and the consultant decides to take her back to theatre. She has had a several doses of opiates to control her pain and is very drowsy.

Answer [ ]

2.34 On the labour ward a new research project is underway comparing two different drugs to treat postpartum haemorrhage. You are called in to put a drip up for a woman who has lost 400 ml of blood already, and the blood loss seems to be ongoing. Although it has not been discussed previously with the patient, the midwife mentions the possibility of the patient being asked to participate in the research project.

Answer [ ]

2.35 A 15-year-old schoolgirl presents to clinic requesting surgical termination of pregnancy accompanied by her 15-year-old boyfriend. She will not tell her parents about the pregnancy, and after much discussion she is thought to be able to understand the risks of the procedure.

Answer [ ]

A	Cancel the operation as it is not the correct procedure for this patient
B	Go ahead with the operation as planned
C	Postpone the operation and arrange counselling
D	Postpone the operation and arrange review in genito-urinary medicine clinic
E	Postpone the operation and arrange routine gynaecology clinic review
F	Postpone the operation and arrange urgent gynaecology clinic review
G	Postpone the operation and organise an USS
H	Postpone the operation until you can arrange further tests
I	Refer her urgently to her GP for a prescription
J	Suggest that the patient has a spinal anaesthetic

The patients that you are seeing in the preoperative clinic are about to undergo gynaecological operations and unfortunately your consultant is not immediately available for advice.

Select the most appropriate management plan for each clinical scenario.

Each option may be used once, more than once, or not at all.

2.36 The waiting list clerk has arranged for a 49-year-old woman to fill a cancelled slot on the operating list at short notice. She is due to have an abdominal hysterectomy in 3 days' time and you are doing her preoperative check. She had a hysteroscopy done under local anaesthetic for irregular heavy bleeding recently but the histology on the endometrium from that operation is not yet available.

Answer [ ]

2.37 A 37-year-old woman presented to clinic with left iliac fossa pain radiating down her left leg several weeks ago and USS revealed a 7 cm simple left ovarian cyst. She was put on the waiting list for an ovarian cystectomy but her symptoms have now disappeared.

Answer [ ]

2.38 A healthy 62-year-old woman is due to be admitted for a prolapse repair. She mentions a family history of 'difficulty waking up' after anaesthetics but is not sure of the clinical details.

Answer [ ]

2.39 A 33-year-old woman is to be admitted for endometrial ablation to treat her menorrhagia. She has turned down the option of a Mirena® intrauterine system because she wishes to have another baby within the next couple of years.

Answer [ ]

2.40 When she was seen in the fertility clinic a couple of weeks ago, a 29-year-old woman had a speculum examination during which some routine swabs were taken. You look up the results before signing her consent form for a laparoscopy and dye test only to discover that the chlamydia swab is positive.

Answer [ ]

A	Acute primary haemorrhage
B	Chest infection
C	DVT
D	Haemolysis
E	Intestinal obstruction
F	Pelvic haematoma
G	Pulmonary embolus
H	Secondary haemorrhage due to vault infection
I	Ureteric injury
J	Urinary tract infection
K	Urinary retention
L	Vault granulations
M	Vault dehiscence

Each of these clinical scenarios describes a woman presenting with complications after hysterectomy; for each patient pick the most likely diagnosis based on the clinical information given.

Each option may be used once, more than once, or not at all.

2.41 You are called to see a morbidly obese 40-year-old woman who had a hysterectomy for endometrial cancer three days ago. She has gradually become more breathless over the previous 24 hours and now seems a little confused. She is hypoxic and expresses discomfort when you ask for deep breaths to auscultate her chest but there is normal air entry. Her temperature is normal and you do not see any abnormality on her chest x-ray.

Answer [ ]

2.42 Three days after a hysterectomy for endometriosis, a 35-year-old woman is found to have a mild pyrexia and a tachycardia of 100 bpm. There is a moderate amount of old blood coming from the vagina and her haemoglobin has dropped from 127 g/l preoperatively to 82 g/l now. The estimated blood loss at operation was described as 250 ml.

Answer [ ]

2.43 A 30-year-old woman had a hysterectomy and left salpingo-oophorectomy for chronic pelvic inflammatory disease. The surgery was described as difficult due to dense adhesions between the hydrosalpinx and the left side of the pelvis. Blood loss during the operation is documented as 900 ml. Two days later she is pyrexial, has a distended abdomen with no bowel sounds, and is complaining of left loin pain.

Answer [ ]

2.44 A woman who had a hysterectomy 10 weeks ago comes to your surgery because she has just started to bleed vaginally again. She has not seen any blood since a week after her hysterectomy but has not been examined following the operation as she did not go to the hospital for her postoperative checkup.

Answer [ ]

2.45 On her fluid balance chart on the first postoperative day, you notice that a woman has apparently not passed urine since she returned from theatre despite having received more than 2 litres of fluid intravenously. She has a pelvic drain in situ which contains 400 mls. The nurses report that she asked for a bedpan twice during the night.

Answer [ ]

A	Advise alternative method of contraception 4 weeks before surgery
B	Continue using current contraceptive method
C	Prescribe full therapeutic anticoagulation therapy
D	Prescribe local vaginal estrogen instead of systemic hormone replacement therapy (HRT)
E	Switch HRT to transdermal method before surgery
F	Stop HRT 4 weeks before surgery
G	Stop HRT 12 weeks before surgery
H	Stopping HRT is not necessary
I	Stop contraceptive method 4 weeks before surgery

These clinical scenarios relate to women seeking advice relating to surgery and the risks of thromboembolism. In each case you should decide on the best course of action regarding her hormonal medication and select the most appropriate advice.

Each option may be used once, more than once, or not at all.

2.46 A 26-year-old woman is on the waiting list for scoliosis surgery and seeks advice about whether she should continue taking her combined oral contraceptive pill.

Answer [   ]

2.47 A 26-year-old woman is being admitted to hospital for scoliosis surgery in 6 weeks' time and seeks advice about whether she should have her next dose of Depo-Provera®, which is now due.

Answer [   ]

2.48 A 26-year-old woman is on the waiting list for diagnostic laparoscopy to diagnose her pelvic pain. She is currently taking Dianette® for contraception and in the hope that it will improve her acne.

Answer [   ]

2.49 A fit 50-year-old woman started on systemic HRT (sequential tablet formulation) 6 months ago because of severe vasomotor and vaginal dryness symptoms. She has felt much better on it but is now on the waiting list for a posterior vaginal repair for prolapse. Apart from the surgery, you do not identify any risk factors for thromboembolism in her medical notes.

Answer [   ]

2.50 A 45-year-old woman is taking tibolone (Livial®) HRT having had a complete pelvic clearance for endometriosis 6 months previously. She is about to undergo carpal tunnel surgery and seeks advice about her tibolone medication.

Answer [   ]

Curriculum Module 3

Antenatal Care

Syllabus

▨ You will be expected to understand and demonstrate appropriate knowledge and attitudes in relation to periconceptional care, antenatal care, and maternal complications of pregnancy.

▨ An awareness of substance misuse, psychiatric illness, and problems of pregnancy at extremes of reproductive age and of domestic violence in relation to pregnancy is expected. An appreciation of emotional and cultural issues is needed too.

▨ You will be expected to have a good understanding of common medical disorders and the effect that pregnancy may have on them, and their effect, in turn, upon the pregnancy. You will be expected to demonstrate your ability to assess and manage these conditions.

▨ Knowledge of therapeutics in antenatal care is expected.

▨ You will need to show understanding of the roles of other professionals, the importance of liaison, and empathic teamwork.

▨ You will be expected to understand the principles of antenatal screening including screening for structural defects, chromosomal abnormalities and haemoglobinopathies, and the effects of relevant infections during pregnancy on the fetus and neonate.

Learning Outcomes

In the past GPs were more involved in provision of antenatal care than they are now. Although few run antenatal clinics now, having delegated this responsibility to midwives, it is not uncommon for midwives to consult the GP for advice when they are dealing with a difficult case or if the patient needs a prescription. When deciding whether to refer a pregnant woman for hospital care, midwives will work to protocols and national guidelines but may consult the GP if they are unsure. Some patients may seek a second opinion if they are unhappy about or need more information about advice given to them by the midwife or the obstetricians.

The 'Confidential Enquiry into Maternal and Child Health Report' has highlighted the important role of the GP where women have preexisting medical disorders. For these reasons the DRCOG exam continues to test knowledge about the antenatal care of pregnant women.

Single Best Answer Questions

3.1 A woman went into hospital at 29 weeks of gestation with fresh vaginal bleeding. An emergency ultrasound scan confirmed that the placenta was not low lying and she was discharged home yesterday.

She is due to fly to Majorca in a week's time and attends surgery for advice about her holiday.

Select the most appropriate advice:

A. Advise against travelling at all whilst pregnant
B. Advise against travel after 32 weeks of gestation
C. Defer the holiday for several weeks
D. Have another scan before leaving on holiday
E. Make sure that she has adequate travel insurance to cover pregnancy complications

Answer [ ]

3.2 A woman books for antenatal care at 12 weeks of gestation in her second pregnancy. In the last pregnancy she developed gestational diabetes that was managed with insulin. The community midwife asks you whether she needs a glucose tolerance test (GTT) arranging.

Select the most appropriate management:

A. Early GTT repeated at 28 weeks
B. GTT at 28 weeks
C. HbA1C instead of GTT
D. Random glucose at this booking appointment
E. Refer straight to diabetic antenatal clinic

Answer [ ]

3.3 A woman has been on antidepressants for years and attends your surgery for advice now that she is pregnant for the first time.

Which of the following statements is correct advice regarding her antidepressant medication during pregnancy and the puerperium?

A. Long-acting selective serotonin re-uptake inhibitors have no adverse neonatal effects
B. Breast-feeding is contraindicated when taking any antidepressants
C. Consider gradual reduction of the antidepressant during the third trimester
D. Stop the antidepressant when the pregnancy reaches 37 weeks of gestation
E. Tricyclic antidepressants do not affect the baby

Answer [ ]

3.4 A care worker is just about to start her first job in an old people's home and is planning a pregnancy next year. She asks occupational health about the possibility of catching chickenpox from a patient with shingles, which seems to be common amongst the elderly residents.

Select the correct information for occupational health to give her:

A. All pregnant women should avoid any contact with chickenpox and shingles
B. Chickenpox cannot be caught from an individual with reactivated zoster (shingles)

C. More than 90 per cent of individuals in the United Kingdom are seropositive for IgG varicella antibodies

D. Pregnant women are routinely tested for immunity to chickenpox at booking

E. Vaccination is available that can be given during pregnancy

Answer [ ]

3.5 In the surgery you see a woman in her first pregnancy who is suffering from hyperemesis. You do not think that she needs admitting to hospital and prescribe an anti-emetic. Her teeth are in poor condition.

Select the main reason for suggesting that she makes an appointment with a dentist:

A. Hyperemesis can result in damage to maternal teeth

B. Periodontitis is a risk factor for low birth weight

C. Pregnant women are entitled to free dental care

D. The immune response to plaque bacteria is altered in pregnancy

E. There is an association between pregnancy and gingival hyperplasia

Answer [ ]

3.6 A woman who was diagnosed with epilepsy many years ago when she was a schoolgirl consults her GP because she is thinking of starting a family. She is taking sodium valproate and has not had a seizure for more than a year.

Select the best advice regarding her medication:

A. It is better to have a fit than to take antiepileptic medication

B. Monotherapy with one drug is the preferred option in pregnancy

C. She should be advised to take 0.5 mg folic acid daily when she gets pregnant

D. Sodium valproate should be continued as it is associated with the least risk of abnormality

E. The increased risk of congenital abnormality will be avoided if she stops taking valproate

Answer [ ]

3.7 A newly pregnant morbidly obese woman in your surgery asks for information about 'the new screening test that can be done looking for the baby's genetic material in her blood'.

Which of the following statements is correct information about noninvasive testing using maternal plasma deoxyribonucleic acid (DNA)?

A. A monochorionic twin pregnancy cannot be tested as the results will be inaccurate

B. It is only used to detect chromosomal abnormalities

C. She does not need to have a scan before the test

D. The test can only be performed in the first trimester

E. The test will be less accurate because of her obesity

Answer [ ]

3.8 A community midwife is concerned about one of the pregnant women on her caseload because she has noted bruises of different ages on the woman's body whilst auscultating the fetal heart during a home visit.

Which of the following situations should also raise concerns about domestic violence?

A. All her older children are brought to antenatal appointments even during school terms

B. Her whole family including her parents come to antenatal appointments

C. Partner is always present at antenatal appointments

D. Poor attendance at antenatal clinic appointments

E. Woman's previous children are all fathered by different men

Answer [ ]

3.9 A multiparous woman with an uncomplicated pregnancy of 24 weeks' gestation is about to go on a long-haul flight. She has a BMI of 42, no medical problems, and is a nonsmoker.

Select the best advice regarding thromboembolism prevention in her case:

A. Aspirin 75 mg oral tablets

B. Graduated compression stockings

C. Hydration and mobilization during flight

D. Low molecular weight heparin injections

E. No special measures needed

Answer [ ]

3.10 A pregnant woman from your GP practice with insulin-dependent diabetes is referred to the hospital diabetic obstetric clinic for antenatal care.

How often should she be scanned for growth and amniotic fluid volume?

A. Fortnightly from 24 weeks of gestation

B. Fortnightly from 28 weeks until term

C. Monthly from 28 weeks of gestation until 36 weeks

D. Monthly from 28 weeks until term

E. No growth scans necessary unless the symphysial-fundal height measures 'small for dates'

Answer [ ]

3.11 Intrahepatic cholestasis of pregnancy is an uncommon but serious complication. Which of the following statements about this condition is correct?

A. Antenatal administration of vitamin K to the mother reduces the itching

B. Meconium in the liquor during labour is to be expected

C. The condition only occurs in primigravid women

D. The problem affects the mother's health but the baby is not at risk

E. The recurrence risk in a subsequent pregnancy is 5 per cent

Answer [ ]

3.12 Which of the following statements concerning HIV in pregnancy is true?

A. In HIV-positive mothers on antiretroviral treatment breast-feeding is safe

B. Infants born to women who are HIV positive should be treated with antiretroviral therapy from birth

C. Interventions can reduce the risk of vertical HIV transmission from 30 per cent to zero

D. Use of short-term steroids to promote fetal lung maturation is inadvisable

E. Women who do not require treatment for their own health do not need to take antiretroviral therapy during pregnancy

Answer [ ]

3.13 A refugee woman from Ethiopia books for antenatal care in her first pregnancy and discloses to the midwife that she has undergone female genital mutilation (FGM) in the past. Which of these statements about FGM is true?

A. FGM can be surgically 'undone' before delivery

B. If her baby is female, she may be at risk of FGM as a teenager in the future

C. She must be delivered by elective caesarean section

D. Usually involves complete closure of the vaginal introitus except for a tiny hole

E. UK law states that the suturing can legally be restored after delivery

Answer [ ]

3.14 You see a pregnant woman in your surgery who has just been to the hospital for a dating scan at 11 weeks of gestation, which reveals that she has monochorionic twins in separate sacs.

Which of the following statements is true about this type of twin pregnancy?

A. Delivery should be planned for 36 weeks if she has not laboured

B. Monochorionic twins are at lower risk of twin-twin transfusion syndrome than dichorionic twins

C. Regular growth scans will be offered from 32 weeks of gestation

D. She should be delivered by caesarean section as there is a risk of cord entanglement

E. She will not be able to have any sort of screening for Down syndrome

Answer [ ]

3.15 You are consulted by a primigravid woman at 24 weeks of gestation who has an unbearable headache. She has a history of severe migraine that she has consulted you about before several times. You do a thorough examination and find epigastric tenderness. Testing her urine reveals proteinuria +++.

Which one of the following statements about her situation is correct?

A. Fundal height is irrelevant as poor growth will not be apparent at this early gestation

B. If her blood pressure is 125/80 mmHg the diagnosis cannot be pre-eclampsia

C. Prescribing antibiotics without awaiting the results of a midstream specimen of urine (MSU) is not advisable

D. She needs assessment by an obstetrician urgently

E. The diagnosis cannot be pre-eclampsia because of the early gestation

Answer [ ]

3.16 Consultant referral is necessary so that antenatal serial growth scans can be arranged to check on fetal growth if the pregnancy is affected by which of the following conditions in the mother:

A. History of polycystic ovarian syndrome

B. 'Slapped cheek' syndrome

C. Previous delivery by caesarean section

D. Recurrent unexplained antepartum haemorrhage

E. Vitamin B12 deficiency

Answer [ ]

3.17 A 14-year-old schoolgirl is brought to your surgery by her mother having been sent home with a note from the school nurse suggesting that she might be pregnant. On examination it is obvious that her abdominal swelling is due to a pregnancy of about 36 weeks of gestation; fetal movements can be clearly seen and the fetal heart auscultated.

Which of the following is true regarding this teenage pregnancy?

A. Her due date can be accurately predicted when she has a scan at the hospital

B. She is no more likely to deliver a small-for-dates infant than mothers aged 20–30

C. She should be offered chlamydia screening

D. There is no point in discussing contraception

E. You should involve the police because her pregnancy must be the result of rape

Answer [ ]

3.18 A 34-year-old woman who has had two uncomplicated pregnancies previously expresses a wish to have a home birth this time. At her 28-week checkup with the midwife she mentions that she has had a couple of minor episodes of vaginal bleeding following intercourse during the previous few weeks. Her blood group is A rhesus negative.

Which one of the following statements about her care is appropriate?

A. A normal 20-week anomaly scan will exclude placenta praevia as a cause

B. Bleeding is unlikely to be caused by cervical cancer if her recent smear is normal

C. Kleihauer testing will help diagnose placental abruption

D. She could still have a home birth if the placenta is not low

E. She should be referred to consultant-led antenatal care for growth

Ansv

3.19 You see a primigravid woman in clinic who has just had a 20-week detailed (anomaly) scan that reveals a low-lying placenta. Her haemoglobin was 107 gm/L at booking and she takes ferrous sulphate 200 mg daily.

Which is the most appropriate advice for her?

A. Admission to hospital will be necessary later in the pregnancy
B. Avoid sexual intercourse
C. Delivery will be by caesarean section at 37 weeks
D. Increase the dose of oral iron to three times daily
E. Take folic acid 5 mg daily

Answer [ ]

3.20 You are looking after a 'grand multip' pregnant with her fifth baby who has had four normal births before.

Which pregnancy complication is she most at risk of?

A. Anaemia
B. Hypertension
C. Low-lying placenta
D. Postpartum haemorrhage
E. Placenta accreta

Answer [ ]

Extended Matching Questions

A	Alpha-fetoprotein level
B	Amniocentesis
C	Chorionic villus sampling
D	Combined nuchal translucency scan and serum screening
E	Cordocentesis
F	Detailed ultrasound scan
G	Karyotype both parents for balanced (Robertsonian) translocation
H	Nuchal translucency scan
I	Serum screening with hCG/alpha-fetoprotein/oestriol levels
J	Third trimester growth scan
K	3-D ultrasound scan

The clinical scenarios that follow relate to prenatal screening and diagnostic tests.
For each woman, select the most appropriate investigation.
Each option may be used once, more than once, or not at all.

3.21 The wife of a prominent politician is referred to a private obstetric clinic at 10 weeks of gestation because she has conceived unexpectedly many years after the birth of her last child and is now aged 42. She wishes to be absolutely reassured that the baby does not have Down syndrome as soon as possible because she feels that it would hamper her contribution to her husband's career.

Answer [ ]

3.22 A patient with a history of a previous pregnancy affected by neural tube defect wishes to have the most sensitive test in this current pregnancy.

Answer [ ]

3.23 A 36-year-old woman has conceived after many years of infertility. She wishes to have a screening test for Down syndrome with the least false positive rate.

Answer [ ]

3.24 A couple who know that they are both carriers of cystic fibrosis present at 9 weeks' gestation requesting prenatal diagnosis.

Answer [ ]

3.25 A 40-year-old woman who has reached 15 weeks of gestation having had three previous first trimester miscarriages wishes to have a diagnostic test for Down syndrome because her partner has a balanced Robertsonian translocation.

Answer [ ]

A	Abruptio placentae
B	Appendicitis
C	Constipation
D	Pancreatitis
E	Pre-eclampsia
F	Red degeneration of a uterine fibroid
G	Torsion of an ovarian cyst
H	Ureteric calculus
I	Urinary tract infection
J	Uterine rupture

These clinical scenarios relate to the emergency presentation of a pregnant woman with abdominal pain.

For each woman select the most likely diagnosis for her pain.

Each option may be used once, more than once, or not at all.

3.26 Two years after a myomectomy operation, a 42-year-old woman has conceived following IVF treatment. At 32 weeks of gestation she is admitted to the obstetric unit with increasing pain in her abdomen for 3 days, which only responds to opiate analgesia. Apart from nausea she has no systemic symptoms. On examination she is apyrexial and normotensive but has a tachycardia. There is localised tenderness only at the fundus of the uterus.

Answer [ ]

3.27 An 18-year-old primigravid woman presents in A&E at 16 weeks of gestation with lower abdominal pain and vomiting. She has foetor oris and a temperature of 37.8°C.

Answer [ ]

3.28 At 32 weeks of gestation a woman pregnant with her second baby is admitted using an ambulance having collapsed in a supermarket due to sudden onset of severe abdominal pain. Her observations are stable apart from a maternal tachycardia. The uterus is tender and unfortunately no fetal heartbeat is detectable.

Answer [ ]

3.29 At 17 weeks of gestation a 38-year-old primigravid woman is rushed in to A&E with severe unilateral colicky loin pain. She was writhing about on the bed but the pain has now subsided following a dose of morphine. Urinalysis reveals haematuria and her temperature is normal.

Answer [ ]

3.30 A primigravid woman on holiday in London attends an NHS 'walk-in' centre with severe epigastric pain and headache. Her pregnancy has been uncomplicated so far and she is now 30 weeks of gestation. On admission, urinalysis reveals that there is a great deal of protein in her urine.

Answer [ ]

A	Aim for vaginal delivery but with a shortened second stage
B	Await spontaneous labour and aim for vaginal delivery
C	Classical caesarean section
D	Elective caesarean section at 39 weeks of gestation
E	Elective caesarean section at 39 weeks of gestation and sterilisation
F	Elective caesarean section at 40 weeks of gestation
G	Emergency caesarean section
H	Induction of labour at 38 weeks of gestation and aim for vaginal delivery
I	Offer external cephalic version and await spontaneous labour
J	Offer external cephalic version and, if successful, induce labour

The following scenarios relate to a woman with a complicated pregnancy or underlying medical condition. How would you counsel her regarding delivery? Each option may be used once, more than once, or not at all.

3.31 Having been delivered by caesarean section in her two previous pregnancies a 30-year-old woman books for antenatal care at 17 weeks of gestation.

Answer [ ]

3.32 Having had a myomectomy operation a few years ago, a 39-year-old woman is followed up carefully in antenatal clinic because she has several more fibroids in the uterus. Serial scans show that the baby is well grown but at 37 weeks the ultrasonographer notes that the fibroid in the lower segment has grown to 8 cm diameter and the baby is lying transversely above it.

Answer [ ]

3.33 A woman with HIV attends antenatal clinic at 36 weeks of gestation. She is on antiretroviral medication and her viral load is extremely low at < 50 copies per ml.

Answer [ ]

3.34 A primigravid woman is referred to hospital antenatal clinic at 37 weeks of gestation because the presentation is found to be breech. Scan confirms that the baby is of average size and the presentation is flexed breech.

Answer [ ]

3.35 Just prior to conceiving, a 34-year-old woman was treated for a cerebral aneurysm, which was successfully clipped leaving no neurological deficit. Her craniotomy wound has healed well and she is now 36 weeks of gestation in her first pregnancy.

Answer [ ]

A	Admit immediately to a psychiatric 'mother and baby' unit
B	Advise that depression is common and resolves after delivery
C	Advise that she should stop medication as it can harm the baby
D	Arrange specialist counselling
E	Ask a psychiatric liaison worker to visit at home
F	Continue medication and seek psychiatric advice
G	Recommence psychiatric medication immediately
H	Refer back to her previous psychiatrist
I	Routine opinion from a specialist obstetric psychiatric clinic
J	Suggest that she considers short-term use of sleeping tablets
K	Suggest that she takes an antidepressant
L	Urgent opinion from a specialist obstetric psychiatric clinic

The following scenarios relate to psychiatric problems in pregnant women. In each case decide the most appropriate course of action.

Each option may be used once, more than once, or not at all.

3.36 Having been diagnosed with schizophrenia at university many years ago, a 34-year-old woman books for antenatal care very late as she had not realised that she was pregnant until the third trimester. She has been off medication for many years and has been psychiatrically well since.

Answer [ ]

3.37 A primigravid woman at 28 weeks of gestation consults you in surgery about feeling very low in mood and having trouble sleeping following the death of her mother. She denies thoughts of self-harm.

Answer [ ]

3.38 A young woman with bipolar disorder has been well controlled on lithium for a few years and seeks preconceptual counselling. She is planning pregnancy soon and has no other medical problems.

Answer [ ]

3.39 The midwife caring for one of your patients contacts you with concerns about a 42-year-old first-time mother who has refused to allow her access to the house for the previous 3 days. The husband reveals on the telephone that his wife has not slept since the baby was born and is making bizarre comments about the health of the baby. Her psychiatric liaison worker has left a written care plan in her obstetric notes.

Answer [ ]

3.40 A woman books for antenatal care at 10 weeks in her second pregnancy. She gives a history of postnatal depression that involved several months of in-patient care following her previous delivery. She is currently well and not on any medication.

Answer [ ]

A	Abdominal ultrasound scan
B	CT scan
C	Doppler measurement of cerebral artery flow
D	Electronic cardiotocograph fetal monitoring
E	Fetal growth scan in 2 weeks
F	Speculum examination of the cervix with fibronectin swab
G	Speculum examination of the cervix with microbiology swabs
H	Transvaginal scan (TVS)
I	Ultrasound scan with umbilical artery Doppler measurement
J	Vaginal examination in theatre with the operating team standing by

These clinical scenarios relate to women in the third trimester of pregnancy, presenting with vaginal bleeding.

In each case, choose the most appropriate initial investigation.

Each option may be used once, more than once, or not at all.

3.41 A woman attends the labour ward at 35 weeks of gestation on account of a small amount of vaginal bleeding that has now stopped. Initially there was some minor abdominal pain, but this has settled and there is no uterine activity. There have been reduced fetal movements since the episode of bleeding. On examination the size of the uterus is compatible with dates.

Answer [ ]

3.42 A primigravid 37-year-old woman presents with a heavy vaginal bleed at 39 weeks of gestation. The uterus is nontender and the baby is well grown but appears to be lying transversely. There are no contractions and the condition of both the mother and the baby is stable.

Answer [ ]

3.43 A primigravid patient is seen in the antenatal assessment unit because of recurrent episodes of antepartum haemorrhage over the previous few weeks. The uterine fundus measures 'small for dates' at 37 weeks of gestation. An ultrasound scan confirms that the baby's abdominal circumference is on the tenth centile of the growth chart and the liquor volume is less than expected.

Answer [ ]

3.44 Having booked late for antenatal care because she tried to conceal her pregnancy, a 15-year-old primigravid woman comes in to labour ward late one evening with a small amount of postcoital bleeding at term. The baby is moving normally and the uterus is nontender.

Answer [ ]

3.45 The emergency ambulance brings a 23-year-old woman to hospital at 34 weeks in her second pregnancy because she experienced sudden onset of abdominal pain and vaginal bleeding an hour ago. On examination the uterus is very tender and feels hard.

Answer [ ]

A	Candida albicans
B	Chlamydia trachomatis
C	Escherichia coli
D	Gardnerella vaginalis
E	Gonococcus
F	Group B streptococcus

G	Listeria monocytogenes
H	Parvovirus B19
I	Rubella
J	Streptococcus faecalis
K	Toxoplasma gondii

The clinical scenarios that follow relate to women with infectious diseases in pregnancy. For each case select the single most likely infecting organism.
Each option may be used once, more than once, or not at all.

3.46 A woman presents in the surgery at 22 weeks of gestation complaining of increasing abdominal discomfort and on examination the uterus is tense and large for dates. She gives a history of a mild flu-like illness 2 weeks previously. The community midwife refers her to hospital for an ultrasound scan, which shows polyhydramnios and fetal hydrops.

Answer [ ]

3.47 A primigravid woman presents at 34 weeks of gestation with a history of feeling increasingly unwell, rigours, and right-upper-quadrant pain. On examination she is flushed, has a tachycardia of 100 bpm, and has a temperature of 38°C. She is tender in the right renal angle.

Answer [ ]

3.48 A 17-year-old woman presents at 30 weeks of gestation in her first pregnancy with a history of recurrent postcoital bleeding. Her booking scan at 20 weeks showed a normally sited placenta. Speculum examination reveals a florid ectropion with contact bleeding on taking swabs.

Answer [ ]

3.49 In antenatal clinic at 17 weeks of gestation a primigravid woman complains of vaginal discharge and soreness. On speculum examination there is a thick, white discharge adherent to the vaginal walls.

Answer [ ]

3.50 A 28-year-old primary school teacher is pregnant for the first time. Several children in her class have 'slapped cheek syndrome' at the start of term and when she comes to hospital for her routine anomaly scan her baby is found to be hydropic.

Answer [ ]

Curriculum Module 4

Management of Labour and Delivery

Syllabus

- You will be expected to have the knowledge, understanding, and judgement to be capable of initial management of intrapartum problems in a hospital and in a community setting.
- This will include knowledge and understanding of normal and abnormal labour; data and investigation interpretation; induction and augmentation of labour; and assessment of fetal well-being and compromise.
- An understanding of the management of all obstetric emergencies is expected. You will need to demonstrate appropriate knowledge of regional anaesthesia, analgesia, and operative delivery including caesarean section.
- You will need to be able to demonstrate respect for cultural and religious differences in attitudes to childbirth.

Learning Outcomes

Times have changed from the days of the family doctor when GPs came into the hospital to look after some of their patients in labour, and few GPs are involved in intrapartum care these days. You might think that there is not much point in acquiring knowledge about what happens on the labour ward and some trainees in O&G posts on the GP training scheme don't enjoy being on duty for labour ward. Nevertheless, patients expect their GP to be aware of what can go wrong during delivery, and many seek the opinion of their GP if they are worried about issues around delivery or after the event if they have had a complication.

This part of the exam will be much easier if you have worked on a labour ward since you were a medical student. However, you will find some useful information on the RCOG website in terms of advice for consent for obstetric procedures, which detail complications and potential problems. In addition, there are several RCOG 'Green-top' guidelines and NICE guidelines relevant to obstetric care that are a good source of information for this part of the syllabus.

Single Best Answer Questions

4.1 In antenatal clinic a woman who was delivered by caesarean section in her last pregnancy is discussing the prospect of vaginal birth after caesarean (VBAC) for her current pregnancy.

In the last pregnancy she had a very slow first stage of labour and got stuck at 9 cm dilatation. The baby was in the occipito-posterior position, but there was no evidence of cephalo-pelvic disproportion.

What is her chance of achieving a vaginal birth this time?

A. 30 per cent
B. 40 per cent
C. 50 per cent
D. 60 per cent
E. 70 per cent

Answer [ ]

4.2 A woman who is considering a VBAC is discussing her birth plan with her community midwife.

Which of these factors increases the chances of rupture of the uterine scar during labour?

A. Fetal distress in the previous labour
B. Having a water birth in this labour
C. Maternal BMI >30
D. Onset of spontaneous labour after the due date in this pregnancy
E. Previous labour complicated by chorioamnionitis

Answer [ ]

4.3 Which of the following obstetric conditions or situations predisposes to cord prolapse during labour?

A. Breech presentation
B. Maternal diabetes
C. Oligohydramnios
D. Placenta praevia
E. Waterbirth

Answer [ ]

4.4 Induction of labour is clinically indicated in which of the following conditions?

A. Maternal urinary tract infection
B. Pathological cardiotocograph (CTG) tracing
C. Pregnancy-induced hypertension
D. Symphysis pubis dysfunction
E. Undiagnosed antepartum haemorrhage

Answer [ ]

4.5 Which of the following is a contraindication to a home delivery?

A. A woman with a BMI of 37 who has had two normal births before
B. Grand multiparity
C. Poor rapport with community midwife
D. Spontaneous labour occurring 10 days postdates
E. Second labour after previous forceps delivery

Answer [ ]

4.6 Which of the following pregnant women should be counselled against planning to labour in a birthing pool in hospital?

A. A primigravid woman whose baby is in the occipito-posterior position at the start of labour
B. A multiparous woman whose pregnancy is complicated by mild rhesus disease
C. A woman with a BMI of 45 and an otherwise uncomplicated pregnancy
D. A woman with an otherwise uncomplicated pregnancy who has had a successful external cephalic version
E. A woman with an uncomplicated postmature pregnancy

Answer [ ]

4.7 An obese woman has just received a spinal anaesthetic for a forceps delivery in theatre and her legs have been raised in the obstetric stirrups. She complains of feeling short of breath and a heavy feeling in both her arms.

What is the most likely cause of her symptoms?

A. Amniotic fluid embolism
B. Hypotension
C. Hyperventilation
D. Myocardial infarction
E. Rising spinal block

Answer [ ]

4.8 Which of these obstetric complications is a recognised indication for assisted vaginal delivery (shortening the second stage of labour with forceps or ventouse)?

A. Macrosomia
B. Maternal cardiac disease
C. Maternal hypotension
D. Prematurity
E. Previous third-degree tear

Answer [ ]

4.9 A previously fit woman is in labour at 36 weeks' gestation and her temperature is noted to be 39°C. The CTG indicates that the baby is becoming distressed and the registrar on call wishes to perform a caesarean section, suspecting chorioamnionitis.

The woman refuses to give consent for the operation and the midwife looking after her thinks that she may be confused on account of her high temperature.

Select the best course of action in this situation:

A.   Ask her husband to sign the consent form
B.   Assess her capacity to understand and process clinical information
C.   Get a court order to force her to have the caesarean
D.   Proceed without consent in the baby's best interests
E.   Use the Mental Health Act to justify proceeding with caesarean delivery

Answer [ ]

4.10 An obstetric anaesthetist will be unwilling to site an epidural until they have seen a recent normal platelet count and clotting screen for a woman whose pregnancy is complicated by:

A.   Induction of labour
B.   Intrauterine fetal death
C.   Maternal diabetes
D.   Previous caesarean section
E.   Twin pregnancy

Answer [ ]

4.11 An ambulance is summoned by a community midwife who is conducting a home delivery for a multiparous woman who has had two normal deliveries before. Halfway through the first stage of labour the patient has become increasingly distressed and is complaining of severe abdominal pain.

The pain continues between contractions, which are occurring every 3 minutes and the midwife has noticed that the uterus is tender and hard on palpation.

Which of the following is the most likely complication?

A.   Chorioamnionitis
B.   Concealed placental abruption
C.   Obstructed labour
D.   Hyperstimulated labour
E.   Uterine rupture

Answer [ ]

4.12 You are in a labour room trying to cope with a severe postpartum haemorrhage whilst waiting for the registrar to arrive. The inexperienced student midwife hands you a selection of drugs to choose from to try and stop the uterine bleeding. Which of these drugs has she picked up in error?

A.   Atosiban
B.   Carboprost

C.   Ergometrine
D.   Misoprostol
E.   Oxytocin

Answer [ ]

4.13 A woman books for antenatal care in her fourth pregnancy. Her obstetric history includes three previous deliveries by caesarean section. She is predisposed to which obstetric complication?

A.   Cord prolapse
B.   Haemorrhage
C.   Placenta accreta
D.   Pre-eclampsia
E.   Unstable lie

Answer [ ]

4.14 The most important reason that administration of ergometrine to control postpartum haemorrhage is contraindicated in a woman with pre-eclampsia is:

A.   It is likely to make her vomit profusely
B.   It does not work as well as oxytocin
C.   It gives a sustained effect rather than a quick onset of action
D.   It is likely to increase her blood pressure
E.   It could decrease her intracranial pressure

Answer [ ]

4.15 As a junior doctor on the labour ward, it often feels as though you are being asked to insert an intravenous line on every woman in labour. Which of the following pregnant women does not need a cannula when she is admitted?

A.   A woman with an uncomplicated pregnancy delivering her sixth baby
B.   A primigravid woman whose haemoglobin was 95 g/l 2 weeks ago
C.   A woman who had a postpartum haemorrhage in her last delivery
D.   A woman who had a forceps delivery for fetal distress in her previous pregnancy
E.   A woman who had an emergency caesarean for fetal distress in her last pregnancy

Answer [ ]

4.16 Having had a massive postpartum haemorrhage following the delivery of her first baby a 34-year-old woman has received 8 units of blood, 2 units of cryoprecipitate, and fresh frozen plasma during the previous couple of hours. She has developed pulmonary oedema with an oxygen saturation of 55 per cent.

Currently, her temperature is 37.5, her pulse is 110 bpm, her blood pressure 90/40 mmHg, and her urine output is reduced to only 5 mls per hour.

The clotting screen is normal and her haemoglobin is currently 95 g/l.

What is likely to be the cause of this clinical situation?

A. Adult respiratory distress syndrome
B. Bacterial contamination of the blood transfused
C. Blood-borne viral infection
D. Delayed transfusion reaction
E. Inadequate transfusion

Answer [ ]

4.17 You are looking after a woman in labour who has had two fetal blood samples done already because of an abnormal cardiotocograph trace, the results of which are normal so far. The obstetric anaesthetist is keen for her to have an epidural inserted thereby avoiding a general anaesthetic if emergency delivery becomes necessary later. The most important reason for avoiding general anaesthetic in labour is:

A. General anaesthetic in an emergency takes longer than topping up an epidural
B. Epidural can lower her blood pressure and improve placental perfusion
C. The mother does not have to be kept 'nil by mouth' in labour
D. The mother is at risk of Mendelssohn's syndrome (aspiration pneumonitis)
E. Ventouse delivery is more difficult under general anaesthetic (GA) because the mother cannot push

Answer [ ]

4.18 When performing a fetal blood sample in the first stage of labour it is preferable to place the mother in the left lateral position for which the following reason:

A. Necessary equipment for the procedure can be placed on the bed within reach
B. Placental perfusion is improved by relieving pressure on maternal vena cava
C. The baby may be lying on the placenta thereby compressing the umbilical cord
D. The cervical os is easier to access with the amnioscope
E. The midwife is more easily able to support the mother's legs

Answer [ ]

4.19 Whilst on labour ward you notice a commotion in one of the delivery rooms and hear someone shouting for help with shoulder dystocia.

Which of the following procedures may help the birth attendants deliver the baby in this life-threatening situation?

A. Delivering the anterior arm of the baby
B. Fundal pressure on the uterus
C. Lovsett's manoeuvre
D. Mauriceau-Smellie-Veit manoeuvre
E. McRobert's manoeuvre to hyperflex the maternal hips

Answer [ ]

4.20 A primigravid woman has been in labour for nearly 20 hours and actively pushing for 90 minutes so a decision is made to perform an assisted vaginal delivery on account of delay in the second stage.

The woman is at increased risk of which complication?

A. Cervical dystocia

B. Fetal distress

C. Inverted uterus

D. Paravaginal haematoma

E. Postpartum haemorrhage

Answer [ ]

Extended Matching Questions

A	Amniotomy
B	Elective caesarean section
C	Electronic fetal monitoring
D	Emergency caesarean section
E	Intermittent auscultation
F	Request a clotting screen
G	Routine elective episiotomy
H	Titrated synthetic Oxytocin infusion
I	Vaginal examination in theatre with the operating team standing by
J	Ventouse delivery

The following clinical scenarios apply to women delivering in a hospital obstetric unit. In each case, select the most appropriate management plan.

Each option may be used once, more than once, or not at all.

4.21 A primigravid 32-year-old woman presents early in the first stage of spontaneous labour at 38 weeks of gestation, contracting once every 10 minutes. Her membranes have just ruptured spontaneously and fresh meconium is seen in the liquor.

Answer [ ]

4.22 During vaginal examination in a woman's third labour, the midwife finds the cervix to be 8 cm dilated and feels a pulsatile cord alongside the fetal head. The head is below the ischial spines and in the occipito-anterior (OA) position.

Answer [ ]

4.23 A primigravid woman has had an uncomplicated pregnancy so far under midwifery care and presents with a heavy vaginal bleed at 39 weeks of gestation. The uterus is nontender and the baby is well grown with a cephalic presentation, four-fifths palpable. The condition of both mother and baby is stable but she is contracting strongly every 3 minutes and the blood continues to trickle from the vagina.

Answer [ ]

4.24 Having been admitted to labour ward 4 hours previously experiencing three contractions every 10 minutes, a low-risk primigravid patient is examined and her cervix is found to be 6 cm dilated with intact membranes. She mobilises in her labour room using nitrous oxide for analgesia and 4 hours later the cervix is 7 cm dilated.

Answer [ ]

4.25 A midwife calls you in to a delivery room because of a small vaginal bleed in a low-risk primigravid woman whose labour has been progressing normally. The midwife is auscultating the baby's heartbeat, which has been 70 bpm for 5 minutes. The mother's pulse is 90, her blood pressure is stable, and the cervix is 8 cm dilated.

Answer [ ]

A	Arrange emergency caesarean section
B	Check airway and administer oxygen by facial mask
C	Check plasma glucose level
D	Commence electronic fetal monitoring
E	Contact the consultant haematologist on call
F	Cross-match blood
G	Counsel about postpartum sterilisation
H	Perform a vaginal examination
I	Rapid IV administration of 1 litre crystalloid
J	Request urgent USS
K	Site IV cannula and check haemoglobin

These clinical scenarios relate to an emergency situation involving a woman on the labour ward in the third trimester of pregnancy. In each case, choose the most appropriate initial management plan.

Each option may be used once, more than once, or not at all.

4.26 A 28-year-old woman with type 1 diabetes attends triage on labour ward early one morning at 30 weeks of gestation because of an antepartum haemorrhage. She collapses in the waiting room, and when you attend to sort out the situation she appears confused and is asking where she is.

Answer [ ]

4.27 A 34-year-old woman is admitted to delivery suite at term in her eighth pregnancy. She has delivered six live children previously. On examination the cervix is 7 cm dilated and she is involuntarily pushing.

Answer [ ]

4.28 The labour ward is very busy when a young primigravid woman is admitted at 38 weeks of gestation with contractions. Earlier, in antenatal clinic she was found to have a breech presentation confirmed by scan and is awaiting a consultant outpatient appointment arranged for tomorrow. On admission she experiences spontaneous rupture of membranes and the cervix is found to be 6 cm dilated.

Answer [ ]

4.29 A woman who has just delivered twins collapses in the delivery room at the end of the second stage. The placenta is still in situ and the midwife tells you that she has just noticed a large amount of blood in the bed. The patient is unresponsive and has a tachycardia of 120 bpm.

Answer [ ]

4.30 Having been admitted with a fresh antepartum haemorrhage, a primiparous patient is diagnosed with a placental abruption at 34 weeks of gestation. Both mother and baby are stable at the moment, but the haematology technician has just contacted you to say that the clotting screen you sent to the lab an hour ago is not normal.

Answer [ ]

A	Cryoprecipitate
B	Iron infusion
C	Iron injections weekly
D	Oral iron
E	Platelet transfusion
F	Recombinant Factor VIIa
G	Transfuse 'O negative' blood
H	Transfuse type-specific blood
I	Transfuse cross-matched blood
J	Transfuse blood from cell saver

Each of these clinical scenarios describes a pregnant woman whose clinical condition is or could be compromised by haemorrhage; for each patient pick the best management option given the information that you are presented with.

Each option may be used once, more than once, or not at all.

4.31 During a routine caesarean section under spinal anaesthetic the consultant you are assisting unexpectedly comes across a low-lying placenta and the woman loses 2,500 ml blood before the baby is delivered and the placenta is removed from the uterus. Her haemoglobin done the previous day is 105 g/l. Her blood pressure has dropped to 70/40 and she has become unresponsive to questions.

Answer [ ]

4.32 A primigravid woman has a blood test at 36 weeks of gestation and is found to have a haemoglobin level of 69 gm/l. She has not been taking the iron tablets prescribed by her GP because of severe nausea, and has tried three different preparations.

Answer [ ]

4.33 A 31-year-old primigravid woman is known to have β thalassaemia and has a haemoglobin level of 80 g/l by the time she reaches 38 weeks of gestation. She is symptomatic, feeling very tired and slightly breathless.

Answer [ ]

4.34 You are the junior doctor on labour ward assisting the registrar dealing with a manual removal of placenta under general anaesthetic. During the last 15 minutes the woman started bleeding heavily and so far has lost 3 litres of blood. The consultant obstetrician has been called and the 2 units of blood stored on the labour ward have already been transfused. Her heart rate is 120 bpm and her blood pressure is 90/50 mmHg.

Answer [ ]

4.35 A 35-year-old woman pregnant with twins attends antenatal clinic at 28 weeks of gestation for a growth scan. She has a routine blood test done and her haemoglobin is 90 g/L.

Answer [ ]

A	Attempt to turn the baby (version) for vaginal delivery
B	Arrange an emergency caesarean section
C	Arrange an elective caesarean section
D	Ask the anaesthetist to site an epidural
E	Conduct an assisted vaginal delivery with ventouse or forceps
F	Conduct a breech extraction
G	Obtain a fetal blood sample from the scalp
H	Obtain a fetal blood sample from the cord
I	Obtain maternal serum for cross-matching blood
J	Obtain maternal serum for a clotting screen
K	Perform a vaginal examination to exclude cord prolapse
L	Put up a syntocinon drip to increase the contractions
M	Rupture the membranes with an amnihook

As the junior doctor on the labour ward you have been called to assist the midwives with the management of labouring women experiencing a complication.

In each scenario, choose the most appropriate immediate action that you think the obstetric team (not necessarily you personally) should take.

Each option may be used once, more than once, or not at all.

4.36 One hour after administration of a prostaglandin pessary to induce labour for postmaturity, a primigravid woman is found to be having more than six contractions in 10 minutes. You are asked to site an intravenous cannula whilst the midwife removes the pessary. Although the contractions lessen in frequency to 3 in 10 minutes, the baby becomes bradycardic and you can hear that the fetal heart rate has been running at 90 bpm for 4 minutes so far.

Answer [　]

4.37 A 21-year-old primigravid woman was admitted in spontaneous labour 6 hours previously when the cervix was 7 cm dilated and has been relaxing in the birthing pool, coping without formal analgesia. The liquor is clear and intermittent auscultation of the fetal heart is reassuring. The cervix is now 8 cm dilated and the baby appears to be lying in the occipito-posterior position.

Answer [　]

4.38 A multiparous woman has delivered her first twin vaginally 15 minutes ago and there is no sign of the second twin appearing although the contractions are continuing every 2 minutes. On examination it is apparent that the second twin is lying transversely in the uterus.

Answer [　]

4.39 A rather frightened 17-year-old primigravid woman is in spontaneous labour and the cervix is 6 cm dilated. The midwife has noted meconium in the liquor and there are late decelerations on the cardiotocograph. The woman has asked for more analgesia and the midwife says that she is becoming more and more uncooperative.

Answer [ ]

4.40 A multiparous woman who has had three previous uncomplicated vaginal births is admitted in advanced labour at term and to everyone's surprise the presentation of the baby is found to be breech, station at the ischial spines, and the cervix 9 cm dilated. The membranes rupture just after the vaginal examination and the liquor is clear. The midwife commences a CTG trace, which shows occasional early decelerations.

Answer [ ]

A	Abruption of the placenta
B	Cervical laceration
C	Disseminated intravascular coagulation
D	Placenta accreta
E	Placenta praevia
F	Retained succenturiate lobe of placenta
G	Rupture of the uterus
H	Uterine atony
I	Vasa praevia
J	Velamentous insertion of the cord

Given the clinical information provided, select the most likely diagnosis for each of these obstetric patients experiencing vaginal bleeding.
Each option may be used once, more than once, or not at all.

4.41 A woman has just delivered her first baby and whilst the midwife is inspecting the placenta she has a brisk vaginal bleed of about 600 ml. Maternal observations are stable and the uterus feels well contracted. The midwife points out to you that there are blood vessels running through the membranes.

Answer [ ]

4.42 A primigravid woman aged 21 presents to labour ward at 39 weeks of gestation because of a brisk painless vaginal bleed of about 100 ml following intercourse. The uterus is nontender with a transverse fetal lie. The fetal heart is steady at 140 bpm.

Answer [ ]

4.43 You are called to see a primigravid woman who has started bleeding half-way through the first stage of labour, losing 200 ml in a couple of minutes. Despite her epidural she seems to be in a great deal of pain and there are unmistakeable signs of severe fetal distress on the cardiotocograph.

Answer [ ]

4.44 During her second labour a 35-year-old woman starts to lose fresh blood per vaginam. Her first baby was delivered by caesarean section because of fetal distress related to chorioamnionitis at 6 cm dilatation in the first stage. This time the cervix has reached 7 cm dilatation but the contractions have stopped.

Answer [ ]

4.45 The midwife looking after a primigravid woman in labour at term ruptured the membranes 5 minutes ago with an amnihook to speed up the progress of the first stage of labour, as cervical dilatation has been stuck at 5 cm for the last 4 hours. You are called because the midwife is concerned that the liquor is very heavily bloodstained. The uterus is nontender, contracting 4 in 10 minutes and the fetal heart rate has risen from a baseline of 120 before amniotomy to 180 bpm with late decelerations.

Answer [ ]

A	Administer oral benzylpenicillin
B	High vaginal swab on admission
C	Induction of labour and intrapartum IV benzylpenicillin
D	Prescribe intrapartum IV benzylpenicillin
E	Prescribe intrapartum IV erythromycin
F	Prescribe intrapartum IV clindamycin
G	Prescribe intrapartum IV metronidazole
H	Reassure the patient that no action is necessary
I	Vaginal cleansing with chlorhexidine on admission in labour

Each of these pregnant women has been found to be carrying group B streptococcus on vaginal swabs at some stage in this or a previous pregnancy. For each patient select the most appropriate management plan to prevent early-onset neonatal group B streptococcal disease.

Each option may be used once, more than once, or not at all.

4.46 A primigravid woman has been admitted to labour ward for elective caesarean delivery for persistent breech presentation. She had a swab taken last week by her GP that has grown group B streptococcus.

Answer [ ]

4.47 A woman is admitted in established labour at term. An MSU done 2 weeks ago when she had abdominal pain grew group B streptococcus.

Answer [   ]

4.48 At 37 weeks of gestation a multiparous woman is admitted with prelabour rupture of the membranes. She was found to have group B streptococcus on a high vaginal swab done a few weeks previously when she was seen in another maternity unit in Skegness on holiday.

Answer [   ]

4.49 A woman presents in spontaneous labour at term with her second baby. In her previous pregnancy she had a swab done in the first trimester that grew group B streptococcus; then she delivered at term and the baby was fine. She has not had any swabs done in this pregnancy.

Answer [   ]

4.50 A woman is admitted in established labour at 38 weeks with ruptured membranes. Her previous baby developed meningitis after delivery that was subsequently found to be due to group B streptococcus. Following that delivery, she developed a rash when she was given penicillin in the puerperium to prevent her developing endometritis.

Answer [   ]

Curriculum Module 5

Postpartum Problems (the Puerperium) Including Neonatal Problems

Syllabus

- You will be expected to understand and demonstrate appropriate knowledge, management skills, and attitudes in relation to postpartum maternal problems including the normal and abnormal postpartum period, postpartum haemorrhage, therapeutics, perineal care, psychological disorders, infant feeding, and breast problems.
- You will be expected to demonstrate an understanding of the investigation and management of immediate neonatal problems including neonatal resuscitation.

Learning Outcomes

Even in the past when women stayed in hospital for days 'lying-in' (and acquiring venous thrombosis!), it has been the remit of the GP to diagnose problems in the puerperium. The management of patients recovering from traumatic deliveries is now an increasing part of the GP's workload as cost and social pressures result in patients spending very little time in hospital after delivery. Some patients are even leaving hospital the following day when they have been delivered by caesarean section. For this reason, we feel that the problems that can occur in the puerperium are core knowledge for a GP working in the United Kingdom, and we continue to expand the bank of questions on this topic.

Single Best Answer Questions

5.1 A woman who delivered her first baby 2 days ago is having problems breast-feeding on account of sore nipples. She is considering bottle feeding instead and the midwife asks you to see her on a home visit.

Which of the following statements is correct advice regarding breast-feeding in her situation?

A. She could give the baby a bottle as well as breastfeeding
B. She should continue to breast-feed to avoid milk stasis
C. She should stop breast-feeding until the soreness has resolved
D. She will need antibiotics to continue breast-feeding
E. Sore nipples mean that she is already developing mastitis

5.2 A baby born to a mother who has used cocaine in pregnancy is at increased risk of which problem?

A. Hypoglycaemia

B. Jaundice

C. Low birth weight

D. Nasal septum defect

E. Neonatal abstinence (withdrawal) syndrome

Answer [ ]

5.3 A woman who delivered her first baby 8 hours ago asks for an urgent home visit from her GP because she is in severe pain and cannot pass urine. She had a normal birth with no stitches and was sent home 6 hours post-partum, when it seemed that all was well. On examination the vulva looks swollen.

Which is the most likely diagnosis?

A. Acute attack of herpes

B. Anaphylactic reaction

C. Paravaginal haematoma

D. Perineal abscess

E. Thrombosed vulval varicosities

Answer [ ]

5.4 For babies born to obese women without diabetes mellitus, which of the following risks is increased?

A. Hypoglycaemia

B. Jaundice

C. Macrosomia

D. Polyhydramnios

E. Transient tachypnoea of the newborn

Answer [ ]

5.5 A woman who is HIV positive has just been delivered of her first baby by caesarean section.

Which of these statements is correct advice regarding the care of the neonate?

A. Cord blood should be sent for viral load

B. She should be advised against breast-feeding the baby

C. The baby should not have any invasive tests such as blood tests

D. The baby does not need antiretroviral therapy

E. The baby should be isolated from the mother until she has stopped bleeding

Answer [ ]

5.6 You are asked to review a woman on the postnatal ward because the mid-wives suspect that she has had a pulmonary embolus 48 hours after an emergency caesarean section for slow progress in labour.

She complains of shortness of breath but no pleuritic chest pain. On examination her legs are of normal size and she is wearing antiembolism stockings.

Which of these statements is correct regarding her management?

A. Anticoagulation should be delayed as it may cause her section wound to bleed
B. Await the results of a lower limb Doppler study
C. Breathlessness is the only symptom so pulmonary embolus is unlikely
D. She cannot breast-feed if you prescribe heparin
E. She should be fully anticoagulated whilst awaiting the results of tests

Answer   [   ]

5.7 When a baby is born to a diabetic mother on insulin, although there is a risk of neonatal hypoglycaemia it is recommended that babies stay with their mothers if possible.

In which circumstance may admission to the special care baby unit be avoided?

A. The baby can be fed every 2 hours on the postnatal ward
B. The baby can be tube fed on the postnatal ward
C. The baby can maintain blood glucose levels >2 mmol/L before feeds
D. The baby feeds well orally
E. The baby has no clinical signs of hypoglycaemia before feeds

Answer   [   ]

5.8 A woman is admitted 2 days after a normal delivery with severe sepsis and the on-call obstetric consultant advises you to institute the 'sepsis six' care bundle.

Which of these statements is correct regarding this clinical pathway?

A. Administer facial oxygen whatever the pO$_2$
B. Intravenous fluids should be used if the woman appears clinically dehydrated
C. Lactate levels > 2 mmol/L mean severe sepsis
D. Oral antibiotics are adequate if she is not vomiting
E. The 'bundle' must be undertaken within 6 hours of diagnosis

Answer   [   ]

5.9 The day after her forceps delivery under epidural anaesthesia, you are asked to see a woman who has a severe continuous headache that has come on gradually and has been worsening over the previous few hours. The midwifery staff on the postnatal ward telephone to expedite your attendance as they are becoming concerned about her condition. She seems to be developing an acute confusional state.

Her pulse, blood pressure (BP) and temperature are all normal and there are no focal neurological signs.

Select the most likely diagnosis for her headache:

A. Cerebral vein thrombosis
B. Dural tap
C. Meningitis
D. Migraine
E. Subarachnoid haemorrhage

Answer [ ]

5.10 You review a postpartum woman at home who has been discharged following a caesarean section 3 days ago. She was given antibiotics in labour and tells you that the baby was admitted to the neonatal intensive care unit shortly after delivery. He is very unwell with meningitis.

What is the most likely infective organism?

A. Candida Albicans
B. E. Coli
C. Group A Streptococcus
D. Group B Streptococcus
E. Staphylococcus Aureus

Answer [ ]

5.11 A woman has just delivered her second baby yesterday and requests sterilisation before she goes home. Her partner is not keen for her to have this done as he is having trouble coping with their toddler and wants her to go home immediately. Whilst you are counselling her about puerperal sterilisation, which of the following statements is correct about this situation?

A. Clip sterilisation is more likely to fail if it is done now as the fallopian tubes are thicker
B. If she is sterilised now it will take longer for the uterus to involute
C. Laparoscopic sterilisation is feasible immediately postpartum
D. Puerperal sterilisation requires the written consent of both partners
E. She should defer the decision 24 hours for further discussion to avoid regret

Answer [ ]

5.12 A woman is recovering on the postnatal ward following an emergency caesarean section. On the third day she complains of discomfort and swelling in her right leg, which is clearly larger than the left leg, with a tender calf. The most appropriate medication whilst awaiting the results of further investigation is:

A. Enoxaparin 20 mg daily
B. Enoxaparin 40 mg daily
C. Enoxaparin 1 mg per kg twice daily
D. Graduated compression stockings
E. Loading dose of Warfarin

Answer [ ]

5.13 A diabetic woman who has been on insulin since the age of 11 years has just delivered her first baby. Which of these statements contains correct advice regarding the management of her diabetes in the puerperium?

A. Breast-feeding is contraindicated because of the risk of hypoglycaemia

B. Glucose tolerance test should be arranged for 6 weeks postpartum

C. Insulin should be stopped for 24 hours in case she becomes hypoglycaemic

D. She needs a sliding scale for 24 hours

E. She should immediately revert to her prepregnant dose of insulin

Answer [ ]

5.14 A community midwife asks you to attend a home delivery because she cannot determine the sex of the baby. On examination the newborn infant is well but the genitalia are ambiguous with a small phallus and some scrotal-like development of the skin. Which is the most appropriate course of action?

A. Advise the parents to choose a name that could be either male or female

B. Reassure the parents that the child is male with undescended testes

C. Send a referral letter to paediatric clinic so karyotyping can be arranged

D. Send the baby into hospital for urgent paediatric review

E. Take the baby's blood for 17-hydroxyprogesterone levels

Answer [ ]

5.15 A woman consults you in surgery about feeling very low in mood for the last 4 weeks. She is experiencing bouts of crying, off her food, and having trouble sleeping. She delivered her first baby 6 weeks ago and is very upset that she has had to give up breast-feeding as she felt unable to cope.

What is the most appropriate course of action to deal with her symptoms?

A. Admit her urgently to a 'mother and baby unit'

B. Inform her that her symptoms are very common and will resolve shortly

C. Inform her that she has a mental illness and should see a psychiatrist

D. Refer to a breast-feeding counsellor

E. Suggest that she takes an antidepressant and monitor her progress

Answer [ ]

5.16 You have just finished assisting at a difficult caesarean section during which the woman sustained a massive haemorrhage. She is at present on the High Dependency Unit having a blood transfusion but her condition seems to have stabilised and her husband is at her bedside looking after the newborn baby.

His mother came into hospital with them but only one person was allowed into the operating theatre with her.

In the hospital cafe you meet the mother-in-law who is anxiously waiting for news and asks you why the delivery is taking so long.

You must deal with her enquiry but what should you tell her?

A. That the mother and baby are both fine

B. That she is not on labour ward but you are not allowed to tell her why

C. That you will send the husband to give her information

D. The delivery has been complicated but everything is alright now

E. To go to the High Dependency Unit to see the new mother and baby

Answer [ ]

5.17 The highest risk factor for puerperal psychosis is:

A. A history of postnatal depression in a previous pregnancy

B. A previous history of bipolar disorder

C. Eating disorder as a teenager

D. Family history of puerperal psychosis

E. Personality disorder

Answer [ ]

5.18 On the evening shift you go to the postnatal ward and find that the midwives have been waiting for you to complete a list of prescribing tasks they have been saving up.

Which task takes priority?

A. A woman who delivered a stillborn baby this morning is waiting for a prescription for cabergoline to suppress lactation.

B. A woman who had a caesarean section 3 days ago is ready to be discharged and is awaiting a prescription for analgesic drugs to take home.

C. A woman who has just been readmitted with puerperal sepsis is waiting for antibiotics. Her temperature is 35.8°C, BP 90/60 mmHg, and pulse 120 bpm.

D. A woman who suffered a major postpartum haemorrhage yesterday is waiting for you to prescribe a blood transfusion. Her haemoglobin is 60g/L.

E. A woman who had an emergency caesarean section 2 hours ago is waiting for a prescription of low molecular weight heparin prophylaxis.

Answer [ ]

5.19 A 34-year-old primigravid Jehovah's Witness signed an advance directive refusing blood transfusion when she first booked for antenatal care. She has just been readmitted a week postpartum with a massive haemorrhage and is on the operating table where the consultant is having difficulty stopping the bleeding. Her haemoglobin is currently 30 g/L and her life hangs in the balance.

Which of the following statements is correct regarding the management of this situation?

A. Her husband can give consent for her to have a blood transfusion

B. Transfuse her without consent because it is in her best interests

C. Get an emergency court order to transfuse

D. Respect advance directive and withhold transfusion

E. Transfuse her own blood from the cell saver

Answer [ ]

5.20 A woman was delivered of her first baby using forceps because of fetal distress in the second stage of labour. The baby is doing fine but the mother sustained a third-degree tear that has been repaired by your consultant. When debriefing her about the third-degree tear, which of the following statements is true?

A. If she has another baby she will need a caesarean section

B. She will be given antibiotics and laxatives postpartum

C. She is very likely to be incontinent of flatus in the future

D. The tear will have involved the anal mucosa as well as the sphincter muscle

E. Third-degree tears do not occur with normal deliveries

Answer [ ]

Extended Matching Questions

A	Combined oral contraceptive pill
B	Condoms
C	Copper intrauterine device
D	Depo-Provera®
E	Diaphragm
F	Female sterilisation
G	Levonorgestrel intrauterine system
H	Progestogen-only pill
I	Spermicide gel
J	Vasectomy

These clinical scenarios describe mothers requesting contraceptive advice in the postpartum period. Select the most appropriate method of contraception for each woman.

Each option may be used once, more than once, or not at all.

5.21 Having just delivered her first baby, a 15-year-old schoolgirl is very keen to avoid getting pregnant again.

Answer [ ]

5.22 A 40-year-old woman who was delivered by caesarean section yesterday has now had two children. She wishes to start secure contraception immediately before she leaves hospital but does not want to rule out having another child in the future.

Answer [ ]

5.23 A 35-year-old woman with a BMI of 45 attends for her postnatal checkup with her first baby. She conceived after IVF treatment because of infertility due to polycystic ovarian syndrome.

She still has some frozen embryos in storage but does not want to conceive again just yet as she has been advised to lose a great deal of weight first.

Answer   [   ]

5.24 Having used the pill with no problems in the past, a 25-year-old wishes to restart contraception after delivering her first baby a week ago. She had a normal delivery, her lochia is normal, and she is successfully breast-feeding.

Answer   [   ]

5.25 A woman who used to suffer from premenstrual syndrome wishes to have a secure form of contraception after delivering her first baby. She has decided that she is very sensitive to hormones and requests a method that does not involve using hormones.

Answer   [   ]

A	Arrange a district nurse to supervise dressings
B	Arrange a visit from a breast-feeding peer-support group
C	Arrange readmission to the obstetric unit for review
D	Arrange urgent admission to the emergency medical ward
E	Ask the community midwife to visit at home
F	Prescribe broad spectrum antibiotics
G	Send her in to A&E
H	Take the sutures out and allow the wound to drain

These clinical scenarios describe recently delivered women who have developed complications. In each case, select the most appropriate management plan. Each option may be used once, more than once, or not at all.

5.26 A woman who had a caesarean section 2 days ago was discharged home yesterday. She has asked for a home visit this morning because there is copious sero-sanguinous fluid discharging from the wound.

Answer   [   ]

5.27 Two days after a normal delivery, a primiparous women telephones the surgery to report heavy vaginal bleeding with clots.

Answer   [   ]

5.28 You are asked to do a home visit to look at the caesarean wound of a patient who has been out of hospital for 4 days. She has an absorbable subcuticular suture in situ in the skin and there is a spreading cellulitis around the scar.

Answer [ ]

5.29 A primiparous patient who delivered 4 days ago is having problems with breast-feeding due to pain. On examination her nipples are cracked and sore, but there is no unusual swelling of the breasts.

Answer [ ]

5.30 The community midwife is doing a home visit for a woman who has been discharged from hospital 2 days after a forceps delivery. She is struggling with breast-feeding and has asked for help. The midwife telephones you because she has noticed that the woman's left leg is swollen.

Answer [ ]

A	Blood transfusion
B	Evacuation of retained products of conception
C	Examination under anaesthetic
D	Full blood count
E	Intravenous antibiotics
F	Norethisterone 5 mg tds
G	Oral antibiotics
H	Pelvic USS
I	Reassure the patient
J	Resuture the perineum

These clinical scenarios relate to women in the puerperium with problems following a vaginal delivery. For each scenario select the most appropriate course of action from the preceding list.

Each option may be used once, more than once, or not at all.

5.31 You are seeing a 24-year-old woman in your GP surgery for her postnatal check. She had a normal vaginal delivery 6 weeks ago with a small second-degree perineal tear. She is breast-feeding and is feeling well. She tells you that she still has a pink loss vaginally but there have been no clots and the loss is not offensive.

Answer [ ]

5.32 You are the junior obstetric doctor on call overnight, and at midnight are asked to see a woman who has been readmitted 3 days after the delivery of her third child. Over the last few hours her lochia has become heavier and she is passing clots vaginally. Her observations are pulse 90 bpm, blood pressure 125/85, temperature 37.5°C, and respiratory rate 14. The midwife has already taken a high vaginal swab.

Answer [ ]

5.33 The midwives ask you to review a woman on the postnatal ward one day after delivery. She had a right medio-lateral episiotomy that was repaired by the registrar and now she is complaining of severe perineal pain so she can't sit comfortably. On examination her temperature is 36.5°C, pulse 75 bpm, and blood pressure 110/65 mmHg. The episiotomy sutures are intact and the perineum is bruised with a 3 cm swelling underlying the sutures. The vaginal sutures are also intact and there is no swelling in the vagina.

Answer [ ]

5.34 Eight hours after delivery a woman who has just arrived on the postnatal ward suddenly starts to bleed heavily per vaginam, losing another 200 ml on top of the 300 ml estimated blood loss at delivery. Her predelivery haemoglobin done on admission in labour was 115 g/L. The notes indicate that the placenta was removed in pieces after the cord came off during controlled cord traction.

Answer [ ]

5.35 A woman is readmitted by her community midwife because she is worried about the appearance of the perineal wound a week after delivery. On examination you find that the wound has broken down and the tissues are covered in a sloughy yellow-green exudate that smells offensive.

Answer [ ]

A	Bimanual pressure to compress the uterus
B	Controlled cord traction (Brandt Andrews method)
C	Ergometrine 500 micrograms IM
D	Evacuation of uterus
E	Inject carboprost (Hemabate®) into the uterus
F	IV infusion of 40 units of oxytocin over 4 hours
G	IV dose of 40 units of oxytocin stat
H	Manual removal of placenta
I	Place a Bakri balloon into the uterine cavity

Each of these obstetric patients has either bled heavily after delivery or is at risk of doing so and this question refers to the prevention or treatment of postpartum haemorrhage. Choose the most appropriate management plan for each woman.

Each option may be used once, more than once, or not at all.

5.36 A 35-year-old woman has just had an emergency caesarean section for failure to progress in labour and the baby weighed 4.8 kg. During the delivery the blood loss was estimated at nearly a litre but she is no longer bleeding actively. As they are suturing the skin at the end of the operation, the registrar asks you to prescribe something to keep the uterus contracted.

Answer [ ]

5.37 A woman has delivered her third baby at home 2 hours ago but the community midwife has transferred her in to hospital because she has not been able to deliver the placenta despite active management of the third stage. There is quite a big blood clot in the bed that amounts to about 600 ml.

Answer [ ]

5.38 A woman is urgently brought back to labour ward 6 hours after a normal delivery because she suddenly bleeds heavily vaginally, losing 500 ml in a couple of minutes. Looking through her previous notes you see that a succenturiate lobe was mentioned on her anomaly scan at 21 weeks of gestation.

Answer [ ]

5.39 You are the only doctor on labour ward when a woman who was being induced for pre-eclampsia unexpectedly starts pushing and rapidly delivers the baby and placenta. She has a brisk postpartum haemorrhage of 500 ml. She has already had 10 units of oxytocin given as the baby was delivering, and you have put up an oxytocin infusion with another 40 units so she is now nearing the maximum dose. The registrar is in the gynaecology emergency theatre dealing with a woman in extremis due to a ruptured ectopic pregnancy and you are waiting for the obstetric consultant to arrive from home. She continues to bleed heavily, so you must select the best course of action to save her life.

Answer [ ]

5.40 The midwives ask you to put up an intravenous infusion on a woman who is bleeding heavily after delivery of her placenta. You are sure the bleeding is coming from the uterus but every time the senior midwife stops massaging the uterus the bleeding starts again. You are having trouble getting a cannula into a vein so you send for the anaesthetist and ask the midwife to continue rubbing the fundus. The registrar is on the way but you need to give something quickly to make the uterus contract.

Answer [ ]

A	Arterial blood gas
B	Blood cultures
C	CT pulmonary angiogram
D	CT brain
E	Chest x-ray
F	D-dimer
G	Electrophoresis
H	Haemoglobin
I	LFT daily until results are normal
J	LFT 10 days after delivery
K	Liver ultrasound
L	Lumbar puncture
M	Pelvic x-ray
N	Pulmonary V/Q scan

These clinical scenarios relate to postpartum women with complicated pregnancies experiencing problems or seeking advice after delivery. For each woman, select the most appropriate initial investigation that will help you make a diagnosis.

Each option may be used once, more than once, or not at all.

5.41 You are asked to see an unwell 27-year-old woman on the postnatal ward who delivered yesterday. She is complaining of a fronto-occipital headache that is so severe that she can hardly move and is associated with nausea. She had an epidural in labour that was initially ineffective and whilst it was being resited the dura was inadvertently punctured. Her temperature is 38°C.

Answer [ ]

5.42 A woman whose labour was induced for obstetric cholestasis has returned home from hospital and you are asked to review her by the community midwife. She asks you what tests she needs now that the baby is safely delivered.

Answer [ ]

5.43 A woman with sickle cell disease is on the postnatal ward after a caesarean section for the delivery of her first baby. She complains of pain at the top of her right leg near the hip joint and cannot stand up comfortably. There is no swelling of either leg on examination.

Answer [ ]

5.44 Following an unsuccessful attempt at induction of labour over 3 days, a primigravid woman has an emergency caesarean section at 42 weeks of gestation. The baby has been admitted to the Special Care Baby Unit (SCBU) with meconium aspiration and you are asked by the SCBU staff to review the mother there the following day because she has become increasingly short of breath.

Answer [ ]

5.45 A primigravid woman has a rather prolonged second stage but achieves a normal delivery of a 4 kg baby after pushing really hard for 2 hours. Shortly after delivery she becomes progressively short of breath and complains of mild left-sided chest pain on inspiration. On examination there is decreased air entry on the left side of her chest. Her midwife brings the saturation probe from theatre and tells you that her oxygen levels are normal.

Answer [ ]

A	Elective caesarean section at 37 weeks
B	Elective caesarean section at 39 weeks
C	External cephalic version
D	Induce labour before term
E	Vaginal birth and consider episiotomy
F	Vaginal birth with CTG monitoring
G	Vaginal birth with oxytocin drip
H	Take low-dose aspirin 75 mg in next pregnancy
I	Terminate the pregnancy

These clinical scenarios relate to women who have recently delivered and have returned to the hospital postnatal clinic for debriefing. In each case, select the most appropriate advice regarding her next pregnancy.

Each option may be used once, more than once, or not at all.

5.46 After being induced for severe pre-eclampsia at 34 weeks of gestation, a primigravid woman is delivered by emergency caesarean section for fetal distress at 8 cm dilatation. She is thinking of embarking on another pregnancy in about a year's time as her husband is keen to have another baby soon.

Answer [ ]

5.47 After a very prolonged first stage of labour, the registrar unsuccessfully attempts a forceps delivery in theatre for a primigravid woman who has been pushing for 2 hours. The position of the baby's head was occipito-anterior at the ischial spines with moulding++. A caesarean section was performed after three strong pulls during which there was no descent of the fetal head. The baby weighed 3.8 kg and was 2 weeks overdue.

Answer [ ]

5.48 Halfway through her labour, when the membranes ruptured at 5 cm dilatation, a primigravid woman was found to have a breech presentation and therefore had her first baby delivered by caesarean section. You observe from the operation notes that there was a bicornuate uterus that might lead to another breech presentation next pregnancy. Choose the best course of action if the next baby is breech too.

Answer [ ]

5.49 During a forceps delivery performed for fetal distress, a primigravid woman sustains a third-degree tear. At her follow-up appointment the perineum has healed well and she has made a full recovery with no symptoms related to the anal sphincter. She wishes to discuss plans for her next birth.

Answer [ ]

5.50 Having reached 8 cm cervical dilation in her first labour, a primigravid woman was delivered by emergency caesarean section because of a fetal bradycardia associated with fresh vaginal bleeding. The labour was progressing well up to that point but unfortunately the bradycardia turned out to be due to placental abruption and the baby did not survive. She does not feel strong enough to contemplate another pregnancy just yet, but is wondering about the mode of delivery next time.

Answer [ ]

Curriculum Module 6

Gynaecological Problems

Syllabus

▨ You will be expected to demonstrate appropriate knowledge, management skills, and attitudes in relation to benign gynaecological problems including urogynaecology, paediatric and adolescent gynaecology, endocrine problems, pelvic pain, and abnormal vaginal bleeding. This will include knowledge of early pregnancy loss, including clinical features, investigation, and management of disorders leading to early pregnancy loss such as miscarriage (including recurrent), ectopic pregnancy, and molar pregnancy.

▨ You will be expected to demonstrate an ability to assess and manage common sexually transmitted infections including HIV/AIDS and be familiar with their modes of transmission and clinical features. You will be expected to understand the principles of contact tracing. You will also be expected to know the basis of national screening programmes and their local implementation through local care pathways.

▨ You will be expected to demonstrate appropriate knowledge of clinical features, investigation, and management of premalignant and malignant conditions of the female genital tract. You will be expected to understand the indications and limitations of screening for premalignant and malignant disease. An understanding of the options available for palliative and terminal care, including relief of symptoms and community support, will be expected.

▨ The examiners will expect you to demonstrate appropriate knowledge and attitudes in relation to subfertility. This includes an understanding of the epidemiology, aetiology, management, and prognosis of male and female fertility problems. You will be expected to have a broad-based knowledge of investigation and management of the infertile couple in a primary care setting and appropriate knowledge of assisted reproductive techniques including the legal and ethical implications of these procedures.

Learning Outcomes

This represents a large part of the workload of a GP with an interest in women's health, and consequently there are many of these questions on the examination bank.

In 'benign gynaecology' areas of knowledge covered (many of which overlap) are menstrual problems; endocrinology, for example, polycystic ovarian syndrome and the menopause; pelvic pain; pelvic inflammatory disease and vaginal discharge; and paediatric/adolescent issues such as delayed puberty.

There is also an area mysteriously called 'issues relevant to a migrant population' that involves subjects such as female genital mutilation, infectious diseases, and ethical problems.

This module of the curriculum also covers sexually transmitted infections, subfertility, early pregnancy loss, and urogynaecology including prolapse and gynaecological oncology. Patients with problems in any of these areas are likely to present initially to the GP so this part of the curriculum features heavily in the actual examination. Questions are likely to concentrate on making a diagnosis and knowing when to refer rather than detailed knowledge of the specialised management once she reaches hospital, although the contents of national guidelines should be referred to in revision as they are likely to be relevant.

Single Best Answer Questions

6.1 A nulliparous 22-year-old woman presents with a 4-month history of inter-menstrual and postcoital bleeding. She is healthy with no other medical problems and is using the withdrawal method for contraception.

Select the most appropriate investigation:

A. Cervical cytology
B. Endocervical chlamydia swab
C. Hysteroscopy
D. Pregnancy test
E. Transvaginal ultrasound scan

Answer [ ]

6.2 An asymptomatic nulliparous 49-year-old woman attends for a routine cervical smear. The practice nurse finds it very difficult to access the cervix because it is pushed backwards and sideways into the left fornix by a 10 cm diameter pelvic mass.

Which is the mass most likely to be?

A. Bowel cancer
B. Diverticular abscess
C. Full bladder
D. Ovarian cyst
E. Uterine fibroid

Answer [ ]

6.3 A 16-year-old woman presents to the surgery with primary amenorrhoea. She has some development of secondary sexual characteristics and is 146 cm tall with a BMI of 28.

Which of these investigations is the most relevant to make a diagnosis for her amenorrhoea?

A. Follicle stimulating hormone (FSH) and luteinizing hormone (LH) levels
B. Karyotype
C. Pregnancy test
D. Serum testosterone
E. USS of pelvis

Answer [ ]

6.4 Some women present to their GP seeking HRT around the time of the menopause to get rid of their vasomotor symptoms. Many of these women are still menstruating.

Which of these statements is correct if HRT is prescribed in these circumstances?

A. HRT is first-line management in a patient at risk of osteoporosis
B. It protects against unwanted pregnancy in perimenopausal women
C. Period-free HRT is the most suitable formulation for menstruating women
D. Prescribe the lowest possible estrogen dose for the shortest possible time
E. The risk of breast cancer is not increased if she only uses HRT for 5 years

Answer [ ]

6.5 Which of the following is a feature of the human papilloma virus (HPV)?

A. Genital warts are associated with HPV subtypes 6 and 11
B. Infection causes intermenstrual bleeding
C. The virus can produce painful ulcers on the vulva
D. There are four different subtypes: HPV 6, 11, 16, and 18
E. Vaccination against HPV completely prevents cervical cancer

Answer [ ]

6.6 A first-year-degree student attends the university GP practice complaining of period pains that are severe enough to prevent her from going to lectures during the first 2 days of each period. Mild analgesic tablets have not helped. She is otherwise healthy and uses condoms for contraception.

Which is most appropriate management option?

A. Co-codamol tablets
B. Combined oral contraceptive pill
C. Prostaglandin synthetase inhibitors
D. Refer for diagnostic laparoscopy
E. Utero-sacral nerve ablation

Answer [ ]

6.7 A 42-year-old woman is diagnosed with a complete hydatidiform mole that was initially treated by surgical evacuation of the uterus. The Regional Trophoblastic Centre then treated her with methotrexate due to rising beta-hCG levels.

She is currently using barrier contraception but is worried about her age and wishes to become pregnant again as soon as possible.

What advice should she be given about when it is safe to discontinue all methods of contraception?

A. She may discontinue at any time
B. She may discontinue when hCG levels normalise

C. She should wait 6 months from the date of evacuation

D. She should wait 6 months from when hCG levels normalise

E. She should wait 12 months from completion of treatment

Answer [ ]

6.8 An 18-year-old student is referred to gynaecology clinic because she has experienced increasingly heavy irregular periods during the previous year. Her menarche occurred aged 14 and her periods were initially normal.

Her BMI is 38 and abdominal examination is unremarkable. She declines pelvic examination because she is a virgin.

Select the most likely diagnosis in her case:

A. Anovulatory cycles

B. Pelvic inflammatory disease

C. Polycystic ovarian syndrome

D. Thrombocytopaenia

E. Von Willebrand disease

Answer [ ]

6.9 A woman having a hysterectomy for fibroids after the age of 45 years may be advised by her gynaecologist to have her ovaries removed at the same time.

Identify the main reason for suggesting that she consider oophorectomy:

A. So that she can have postoperative estrogen-only replacement therapy

B. To avoid ovarian cysts in the future

C. To eliminate premenstrual syndrome

D. To prevent metabolic effects of polycystic ovarian syndrome, for example, diabetes

E. To prevent ovarian cancer

Answer [ ]

6.10 A woman telephones your surgery for advice about vomiting in pregnancy. She thinks that she is 6 weeks pregnant and is just starting to feel nauseous. She is very worried because she had her last pregnancy terminated at 10 weeks because of severe hyperemesis.

Regarding her situation, which is the best advice to give her?

A. Antiemetics are not available without a prescription in the United Kingdom

B. It is better to try and manage symptoms by dietary manipulation

C. Preemptive prescription of antiemetics has been shown to reduce the incidence of hyperemesis

D. Risk of recurrence of hyperemesis is less than 1 per cent

E. She needs a higher dose of folic acid than normal

Answer [ ]

6.11 A 68-year-old woman with a BMI of 30 presents to her GP with a history of urinary urgency and frequency almost every hour with occasional urge incontinence. She must wear a pad all the time and rarely leaves the house as a result. Vaginal examination reveals no prolapse and urinalysis is negative.

Which one of the following management options is most likely to ameliorate her symptoms?

A. Colposuspension operation
B. Electrical stimulation of pelvic floor muscle
C. Weight loss
D. Prescription of duloxetine
E. Bladder drill (retraining)

Answer [ ]

6.12 A 38-year-old woman attended for a routine cervical smear during which an asymptomatic polyp is noted on the surface of the cervix. The result of the smear was normal.

In counselling her about the polyp, which one of the following statements is true?

A. It could be caused by chlamydia
B. It is unlikely to be associated with endometrial pathology
C. It is most likely to be a nabothian follicle
D. It is associated with HPV infection
E. It should be removed because it is likely to be malignant

Answer [ ]

6.13 When you are on call for gynaecological emergencies in your hospital, you are frequently asked to organise management for women attending the Early Pregnancy Clinic. Which one of these statements is correct regarding the management of miscarriage?

A. Expectant management is the treatment of choice if the uterus is septic
B. Histological proof that the uterus contained trophoblastic tissue will always exclude ectopic pregnancy
C. Medical management is associated with an increased incidence of pelvic infection
D. Perforation of the uterus during surgical evacuation is more likely in incomplete rather than missed miscarriage
E. Women having a surgical evacuation should be screened for chlamydia

Answer [ ]

6.14 A woman has been fully investigated after her third first trimester miscarriage and all the results are normal. In this situation in which there is unexplained recurrent miscarriage, which of the following interventions have been shown to be effective in reducing the risk of further miscarriage?

A. Cervical cerclage
B. HCG injections

C. Metformin treatment

D. Progesterone supplements

E. Psychological support and regular scans

Answer [ ]

6.15 A routine 'dating' scan arranged by the midwife at 11 weeks of gestation shows that a primigravid woman has suffered a missed miscarriage. The sac contains a fetus about 9 weeks' size but there is no fetal heart pulsation seen. She was not expecting this as she has not had any bleeding at all during the pregnancy, so is extremely upset and would like to deal with the problem as quickly as possible.

Select the best management plan in her case:

A. Admit to hospital for medical management with methotrexate

B. Evacuate the uterus with cervical preparation

C. Expectant management with another scan in 2 weeks to see if she has miscarried

D. Give 800 micrograms of misoprostol

E. Prescribe mifepristone orally and follow up after 2 weeks

Answer [ ]

6.16 A 24-year-old woman whose scan reveals polycystic ovarian syndrome (PCO) consults you about management of her facial hirsutism. Her serum testosterone is within normal limits and she does not wish to conceive.

Which of these treatments for PCO is the most appropriate management option?

A. Clomifene citrate

B. Co-cyprindiol combined oral contraceptive pill

C. Cyproterone acetate

D. Metformin

E. Ovarian drilling

Answer [ ]

6.17 In your GP surgery you see a diabetic woman aged 49 years who seeks treatment for irregular heavy menstrual bleeding. Her pelvis feels normal on examination and speculum reveals a healthy cervix.

Which of the following statements about her management is correct?

A. LH/FSH levels are a useful investigation

B. Serum ferritin should be measured as well as haemoglobin at the first visit

C. She should be referred to gynaecology clinic

D. Testing for coagulation disorders should be done prior to commencing treatment

E. Tranexamic acid can be prescribed as first line therapy

Answer [ ]

6.18 You are seeing a 48-year-old woman for a preoperative checkup. She is due to have a hysterectomy for fibroids next week and is thinking of having her normal ovaries removed at the same time as the uterus. She wishes to discuss the possible benefits and problems associated with a surgical menopause. Which one of her ideas about the bilateral oophorectomy operation is actually correct?

A.   Oophorectomy will not affect her libido

B.   She will need sequential HRT to get rid of her menopausal symptoms

C.   It will completely prevent her from getting any gynaecological cancer in later life

D.   She should consider oophorectomy if her mother had ovarian cancer

E.   Oophorectomy will increase the operating time substantially

Answer   [   ]

6.19 A 23-year-old woman with a BMI of 50 attends your GP surgery to discuss her fertility problems because she and her husband have been trying to conceive for 18 months. She has irregular periods with a cycle varying from 35 to 42 days, and the ovulation predictor kits she has purchased from the chemist indicate that she is not ovulating. Her husband has two children from his previous marriage.

Which of the following is the most appropriate piece of advice?

A.   Continue trying for six more months; then you will refer her to infertility clinic

B.   Commence taking folic acid 10 mcg daily

C.   Make an appointment for her husband to arrange a semen analysis

D.   Prescribe clomifene citrate to be taken on days 2 to 6 of the cycle

E.   To avoid pregnancy until she has lost weight

Answer   [   ]

6.20 A young woman attends her GP's surgery with a positive pregnancy test after 7 weeks of amenorrhoea. She is anxious because has suffered two previous early pregnancy losses; a miscarriage at 10 weeks followed by an ectopic pregnancy that was managed surgically. Which course of action is most appropriate?

A.   Admit to gynaecology ward

B.   Arrange midwifery booking

C.   Refer for early scan

D.   Refer to antenatal clinic

E.   Take blood for serum hCG in the surgery

Answer   [   ]

Extended Matching Questions

A	Ascorbic acid
B	Clomifene citrate
C	Danazol
D	Depo-Provera®
E	Dianette®
F	Luteinizing hormone releasing hormone (LHRH) analogues
G	Medroxyprogesterone acetate
H	Mefenamic acid
I	Tamoxifen
J	Tibolone
K	Tranexamic acid

Each of these clinical scenarios describes a woman presenting to her GP requesting help with menstrual problems; for each patient pick the most appropriate treatment option given the information that you are presented with.

Each option may be used once, more than once, or not at all.

6.21 A 22-year-old nulliparous lady who is not currently sexually active seeking treatment for menorrhagia and primary dysmenorrhoea

Answer [ ]

6.22 An obese teenager with acne and frequent heavy periods seeking secure contraception

Answer [ ]

6.23 A 34-year-old overweight woman with irregular heavy bleeding whose endometrial biopsy reveals cystic hyperplasia with no atypia

Answer [ ]

6.24 A 30-year-old woman with three children has just undergone a third termination of pregnancy without complications. She has attended the surgery twice in the past for help with her menorrhagia and dysmenorrhoea.

Answer [ ]

6.25 A sterilised 32-year-old woman whose menorrhagia has not responded to treatment with nonsteroidal anti-inflammatory drugs.

Answer [ ]

A	Anterior colporrhaphy operation
B	Antibiotics
C	Biofeedback
D	Bladder drill (retraining)
E	Helmstein bladder distension
F	Injection of phenol into the bladder trigone
G	Sacrocolpopexy operation
H	Supervised pelvic floor physiotherapy
I	Tension-free vaginal tape (TVT) operation

Each of these scenarios describes a woman presenting to gynaecology clinic with urinary incontinence; for each patient pick the most appropriate treatment option given the clinical information.

Each option may be used once, more than once, or not at all.

6.26 Eighteen months after a colposuspension operation for stress incontinence, a 60-year-old woman presents with a recurrence of her incontinence. She brings with her the results of a private urodynamic study that she had done after surfing the Internet. This shows that she has a compliant bladder on filling in a sitting position, but when she stands up there is demonstrable leakage of urine associated with spikes of high detrusor pressure measurements >30 cm water.

Answer [ ]

6.27 Less than a week after her bladder pressure study where she was diagnosed as having detrusor instability, a 51-year-old postmenopausal woman comes to the surgery seeking treatment on account of a marked deterioration in her symptoms of dysuria, urinary frequency, and urgency with urge incontinence.

Answer [ ]

6.28 Six months after the normal vaginal birth of her first child, a 37-year-old teacher complains of urinary incontinence when doing her aerobic classes. On examination she does have a moderate cystocoele and minor rectocoele but no uterine descent.

Answer [ ]

6.29 A bladder pressure study excludes detrusor instability in a 55-year-old woman with a mixed picture of stress and urge urinary incontinence. Her symptoms are getting worse with frequent leakage despite intensive supervised pelvic floor physiotherapy.

Answer [ ]

6.30 A fit 62-year-old woman has had a vaginal hysterectomy done years ago for menorrhagia. She presents with 'something coming down' and on examination of the external genitalia you can see the vaginal vault protruding.

Answer [ ]

A	Appendicitis
B	Ectopic pregnancy
C	Haemorrhage into an ovarian cyst
D	Incomplete miscarriage
E	Missed miscarriage
F	Normal intra-uterine pregnancy
G	Partial hydatidiform mole
H	Threatened miscarriage
I	Urinary tract infection

These clinical scenarios describe women presenting with pain in early pregnancy. For each case select the most likely diagnosis.

Each option may be used once, more than once, or not at all.

6.31 A 23-year-old woman comes in to the Gynaecological Admission Unit complaining of left iliac fossa pain. She is very tender on the left side of her abdomen and on pelvic examination you find cervical excitation. She has had 7 weeks of amenorrhea and her serum βhCG is 5,000 IU/ml. The transvaginal ultrasound scan shows a small, empty, rounded structure (thought to be a gestational sac) in the uterus.

Answer [ ]

6.32 A week after her 12-week dating scan, a 24-year-old woman presents to A&E with an acute onset of central abdominal pain and nausea. On examination you find severe lower abdominal tenderness with generalised guarding and rebound. Her white cell count is $14 \times 10^6/l$, and urinalysis is negative.

Answer [ ]

6.33 An obese 35-year-old who had her Mirena® intrauterine system removed 5 months ago on account of breast tenderness attends her GP to complain of lower abdominal discomfort and that her breast tenderness persists. She remains amenorrhoeic. On examination you can feel a mass in her lower abdomen above the symphysis pubis.

Answer [ ]

6.34 A 21-year-old woman is admitted to A&E by ambulance having collapsed while out shopping. On arrival at hospital she is complaining of shoulder tip pain, and examination shows a tender abdomen with guarding. She had a copper coil fitted just after the delivery of her 2-year-old son, and thinks her last menstrual period was 2 weeks ago although it was lighter than usual.

Answer [ ]

6.35 A primigravid woman presents to the Early Pregnancy Unit with a history of 11 weeks' amenorrhea, minor lower abdominal discomfort, and a small amount of vaginal bleeding. A urine pregnancy test is positive. Pelvic examination reveals no tenderness and the uterus is the correct size with a closed cervical os.

Answer [ ]

A	Adenomyosis
B	Appendicitis
C	Chronic pelvic inflammatory disease
D	Endometriosis
E	Interstitial cystitis
F	Irritable bowel syndrome
G	Ovarian cyst
H	Polycystic ovarian syndrome
I	Urinary tract infection
J	Uterine fibroids

These clinical scenarios describe nonpregnant women presenting in the gynaecology clinic with lower abdominal or pelvic pain. For each case select the most likely diagnosis.

Each option may be used once, more than once, or not at all.

6.36 A 22-year-old student with an 18-month history of noncyclical intermittent lower abdominal pain and deep dyspareunia. She is tender in both adnexae and the uterus is retroverted.

Answer [ ]

6.37 As well as experiencing deep dyspareunia for 6 months, a 48-year-old woman has pain when her bladder is full, which is associated with urinary frequency and nocturia.

Answer [ ]

6.38 After years of being on the pill, a 35-year-old woman has developed gradually increasing severe dysmenorrhoea, intermittent pelvic pain, and dyspareunia in her first pill-free year. On examination her uterus is normal size but both adnexae are tender.

Answer [ ]

6.39 A woman who has had five normal deliveries complains of increasingly severe secondary dysmenorrhoea. Her periods are regular but becoming heavier. The uterus is bulky and very tender on pelvic examination.

Answer [ ]

6.40 A 24-year-old woman has been using the pill since her teenage years to control her heavy periods as well as for contraception. She seeks help on account of intermittent pain in both iliac fossae associated with abdominal bloating and deep dyspareunia.

Answer [ ]

A	Reassurance only
B	Repeat pelvic ultrasound at beginning of next cycle
C	Repeat pelvic ultrasound in 3 months
D	Repeat serum CA125
E	Routine referral to a gynaecological oncologist
F	Routine referral to a gynaecologist
G	Serum CA125 and repeat pelvic USS
H	Serum CA125 and urgent (2-week wait) referral to gynaecologist
I	Urgent (2-week wait) referral to gynaecological oncologist
J	Urgent (2-week wait) referral to gynaecologist

Each of these clinical scenarios relates to a woman presenting in a general practice surgery with an ovarian cyst. In each case select the most appropriate management plan for that patient.

Each option may be used once, more than once, or not at all.

6.41 A 54-year-old postmenopausal woman presents to your surgery with irregular vaginal bleeding over the last 6 months. An USS shows an endometrial thickness of 8 mm and large bilateral multiloculated ovarian cysts. There are no other abnormal features on the scan.

Answer [ ]

6.42 A 27-year-old woman gives a history of long-standing dysmenorrhoea and deep dyspareunia. A pelvic ultrasound shows a unilocular 4 cm diameter cyst on the left ovary consistent with a 'chocolate cyst'.

Answer [ ]

6.43 A 19-year-old woman attends surgery with right iliac fossa pain, nausea, and vomiting. Her last menstrual period was 3 weeks before and an USS shows a 3 cm diameter right ovarian cyst with internal echoes consistent with haemorrhage. Her pain settles with simple analgesia.

Answer [ ]

6.44 A 39-year-old woman complains of left iliac fossa pain radiating down her left leg. The ultrasound shows a 9 cm diameter complex cyst on her left ovary and her CA125 level is 470.

Answer [ ]

6.45 A 65-year-old woman presents to the surgery with loss of appetite and abdominal distension, 12 years after her menopause. It started with a bout of 'gastroenteritis', which has just settled. You organise a CA125 level, which is slightly raised at 55, and an ultrasound scan of the pelvis, which is normal.

Answer [ ]

A	Ergometrine infusion over 4 hours
B	Evacuation of uterus on routine consultant list tomorrow
C	Evacuation of uterus immediately on emergency list
D	Evacuation of uterus after cervical priming
E	Gemeprost pessaries
F	Intravenous antibiotics
G	Methotrexate injection
H	Mifepristone and misoprostol
I	Oxytocin infusion over 4 hours
J	Repeat βHCG level in 48 hours

These clinical scenarios describe women experiencing complications in the first trimester of pregnancy. For each case, select the most appropriate management plan for that patient.
Each option may be used once, more than once, or not at all.

6.46 Having developed hyperemesis, a 39-year-old primigravid patient has an USS during her hospital admission that shows a 'snowstorm appearance'. You are asked to review the scan and plan management when you take over the night shift at 8 pm.

Answer [ ]

6.47 A 20-year-old shop assistant presents to early pregnancy unit at 7 weeks gestation in her second pregnancy complaining of left-sided abdominal pain. She had an ectopic pregnancy a year ago that was treated by laparoscopic right salpingectomy. Her BP and pulse are normal and scan shows an empty uterus with a mixed echo mass in the left adnexa that is 2 cm in diameter. The βhCG level is 2,150 iu/ml and haemoglobin is 117 g/L.

Answer [ ]

6.48 A routine 'dating' USS shows that a 21-year-old woman, who had a ventouse delivery for her previous child 9 months ago, has suffered a missed miscarriage.

Answer [ ]

6.49 On admission to the gynaecology ward, you note that a young woman admitted with bleeding at 10 weeks of gestation has a temperature of 38.5°C and a tender uterus. There is a small amount of bleeding on speculum examination but the cervical os is open and you can see what looks like a gestation sac protruding through.

Answer [ ]

6.50 At 2 am you are summoned to A&E urgently to see a 23-year-old woman who is having a miscarriage. There is a great deal of blood all over the bed and someone has initiated an intravenous infusion as she is hypotensive. On speculum examination you have to remove clots from the vagina to visualise the cervix and find that the cervical os is wide open.

Answer [ ]

Fertility Control (Contraception and Termination of Pregnancy)

Syllabus

▪ You will be expected to demonstrate appropriate knowledge, management skills, and attitudes in relation to fertility control and termination of pregnancy (TOP).

▪ You will be expected to understand the indications, contraindications, complications, mode of action, and efficacy of all reversible and irreversible contraceptive methods.

▪ You will be expected to demonstrate appropriate knowledge of abortion and should be familiar with the accompanying laws related to abortion, consent, child protection, and the Sexual Offences Act(s).

▪ There may be conscientious objection to the acquisition of certain skills in areas of sexual and reproductive health but knowledge and appropriate attitudes as described previously will be expected.

Learning Outcomes

This module covers contraception including emergency contraception (EC) and TOP. Questions on this part of the syllabus test clinical knowledge and understanding of the law relating to TOP and assessing Lord Fraser competency for girls under the age of 16 years requesting contraception or TOP. The questions in the exam may also test attitudes and behaviours in terms of medical ethics as applied to fertility control. The RCOG recognises the relevance of fertility control to everyday general practice hence it is part of the DRCOG curriculum in addition to the option of studying for the Diploma of Sexual and Reproductive Health.

Single Best Answer Questions

7.1 If a 15-year-old schoolgirl consults you in the surgery for contraception provision; select the most appropriate statement:

A. She should be advised to have a cervical smear as she has become sexually active

B. She cannot attend a family planning clinic until she reaches the age of 16 years

C. There are unlikely to be child protection issues if she is deemed competent to give consent for treatment

D. You must inform her parents or legal guardians before prescribing

E. You should enquire about her sexual history regarding partners

Answer [ ]

7.2 Which of these statements is correct regarding the health of women who are using the combined pill for contraception?

A. An alternative method should be used if they are planning a long high-altitude trek

B. A family history of breast cancer is a contraindication

C. The risk of mortality from large bowel cancer is increased

D. The failure rate in typical use rather than in ideal use is <1 per cent

E. The risk of venous thromboembolism is about the same as in pregnancy

Answer [ ]

7.3 A woman comes to the GP surgery requesting referral for female sterilisation as she has had trouble with various other forms of contraception. She is not in a stable relationship currently but has had six pregnancies: five children and one ectopic pregnancy.

Which of these statements is correct regarding sterilisation?

A. A history of previous ectopic pregnancy is a contraindication to laparoscopic sterilisation

B. If she regrets her decision, reversal involves laparoscopic clip removal

C. Mirena® intrauterine system (IUS) has a much lower Pearl index than sterilisation

D. Sterilisation carries a lifetime failure rate of 1 in 2,000

E. There is a future risk of ectopic pregnancy

Answer [ ]

7.4 Which three compounds can be found as the estrogen component in combined oral contraception formulations?

A. Conjugated equine estrogen, estriol, estradiol valerate

B. Estriol, estradiol valerate, ethinylestradiol

C. Mestranol, estriol, estradiol valerate

D. Mestranol, estradiol valerate, ethinylestradiol

E. Mestranol, estriol, ethinylestradiol

Answer [ ]

7.5 A 15-year-old girl attends the GP surgery requesting contraception as she is sexually active using condoms but is very worried about pregnancy and wishes to use something much more secure. She has no relevant past medical history and you deem her to be Fraser competent to make decisions on her own behalf.

Select the best first-line contraception for her:

A. Combined pill

B. Depot medroxyprogesterone acetate

C.   Etonogestrel implant
D.   Levonorgestrel IUS
E.   Progestogen-only pill

Answer [ ]

7.6   A 52-year-old woman had a Mirena IUS® inserted 5 years ago for treatment of menorrhagia as well as contraception. She has been amenorrhoeic since it was inserted and is requesting HRT for menopausal symptoms.

What is the most appropriate advice to give her regarding her Mirena IUS® and contraception?

A.   If her Mirena IUS® is removed she should use barrier contraception for another 2 years
B.   In terms of her contraceptive needs the Mirena IUS® is effective for another 2 years
C.   Remove the Mirena IUS® as it will have run out of levonorgestrel
D.   The Mirena IUS® can be removed as HRT is adequate contraception
E.   The Mirena IUS® should be left in place so she can use estrogen-only HRT

Answer [ ]

7.7   You are asked to review a woman on the Day Case Unit who had a laparoscopic sterilisation yesterday. She has had four children between the ages of 6 months and 4 years, all delivered by caesarean section.

The nurses are concerned because she maintains that she is still not well enough to go home, although your consultant saw her last night after the operating list had finished and discharged her. When you examine her, you notice that the dressing on her suprapubic incision is wet.

Select the most appropriate course of action:

A.   Arrange an ultrasound
B.   Enquire sensitively about home circumstances
C.   Increase her analgesia
D.   Prescribe antibiotics
E.   Request a cystogram

Answer [ ]

7.8   A woman who has had two children has a Mirena IUS® fitted at the hospital. She attends the surgery for a checkup 6 weeks later but on speculum examination you cannot find the coil strings.

Which of the following statements is correct regarding counselling her about the situation?

A.   An x-ray is better than an USS to locate the coil
B.   She cannot be pregnant if the coil is in the uterus
C.   She is not currently covered for contraception
D.   The coil could not have been extruded per vaginam without her noticing
E.   The next step is to try and retrieve the coil strings with a thread retriever

Answer [ ]

7.9 In the surgery you are counselling a woman who is considering using a progesterone-only pill (POP) for contraception. Which is correct information about these preparations?

A. Additional measures are not required if the method is initiated on days 1 to 5 of the menstrual cycle

B. She can expect a couple of kilos weight gain associated with POP use

C. She should stop taking POP prior to major surgery to avoid thromboembolism

D. There is a link between POP use and breast cancer

E. The window for missed pill taking is only 3 hours for all formulations

Answer [ ]

7.10 When advising women about methods of postcoital emergency contraception, which statement is correct?

A. The copper device should be fitted within 10 days of unprotected intercourse

B. The levonorgestrel pill (Levonelle®) can only be used once in a cycle

C. Ulipristal (EllaOne®) works primarily by altering the endometrium to prevent implantation

D. Use of the coil may predispose to ectopic, but not the oral methods

E. Women with poorly controlled asthma should avoid ulipristal (EllaOne®)

Answer [ ]

7.11 Which is the single best course of action if a woman presents to your surgery at 12 weeks of gestation having conceived with an intrauterine contraceptive device (IUCD) in situ?

A. Do serial βHCG estimations to exclude ectopic pregnancy

B. Repeat the pregnancy test to check for miscarriage

C. Remove the coil if the strings can be visualised

D. Request an x-ray to localise the coil

E. Take triple swabs as infection is likely in this situation

Answer [ ]

7.12 A woman whose pelvic USS indicates that she has polycystic ovarian syndrome consults you because she does not wish to conceive for a couple of years. She has sought help previously for management of her facial hirsutism and her serum testosterone is within normal limits.

Select the most appropriate management option in her case from the following list:

A. Clomifene citrate

B. Co-cyprindiol (cyproterone acetate and 35 mcg ethinylestradiol)

C. Cyproterone acetate

D. Levonorgestrel releasing intrauterine system

E. Metformin

Answer [ ]

7.13 Which one of the following statements about laparoscopic female sterilisation is correct?

A. Applying two clips to each tube is advisable to improve efficacy
B. Diathermy sterilisation increases the chances of successful reversal
C. The clips are made of nickel so can't be used if a woman is allergic to base metal
D. The operation is usually done under local anaesthetic
E. The patient should regard it as an irreversible method of contraception.

Answer [ ]

7.14 A 28-year-old woman who is virgo intacta wishes to start contraception in advance of her marriage, which is arranged to happen in a few months' time. She has polycystic ovarian syndrome, which was diagnosed when she saw a gynaecologist with oligomenorrhea, and she is worried that she will develop hirsutism, which would spoil her wedding photographs.

From the list given in the following text, select the most appropriate form of contraception for her in these unusual circumstances:

A. Cerazette®
B. Dianette®
C. Marvelon®
D. Nexplanon®
E. NuvaRing®

Answer [ ]

7.15 A woman has unprotected intercourse with a stranger at a party 2 days before she consults you for emergency contraception (EC). She has since heard that he is HIV positive and she has made herself an appointment with the local GUM Clinic this afternoon.

Choose the best option for EC in her case:

A. EllaOne®
B. Levonelle 1500®
C. Marvelon®
D. Mirena®
E. Multiload Cu 375®

Answer [ ]

7.16 A woman who is using a copper intrauterine device (IUD) for contraception has had a cervical smear that shows the presence of actinomyces-like organisms. She has no pelvic pain or vaginal discharge and on examination her pelvis is normal. Her last menstrual period (LMP) was 2 weeks ago and she had sexual intercourse yesterday.

Which is the most appropriate management option for this woman?

A. Leave the IUD in place and arrange an USS to exclude pelvic abscess
B. Leave the IUD in place and reassure

C. Remove the IUD and prescribe EC
D. Remove the IUD and prescribe penicillin
E. Remove the IUD and repeat the smear

Answer [ ]

7.17 A neurology consultant colleague has written to you about an epileptic patient on your surgery list whose compliance with her phenytoin medication is poor so that she is having frequent fits. She attends surgery asking for contraceptive advice, having found a new partner.

What is the best method of contraception for her?

A. Cerazette®
B. Evra®
C. Marvelon®
D. Mirena®
E. NuvaRing®

Answer [ ]

7.18 Which of the following statements is true of abortions performed in the United Kingdom?

A. More than 90 per cent of terminations are performed in the first trimester below 13 weeks of gestation
B. Patients are not usually screened for sexually transmitted infections (STIs) if undergoing medical rather than surgical termination
C. Patients are routinely scanned to check the gestational age of the pregnancy
D. Simultaneous sterilisation should be carried out on request if the patient is having a general anaesthetic
E. Subsequent subfertility can be reliably prevented by administering routine antibiotic prophylaxis effective against chlamydia

Answer [ ]

7.19 A 40-year-old woman with mild learning difficulties needs contraception because she is having a sexual relationship with another patient in the same residential accommodation. An USS is requested because her periods are known to be heavy, and this reveals multiple small submucosal fibroids distorting her uterine cavity.

Select the most appropriate form of contraception in her case:

A. Copper IUD
B. Hysterectomy
C. Mercilon®
D. Mirena®
E. Nexplanon®

Answer [ ]

7.20 Which of the following statements is not true about the use of the combined oral contraceptive pill?

A.   It will reduce primary dysmenorrhoea
B.   It ameliorates the symptoms of premenstrual syndrome
C.   It is associated with an increased risk of pelvic inflammatory disease
D.   It reduces the incidence of benign breast disease
E.   It reduces the risk of ovarian cancer in later life

Answer [ ]

Extended Matching Questions

A	Combined oral contraceptive pill
B	Depot medroxyprogesterone acetate
C	Etonogestrel subdermal implant
D	Female sterilisation
E	Intrauterine contraceptive device
F	Levonelle®
G	Levonorgestrel intrauterine system
H	Male condom
I	Progestogen-only pill
J	Vasectomy

These clinical scenarios relate to women attending your surgery for contraceptive provision. In each case select the most appropriate method for her.
  Each option may be used once, more than once, or not at all.

7.21 An 18-year-old student is about to go abroad on a 'gap year' and wishes to organise effective contraception whilst she is away. She has regular periods and no relevant medical or family history.

Answer [ ]

7.22 The development of a latex-allergy rash on the vulva results in a 38-year-old woman requesting a change in her contraceptive plans. She has four children and has consulted you recently for heavy periods.

Answer [ ]

7.23 A 17-year-old hairdresser has just had her second TOP. Both pregnancies occurred as a result of running out of supplies of the pill.

Answer [ ]

7.24 At her postnatal appointment, a 38-year-old mother of three children seeks advice about a reliable method of contraception. She had severe breast tenderness on the progestogen-only pill and is therefore not keen on taking any hormones.

Answer [ ]

7.25 A 32-year-old woman attends gynaecology clinic, having been referred by her GP for sterilisation. She reveals that her husband and father of her two children has just found out about her extramarital affair and left the family home. Her lifestyle is rather chaotic and she needs a very secure method of contraception.

Answer [ ]

A	3 months
B	6 months
C	12 months
D	24 months
E	5 years
F	7 years
G	10 years
H	15 years
I	20 years

These statements refer to a 47-year-old woman seeking contraceptive advice. Choose the most appropriate time option given the clinical information in each scenario.

Each option may be used once, more than once, or not at all.

7.26 If the 47-year-old woman chooses the Mirena® how long will it be effective as a contraceptive in her particular case?

Answer [ ]

7.27 If the 47-year-old woman chooses a nonhormonal method, how long should she continue to use the method if she has her menopause (last ever period) next year?

Answer [ ]

7.28 The 47-year-old woman makes an informed decision to choose the combined pill as she has no cardiovascular risk factors. When she eventually stops taking the pill, for how long after cessation could she expect a protective effect against ovarian cancer?

Answer [ ]

7.29 If the 47-year-old woman makes an informed decision to choose the combined pill, how soon should you check her blood pressure after initiating the prescription?

Answer [ ]

7.30 If the 47-year-old woman makes an informed decision to choose the combined pill, how often should she attend for blood pressure checks?

Answer [ ]

A	Administer a GnRH analogue
B	Commence antibiotics
C	Commence the combined oral contraceptive pill (COC)
D	Commence oral progestogens for 25 days
E	Continue with the next pack of the COC without a pill-free period
F	Insert an IUD
G	No intervention is required
H	Remove the IUD
I	Use condoms as an additional form of contraception

These clinical scenarios relate to women seeking advice in the Family Planning Clinic in your surgery. For each case, select the most appropriate management plan.

Each option may be used once, more than once, or not at all.

7.31 A 26-year-old woman using Depot medroxyprogesterone acetate who has a BMI of 27 kg/m^2 is suffering from breakthrough bleeding. This is now causing relationship difficulties as she does not want to have intercourse when she is bleeding and she is annoyed that she needs to carry pads around with her all the time. She wishes to control the bleeding if possible.

Answer [ ]

7.32 A 32-year-old woman attends surgery because she is feeling unwell and on examination she has a large boil in her left armpit after shaving. You prescribe flucloxacillin 500 mg qds for 7 days. She is using Microgynon® for contraception and has five pills left in her pack.

Answer [ ]

7.33 A 29-year-old woman attends surgery. She has a BMI of 34 kg/m^2. She has bought the antiobesity drug orlistat over the counter at a chemist and is worried as she has developed severe diarrhoea since taking it. You discover that she is using Mercilon® for contraception but she has not had sexual intercourse since the commencement of orlistat.

Answer [ ]

7.34 A 27-year-old woman attends surgery because she has discovered that she is 8 weeks pregnant having had a scan in the local hospital department where she went complaining of severe nausea. This confirmed an intrauterine pregnancy and she has a Multiload Cu 375® in place. She is shocked to find herself pregnant but wishes to continue with the pregnancy.

Answer [   ]

7.35 A 34-year-old woman attends your surgery. She has a Nova T 380® copper IUD in situ for contraceptive purposes. She had a casual sexual encounter with a stranger 4 days ago and now she is suffering from abdominal pain. On examination she is apyrexial, a yellow discharge is noted, and the uterus is tender to palpate.

Answer [   ]

A	At any time in the menstrual cycle
B	After 3 weeks
C	After 6 weeks
D	After 8 weeks
E	After 12 weeks
F	After 3 months
G	After 3 years
H	After 5 years
I	After 7 years
J	Day 1–5 of cycle
K	Day 19 of cycle
L	Day 21 of cycle

Each of these clinical scenarios relate to women requesting contraceptive advice. For each patient select the single most appropriate advice to give from the list above.

Each option may be used once, more than once, or not at all.

7.36 An 18-year-old woman attends for repeat emergency contraception having had a second episode of unprotected intercourse in this menstrual cycle. You offer her levonorgestrel 1.5 mg orally and counsel her about the need for more reliable contraception. She is keen to have the etonogestrel implant (Nexplanon®) inserted and asks you when is the most appropriate time that this can be done.

Answer [   ]

7.37 A 23-year-old woman has opted to use medroxyprogesterone acetate injection (Depo-Provera®) for contraception. She enquires when she will need her second injection.

Answer [ ]

7.38 A 45-year-old woman attends for replacement of her levonorgestrel IUS (Mirena ®), which she uses both for contraception and control of her heavy menstrual bleeding. She is currently amenorrhoeic with the IUS in place. She asks you when she will need the next IUS if she hasn't gone through the menopause.

Answer [ ]

7.39 A 25-year-old woman is requesting the COC for contraception postnatally. She had a normal vaginal delivery and is bottle feeding her baby. When should she commence the COC?

Answer [ ]

7.40 A 25-year-old woman attends your surgery requesting to commence the COC for the first time. She has been amenorrhoeic for some time but her pregnancy test is negative. When can she commence her pill?

Answer [ ]

A	Copper IUCD delayed until chlamydia swab results available
B	Copper IUCD with chlamydia antibiotic prophylaxis
C	Depot medroxyprogesterone acetate injection
D	Levonorgestrel (Levonelle®) 1.5 mg oral dose
E	Levonorgestrel IUS (Mirena®)
F	Nexplanon® etonogestrel implant
G	No prescription needed; reassure
H	Ulipristal acetate (EllaOne®) 30 mg oral dose
I	Repeat ulipristal acetate (EllaOne®) 30 mg oral dose

These clinical scenarios relate to women seeking emergency contraception. For each case, select the most appropriate method.

Each option may be used once, more than once, or not at all.

7.41 A 35-year-old woman presents to her local police station the morning after an alleged rape and is seen at the Sexual Assault Referral Centre (SARC). She has had a full infection screen done and thinks that her last period was about 12 days ago. She does not usually use contraception as she has never been sexually active and is very distressed at the thought of possible pregnancy as a result of the attack.

Answer [ ]

7.42 The same 35-year-old woman returns to the SARC 3 hours later having just vomited in the car on the way home.

Answer [ ]

7.43 Three months after her first delivery, a woman is still fully breast-feeding her baby. She has not had a period yet and thought that she didn't need to use contraception at all so had unprotected intercourse 2 days ago. It took her a long time to get pregnant and you suspect that her subfertility might have been due to previous episodes of pelvic inflammatory disease related to proven chlamydia infection.

Answer [ ]

7.44 A 24-year-old woman normally uses Depot medroxyprogesterone acetate for contraception but has forgotten to return for her usual injection, which is now over a month overdue. She has been amenorrhoeic since she started on Depot medroxyprogesterone acetate 3 years ago and she is keen to continue using it because her periods had been heavy previously. She had unprotected intercourse 3 days ago.

Answer [ ]

7.45 On return from her holidays, a teenage woman seeks help 4 days after a condom failure abroad. She is now on day 18 of an irregular cycle and uses a Ventolin inhaler several times a day for her asthma (which has been severe enough to necessitate hospital admission in the past).

Answer [ ]

A	24 hours
B	72 hours
C	120 hours
D	Anytime in the cycle
E	Day 1–5 of the menstrual cycle
F	Day 1–7 of the menstrual cycle
G	Five days after expected ovulation
H	Immediately
I	Next expected menses
J	2 weeks
K	3–4 weeks

These clinical scenarios relate to timing of commencement of contraceptive methods. For each scenario select the most appropriate option.
Each option may be used once, more than once, or not at all.

7.46 A 19-year-old drug user had a vaginal delivery yesterday and the baby has been taken into care. She has a chaotic lifestyle and this was her third unplanned pregnancy. She is happy to have an etonogestrel implant but is keen to leave hospital and asks you when is the soonest that the device can be inserted.

Answer [ ]

7.47 A 19-year-old woman has just completed the second part of a medical abortion. Following counselling she has requested the etonogestrel sub-dermal implant (Nexplanon®) for ongoing contraception. When should she have this inserted?

Answer [ ]

7.48 A woman using medroxyprogesterone acetate (Depot medroxyprogester-one acetate) for contraception has forgotten to attend her appointment for her next injection. She telephones the surgery to make another appoint-ment and asks how much time she has before she cannot rely on the injec-tion for effective contraception.

Answer [ ]

7.49 A 32-year-old woman has been using a POP for a year following the birth of her second child. She has stopped breast-feeding now and is unhappy with the intermenstrual bleeding that she has with the POP. She is keen to switch to the COC and asks how long after finishing her POP packet she should start the COC.

Answer [ ]

Curriculum Module 1

Answers

Single Best Answer Questions

1.1 Pelvic pain is a common problem in women of childbearing age. When taking a history, which of the following symptoms suggests that the diagnosis might be endometriosis?

A. Abdominal distension
B. ***Dyschezia**
C. Pain throughout the menstrual cycle
D. Primary dysmenorrhoea
E. Superficial dyspareunia

Dyschezia means pain on defaecation and suggests that there is endometriosis in the recto-vaginal septum. Primary dysmenorrhoea starts at puberty or shortly afterwards and is not due to pelvic pathology, as opposed to secondary dysmenorrhoea.

1.2 Pregnancy is known to provoke episodes of domestic violence and GPs, midwives, and obstetricians are encouraged to be aware of the possibility.

Which of the following might raise the suspicion of domestic abuse?

A. All the family turn up for every antenatal appointment
B. ***Repeated failure to attend antenatal appointments**
C. The woman always brings a female relative to translate for her
D. There is a linear burn across the patient's abdomen that occurred during ironing
E. The woman seems unsure about her request for termination of unwanted pregnancy

Domestic abuse is intentional abuse inflicted on one partner by another whilst in an intimate relationship. It includes physical, sexual, emotional, psychological, or financial abuse.

One would assume that pregnancy would be protective but it appears to provoke attacks rather than prevent them. Domestic violence knows no boundaries of social class or race. It could be happening to a colleague in a hospital residence near you, and community midwives are trained to ask the question of every pregnant woman, whatever their social class.

'Repeated termination' is recognised as a marker for domestic violence and some victims of abuse may be coerced into requesting TOP against their will. However, being unsure of the decision is relatively common.

1.3 Which of these conditions causes primary rather than secondary amenorrhoea?

A. Asherman syndrome
B. Anorexia nervosa
C. Polycystic ovarian syndrome
D. *Rokintansky syndrome
E. Sheehan syndrome

Asherman syndrome is the formation of intrauterine adhesions that typically develop after intrauterine surgery. Anorexia nervosa usually develops as puberty progresses and will result in secondary amenorrhoea as the condition worsens. Polycystic ovarian syndrome also usually develops after puberty.

Rokitansky syndrome is also known as Mullerian agenesis and there are no periods because there is no uterus (and sometimes no vagina either).

Sheehan syndrome typically happens after a massive postpartum haemorrhage with persistent hypotension that causes avascular necrosis of the pituitary in a pregnant woman.

1.4 A 27-year-old woman attends the surgery for booking in her fourth pregnancy. She has a BMI of 38 and has had three previous caesarean sections, delivering babies of more than 4 kg each time.

Which complication is a recognised extra risk factor for her in this pregnancy?

A. Antepartum haemorrhage
B. *Placenta accreta
C. Postpartum haemorrhage
D. Intrauterine growth restriction
E. Pre-eclampsia

With every successive caesarean section, the chance of having placenta praevia increases and the risk of the low-lying placenta also being accreta increases exponentially. This situation could result in emergency hysterectomy and is one of the reasons obstetricians like to limit caesarean sections to three.

On the fifth and subsequent babies, we label a mother as being a 'grand multip' whatever the mode of delivery for her previous babies; the significance being that grand multips are more at risk of postpartum haemorrhage.

Pre-eclampsia usually occurs in women on their first pregnancy and rarely in multiparous women.

1.5 When a woman presents with an ovarian cyst, the gynaecologist works out the risk of malignancy index (RMI), which helps to evaluate the likelihood of the ovarian cyst being malignant.

Which of the following contributes to the RMI?

A. Solid areas in the cyst on CT scan
B. The age of the woman
C. The CA15-3 tumour marker level
D. *The menopausal status of the woman
E. A family history of ovarian cancer

The RMI is worked out using the woman's menopausal status, the CA125 level, and the ultrasound findings. The score predicts the likelihood of malignancy (which guides subsequent investigations, identifies those patients that should be referred to the gynae-oncology MDT, and helps to plan treatment).

1.6 **About 15 per cent of pregnant women will be rhesus negative.**

When they suffer an early pregnancy complication, which one of these nonsensitised, rhesus negative patients does not need anti-D immunoglobulin?

A. Miscarriage less than 12 weeks when the uterus is evacuated surgically or medically

B. Ectopic pregnancy

C. Incomplete miscarriage more than 12 weeks

D. Complete miscarriage less than 12 weeks when bleeding is heavy

E. ***Threatened miscarriage less than 12 weeks when the fetus is viable**

The rules for administration of anti-D have changed recently to avoid giving it to women who are less than twelve weeks of gestation and have had a spontaneous miscarriage with conservative management or a threatened miscarriage, as the risk of sensitisation is very low.

British Committee for Standards in Haematology (BSCH) guideline on anti-D administration in pregnancy (2014) accessible via RCOG website www.rcog .org.uk

1.7 **Maternal deaths in the United Kingdom are reported nationally and the World Health Organisation keeps records of the rates worldwide.**

With relation to maternal death, which of these statements is correct?

A. ***Every maternal death in the United Kingdom is scrutinised to look for substandard care**

B. Reducing the number of maternal deaths worldwide by the year 2050 is a 'millennium development goal'

C. The maternal mortality rate is lower in the United States than in the United Kingdom

D. The maternal mortality ratio is defined as the number of maternal deaths per hundred thousand pregnancies

E. There were no maternal deaths from swine flu in the last epidemic

Surprisingly the chance of dying in pregnancy is much higher in the United States and the rate is increasing. Perhaps this reflects access to health care but the reasons remain obscure. Millennium development goal number 5 was to achieve a 75 per cent reduction in the worldwide maternal mortality ratio by 2015, but this was not realised. The maternal mortality ratio is the number of deaths per hundred thousand maternities (which is the number of pregnancies that result in either a live birth or stillbirth occurring from 24 weeks of gestation onwards).

Stillbirths at or after 24 weeks must be reported by law and the number of pregnancy losses before this time is unknown: therefore, using maternities rather than pregnancies as a denominator is more accurate and allows comparison between time periods.

The most recent maternal mortality report (MBRRACE-UK) can be accessed using the RCOG website.

1.8 A nulliparous 22-year-old woman presents with a 3-month history of inter-menstrual bleeding. She is healthy with no other medical problems and is using the withdrawal method for contraception.

Select the most likely diagnosis:

A.   Cervical cancer
B.   ***Chlamydia infection**
C.   Endometrial polyp
D.   Nabothian follicle on the cervix
E.   Ovarian granulosa cell tumour

Chlamydia causes cervicitis, which can make the cervix bleed. In this age group, this is the most likely diagnosis.

Cervical cancer is possible but unlikely at this age.

Endometrial polyps are affected by the hormonal changes of the menstrual cycle but tend to be a bit more fragile than normal endometrium and can bleed at any time, but again are unlikely at this age.

Nabothian follicles are mucous retention cysts on the cervix and are covered with normal epithelium, so they don't bleed.

The ovarian granulosa cell tumour secretes estrogen that can cause the endometrium to become unstable or even hyperplastic so that the woman bleeds erratically, but they are not very common (5 per cent of all ovarian cancers).

1.9 A primigravid woman who is 33 weeks pregnant has just arrived in the United Kingdom from Africa to visit her family. She presents to the surgery feeling ill with joint pains and diarrhoea. She has a temperature and may be infected with the Ebola virus.

Which of the following statements is correct regarding Ebola infection in pregnancy?

A.   If she delivers whilst she is ill, she will be able to breast-feed her baby
B.   ***The main Ebola viral load is concentrated in the fetus and placenta**
C.   The fetus is likely to survive if delivered now because she is in the third trimester
D.   The maternal mortality rate is around 10 per cent
E.   Viral spread is by inhaled airborne droplets

The chance of the baby surviving is virtually zero whatever the gestation as the virus is concentrated in the fetus and placenta.

Transmission is by bodily fluids and health care workers are particularly at risk whilst looking after women during delivery because of the massive viral load. She would not be advised to breast-feed for the same reason, although it is not likely that the baby will survive to be breast-fed.

Pregnant women do very badly compared with nonpregnant women and the chance of death is about 95 per cent.

Source: `Ebola in pregnancy: information for healthcare workers' Public Health England publications gateway number: 2014 421; published (version 3) 20 November 2014, reviewed May 2015; accessible from www.gov.uk.

1.10 A 43-year-old smoker attends the emergency department at 35 weeks of gestation complaining of sudden onset of central chest pain. On examination she is pale and sweaty with a tachycardia of 120 bpm. Her temperature and blood pressure are normal.

She has had three normal births in the past. Her BMI is 35 but she is otherwise fit and well and this pregnancy has been straightforward so far.

Which is the most likely diagnosis?

A. ***Cardiac ischaemia**
B. Chest infection
C. Pneumothorax
D. Pulmonary embolus
E. Reflux oesophagitis

The symptoms suggest cardiac ischaemia and the most appropriate investigation is coronary angiography because there is an increased incidence of coronary artery dissection in the pregnant population, which will not be relieved by thrombolysis

1.11 Taking over the gynaecology on-call duties one evening, you are given this list of tasks to be done on the ward.

Select the task that takes priority:

A. Site an intravenous infusion for a severely dehydrated patient with hyperemesis
B. Sign a death certificate as a patient's husband is waiting on the ward for it
C. Review the scan report of a woman with a suspected ectopic pregnancy
D. ***Review a woman who has just miscarried an 18-week fetus but not delivered the placenta**
E. Clerk a new patient that a GP has sent in to hospital with a suspected torted ovarian cyst

The reason for choosing the 18-week miscarriage patient first is that she is likely to bleed heavily as she has a retained placenta. If you cannot remove the placenta easily on the ward she needs to go to theatre. The later in a pregnancy that the miscarriage happens, the greater the bulk of the placenta and the more bleeding you get. With a second trimester miscarriage it is likely to be very heavy indeed. In addition, there could well be an element of infection here that puts her at increased risk of haemorrhage.

The patient with a possible torted ovarian cyst is likely to be in severe pain, but a potential haemorrhage takes precedence over that.

The patient with a possible ectopic has already been clerked and is likely to have established IV access; she only goes to the top of the list if she drops her blood pressure.

1.12 You are trying to persuade a postoperative woman with a haemoglobin of 55 g/L that she would not be so breathless if she had a blood transfusion, but she is concerned about the risk of acquiring HIV. The chance of acquiring HIV infection as a result of blood transfusion in the United Kingdom is approximately:

A. 1 in 6 thousand
B. 1 in 60 thousand
C. 1 in 600 thousand
D. ***1 in 6 million**
E. 1 in 60 million

This is useful information to have at your fingertips if you are counselling a woman who needs a blood transfusion.

Source: RCOG Green-top Guideline, 'Blood Transfusion in Obstetrics' (2008).

1.13 The community midwife doing an antenatal clinic in your GP surgery asks you to see a 37-year-old obese woman who has come for a routine checkup at 32 weeks of gestation in her first pregnancy. Her booking blood pressure in the first trimester was 130/88 mmHg, but it is now 160/95 mmHg and the midwife has checked the blood pressure twice. The woman is asymptomatic. Which is the most appropriate course of action?

A. Urinalysis and prescribe antihypertensives if no proteinuria

B. Send urgent full blood count, urate, and liver function tests

C. ***Refer her urgently to hospital for further investigation and treatment**

D. Urinalysis and request urgent antenatal appointment if no proteinuria

E. Twenty-four-hour urine collection for protein analysis

This woman probably has underlying essential hypertension. However, it is irrelevant to your immediate decision whether she has proteinuria or not (and therefore superimposed pre-eclampsia) because her blood pressure is at a level where cerebro-vascular accident is a real possibility. The maternal mortality reports stress that a systolic of 160 mmHg is a critical level where treatment must be instituted to prevent this complication. There is also a need for fetal assessment to check for placental insufficiency so referral to hospital is a sensible solution rather than treating the hypertension in primary care.

1.14 A 52-year-old woman presents to your surgery with a very sore vulva. On examination you find thickening of both labia minora with a couple of shallow ulcers on both sides and a split area at the fourchette. What is the most likely diagnosis in her case?

A. Eczema

B. Genital herpes

C. Lichen planus

D. ***Lichen sclerosus**

E. Vulval intraepithelial neoplasia (VIN)

Lichen sclerosus is the most common cause of these findings on the vulva. Women of this age do not usually get genital herpes and lichen planus and VIN are rare.

1.15 The clinical scenarios detailed in the following text describe gynaecological patients admitted as an emergency. Which patient is most likely to have a diagnosis of ectopic pregnancy?

A. Acute onset of central abdominal pain and nausea at 12 weeks of gestation. On examination severe lower abdominal tenderness with generalised guarding and rebound, also foetor oris. White cell count is $18 \times 10^9/l$ and urinalysis is negative.

B. History of 11 weeks' amenorrhea and brown vaginal discharge but no pain. Pelvic examination reveals no tenderness but uterus is small for dates and the cervical os is closed. Serum βhCG is 2,010 IU/ml and scan is awaited.

C. Seven weeks' amenorrhea and vaginal bleeding. Pelvic examination reveals no tenderness. Uterus is soft and slightly enlarged with an open cervical os.

D. Admitted with bleeding and lower abdominal pain at 8 weeks of gestation. Transvaginal ultrasound scan shows an intrauterine sac with a fetal pole but no heart pulsation detected. Serum βhCG is 150 000 IU/ml.

E. ***Patient with lower abdominal and shoulder tip pain who has a copper coil fitted. Last menstrual period was 2 weeks ago and on examination has a tender abdomen with guarding. Urinary hCG test positive in A&E.**

Patient A probably has appendicitis and ectopic pregnancies usually present before 12 weeks of gestation. Patient B probably has a missed miscarriage as the uterus is small for dates. Patient C either has an inevitable or incomplete miscarriage as the os is open. Patient D's pregnancy has come to grief and it may be a partial hydatidiform mole as the hCG is so high. Patient E is most likely to have an ectopic because of the shoulder tip pain and the coil. Many patients presenting with ectopic pregnancies do not have a history of amenorrhoea (although the bleeding a couple of weeks before is not a normal 'period' but uterine decidua being shed).

1.16 A 46-year-old woman presents to her GP seeking help with her period problems, which date back almost a year. Her cycles are still regular with a cycle of 26 days but the bleeding is now very heavy with clots. She complains of severe secondary dysmenorrhoea but no other pelvic pain. On examination there are no masses palpable in the pelvis. The uterus is enlarged to the size of an orange, smooth, and very tender but mobile with no adnexal tenderness.

Select the most likely gynaecological cause of this clinical picture:

A. ***Adenomyosis**
B. Chronic pelvic inflammatory disease
C. Endometriosis
D. Endometrial hyperplasia
E. Fibroids

The enlargement of the uterus combined with tenderness suggests the diagnosis of adenomyosis. Fibroids are not usually tender and you would not suspect endometriosis without some other pelvic pain and/or tenderness. If she had chronic pelvic inflammatory disease it would have presented before the age of 46 and endometrial pathology causes irregular bleeding.

1.17 A 39-year-old woman asks for a hospital referral so that she can be investigated for recurrent miscarriage, having suffered three first trimester pregnancy losses. She believes that her miscarriages are due to stress. She works long hours as a computer programmer and smokes fifteen cigarettes a day. Which of the following factors is the most likely cause of her recurrent miscarriages?

A. Working with visual display units
B. Smoking
C. ***Advanced maternal age**
D. Natural killer cells
E. Bacterial vaginosis

Maternal age over 35 is associated with a 25 per cent risk of miscarriage.

Source: RCOG Green-Top Guideline, No. 17, 'The Investigation and Treatment of Couples with Recurrent First-Trimester and Second-Trimester Miscarriage'. Published 2011.

1.18 In your GP surgery the practice nurse asks you to see a 25-year-old woman who is unable to tolerate speculum examination for her first smear test. The patient tells you that she has experienced severe dyspareunia since her marriage 2 years ago and discloses that she was sexually abused as a child. Which of the following statements about child abuse is untrue?

A. *Abuse in childhood predisposes to depressive illness in later life that does not respond to treatment

B. Child abuse encompasses neglect as well as physical and sexual abuse

C. Somatisation as an adult can be a result of child abuse

D. Women who have been abused as children rarely disclose such a history

E. Abuse in childhood is known to be associated with illicit drug use as an adult

Childhood sexual abuse is known to result in sexual problems in later life such as vaginismus but could also lead to behaviour such as promiscuity, early pregnancy, and STIs. There is also an association with psychiatric problems, but they can be treated.

1.19 The mother of a 13-year-old girl attends the surgery for advice. Her daughter has been offered the human papilloma virus (HPV) vaccine at school but did not bring an information leaflet home, so she wants to know more about it.

Which one of these statements about the quadrivalent vaccine (Gardasil®) is correct?

A. She will require three doses of the vaccine over 6 months

B. *The vaccine will reduce the chance of her developing genital warts as well as cervical intraepithelial neoplasia

C. If she completes the course of vaccinations she will not need cervical smears in the future

D. The vaccine is not appropriate if she is already sexually active

E. The vaccine is made from live attenuated HPV

The quadrivalent vaccine contains particles of HPV viruses 6, 11, 16, and 18, which are associated with more than 70 per cent of cases of cervical cancer as well as cervical intraepithelial neoplasia (CIN) and genital warts too. As it does not prevent all cases of CIN and cancer, women do need to stay on the smear programme, although this is now developing into HPV typing rather than just cytology. The vaccine is given as a course of two doses over 6 to 12 months in girls less than 15 years, but we are still not sure how long the antibody levels will persist in vivo. Girls older than 15 years seem to have a poorer antibody response and are still offered a three-dose course.

Source: NHS Choices website information about HPV vaccine (www.nhs.uk) and patient information leaflets about vaccination (www.gov.uk).

1.20 Which one of the following statements is true in relation to women with Turner syndrome?

A. They have no problems with learning difficulties

B. Estrogen therapy may result in spontaneous fertility

C. *There is a high prevalence of left-sided congenital heart malformation

D. Administration of growth hormone at puberty will not produce any extra height

E. They all have karyotype 46XO

The prevalence of bicuspid aortic valve is up to 17 per cent and aortic coarctation is up to 10 per cent. When the diagnosis of Turner syndrome is made, the woman should have investigations as cardiovascular malformations are responsible for much of the reduced life expectancy on these women.

If they are given growth hormone and oestrogen at puberty, they can achieve normal height. HRT will prevent osteoporosis but does not make Turner syndrome patients ovulate.

Turner syndrome does not cause mental retardation but they can have difficulties with nonverbal learning disorders (problems with spatial relationships and mathematics, problems with motor control).

The karyotype is 45XO although it is also possible to have a mosaic karyotype.

Extended Matching Questions

A	CT scan of the pelvis
B	Cystoscopy
C	Diagnostic laparoscopy
D	Dye laparoscopy
E	High vaginal swab for chlamydia
F	Hysterosalpingogram
G	MRI scan of the pelvis
H	Serum CA125 level
I	Transvaginal ultrasound scan
J	Urodynamic study

Each of these clinical scenarios describes a woman presenting with symptoms of pelvic pain; for each case pick the most appropriate initial investigation given the information that you are presented with.

Each option may be used once, more than once, or not at all.

1.21 Secondary dysmenorrhoea in a 40-year-old nulliparous woman with a BMI of 48. Over the last year her periods have become heavier and she is not currently sexually active.

I. Transvaginal ultrasound scan

Possible causes of secondary dysmenorrhoea in this woman include fibroids, adenomyosis, and endometriosis. Chronic pelvic inflammatory disease (PID) is less likely in a woman of this age especially as she is not sexually active. The choice is between laparoscopy and scan to investigate this. Laparoscopy might be difficult in view of her BMI and an ultrasound is an easier option initially although it will not diagnose nonovarian endometriosis.

1.22 A 38-year-old woman complains of premenstrual pain, severe secondary dysmenorrhoea, and dyschezia

C. Diagnostic laparoscopy

Dyschezia means pain on opening bowels, and this lady is likely to have endometriosis with this collection of symptoms. Ultrasound will show endometriomas on her ovaries but may be normal if the ovaries are unaffected.

1.23 A 24-year-old secretary with noncyclical pain and deep dyspareunia who has been trying to get pregnant for 2 years

D. Dye laparoscopy

The most likely diagnosis here is pelvic inflammatory disease and an USS; whilst it will show hydrosalpinges and ovarian cysts it will not help much with the diagnosis as much as a laparoscopy – and the dye to investigate the fertility aspect instead of just doing a diagnostic laparoscopy. Although chlamydia swabs are indicated, especially prior to flushing dye through the fallopian tubes, you take cervical swabs for chlamydia not high vaginal.

1.24 A postmenopausal woman with left iliac fossa pain radiating down her leg, whose abdominal USS shows a 9 cm septated cyst adjacent to the uterus on the left side with free fluid around it

H Serum CA125 level

There are a couple of worrying features about this cyst – the free fluid and the fact that it is not simple. Also it is quite large and she is postmenopausal so it is not likely to be an ovulatory cyst. The CA125 level will help to calculate the RMI which will aid the management decision regarding surgery, that is, to remove the cyst only or to perform a hysterectomy and bilateral salpingo-oophorectomy in case it is malignant on histology. Serum CA125 is raised in more than 80 per cent of ovarian cancer cases and, if a cutoff of 30 u/ml is used, the test has a sensitivity of 81 per cent and specificity of 75 per cent. In routine practice, the value of 35 u/ml is used as the cutoff for ordering an USS in a symptomatic woman.

Although she might have a CT scan done later if the risk of malignancy index is high and she is referred to gynae-oncology, this would not be an initial investigation.

Sources: RCOG Green-top Guideline number 34, 'Ovarian Cysts in Postmenopausal Women' (updated 2016) and NICE clinical guideline number CG122, 'Ovarian Cancer; Recognition and Initial Management' (2011, under review).

1.25 A 62-year-old woman with severe urinary frequency for 8 weeks associated with dyspareunia

B. Cystoscopy

This woman is in the right age group for a transitional cell carcinoma of the bladder and her symptoms have persisted for many weeks. We have not given you an MSU option and it is important not to miss a cancer. If the bladder is normal at cystoscopy, urodynamics may help you establish a diagnosis eventually.

A	Bleeding corpus luteum cyst
B	Ectopic pregnancy
C	Gastroenteritis

D	Heterotopic pregnancy
E	Ovarian hyperstimulation syndrome
F	Ovarian torsion
G	Pelvic sepsis
H	Pulmonary embolism
I	Threatened miscarriage

These women have all undergone assisted conception treatment with IVF and have developed complications. For each clinical scenario select the most likely diagnosis.

Each option may be used once, more than once, or not at all.

1.26 Following a cycle of IVF, a young woman is pregnant for the first time. She presents to A&E with increasing lower abdominal pain and diarrhoea. She has had brown vaginal loss for a couple of days. On examination she is pale with a tachycardia of 100 bpm but her blood pressure is normal. An urgent USS shows an endometrial thickness of 12 mm but no gestation sac seen.

B. Ectopic pregnancy

The diarrhoea might lead you to think that she has gastroenteritis but diarrhoea can also be caused by blood in the pelvis irritating the bowel. Her tachycardia may be due to sepsis but the overall picture suggests ectopic pregnancy with intra-abdominal bleeding.

1.27 A slightly obese woman with polycystic ovarian syndrome is admitted a week after an IVF cycle during which 12 oocytes were collected. She had an embryo transfer 5 days previously and now has shortness of breath, nausea, and abdominal pain. Her abdomen is distended on examination.

E. Ovarian hyperstimulation syndrome

The combination of her breathlessness and abdominal distension are the key to the diagnosis of hyperstimulation syndrome. Pulmonary embolus will also cause breathlessness and several of the other diagnoses will cause abdominal pain (gastroenteritis, heterotopic pregnancy, bleeding corpus luteum, torsion, sepsis, ectopic, miscarriage, and perforation), but they should not cause breathlessness.

PCO patients are more at risk of hyperstimulation during IVF treatment.

1.28 A 27-year-old woman is admitted to the gynaecology ward as an emergency with severe abdominal pain and vomiting. She is unable to lie still and scores her pain 9 out of 10. On examination she is apyrexial, tachycardic, and normotensive. She has a tender mass on the left side of the pelvis. She had a cycle of IVF recently with oocyte recovery 10 days previously, followed by embryo transfer 2 days later.

F. Ovarian torsion

The severe pain in combination with vomiting suggests torsion, and it is too early in the process for it to be an ectopic pregnancy. Sepsis unlikely because she is apyrexial and gastroenteritis should not produce a tender mass in the pelvis.

1.29 Three weeks after a cycle of IVF a 34-year-old woman presents to her GP with increasing pain in the lower abdomen and rigors. She only had one embryo replaced in the uterus because only one of the oocytes that were retrieved actually fertilised.

G. Pelvic sepsis

Pain and rigors suggest infection and pelvic sepsis is a possible consequence of oocyte retrieval as it is usually done by inserting a catheter into the ovarian follicles individually, transvaginally under ultrasound control.

1.30 A pregnant woman is rushed to A&E in the United Kingdom having collapsed at the airport. She had a cycle of IVF in another country 7 weeks ago, during which three embryos were replaced in the uterus. She has a scan picture with her, showing an intrauterine pregnancy with a viable 6-week fetus.

Her blood pressure is 85/45 mmHg, her pulse is 120 bpm, her temperature is 36.5°C, and on abdominal examination she has rigidity, rebound tenderness, and guarding. Pelvic examination reveals tenderness in the left adnexa and she has cervical excitation. Her haemoglobin is 95 g/l and her white cell count is 8×10^9/l.

D. Heterotopic pregnancy

The abdominal and pelvic examinations suggest a diagnosis of ectopic, sepsis, or ovarian cyst accident. An ovarian cyst would have been noted on her scan and her normal temperature and white cell count rule out sepsis. Although there is an intrauterine pregnancy on the scan, it is possible that there is another one in her left fallopian tube especially as more than one embryo was replaced.

A	Bacterial vaginosis
B	Beta-haemolytic streptococcus
C	Candida
D	Chlamydia
E	Gonorrhoea
F	Herpes genitalis
G	Primary syphilis
H	Streptococcus A (streptococcus pyogenes)
I	Trichomonas vaginalis

These clinical scenarios relate to women presenting to a hospital clinic or general practice surgery. Select the most likely infecting organism given the clinical information for each woman.

Each option may be used once, more than once, or not at all.

1.31 A 23-year-old woman is admitted two days postpartum with severe sepsis. Her temperature is 38°C, pulse 110 bpm, her respiratory rate is raised, and her uterus is enlarged and tender. She has a sore throat with a red pharynx and white spots on her tonsils on examination.

H. Streptococcus A

In the 2006–2008 maternal mortality report, the leading cause of maternal death was sepsis with Group A strep mentioned as the causative organism for the first time. Women seem to become very sick very quickly, and every hospital has since introduced a sepsis protocol as timely antibiotics save lives. It is also possible to acquire chlamydial pharyngitis through sexual activity.

1.32 A 55-year-old diabetic woman presents to her GP with a 6-week history of a sore vulva. On examination her vulval skin is red and excoriated.

C. Candida infection

These sorts of changes on the vulva are sometimes described as 'diabetic vulva' and often thrush infection is underlying the problem, although diabetic women can look like this with negative swabs if their control is poor.

1.33 A 19-year-old presents to the practice nurse with postcoital bleeding and on speculum examination her cervix bleeds on contact.

D. Chlamydia

The most likely cause of postcoital bleeding in teenagers is cervical infection, with Chlamydia being the likely organism (although most Chlamydial infections are asymptomatic).

1.34 A primigravid woman is admitted in labour at term. Her uterus is tender and a diagnosis of chorioamnionitis is made. Postnatally the baby develops meningitis.

B. Beta-haemolytic streptococcus

The chorioamnionitis is likely to have resulted from ascending infection from the vagina and in combination with the neonatal meningitis, group B strep is the most likely organism on this list.

1.35 A 22-year-old woman is admitted to the gynaecology ward with acute retention of urine. On examination she has a sore vulva.

F. Herpes genitalis

Very few conditions cause urinary retention especially in young women but a primary attack of genital herpes will do this. The key to the diagnosis is finding herpetic ulcers on the vulva that are often secondarily infected too.

A	Colposcopy
B	Colposcopy and cervical biopsy
C	Dilatation and curettage
D	Endometrial biopsy using sampling device
E	Hysteroscopy and endometrial biopsy
F	HPV typing

G	Liquid-based cervical cytology
H	MRI scan of abdomen and pelvis
I	Transvaginal ultrasound scan

These scenarios described relate to women whose GP suspects that they might have cancer so they have been referred to gynaecology clinic with an urgent '2-week wait' appointment. For each patient select the most appropriate investigation given the clinical information described in each case.

Each option may be used once, more than once, or not at all.

1.36 A 48-year-old diabetic woman with a BMI of 48 presents with a history of irregular periods and intermenstrual bleeding. She is nulliparous.

E. Hysteroscopy and endometrial biopsy

There is a good chance that this woman will have endometrial cancer because of her obesity and diabetes. Although you might be able to get a diagnosis from sampling the endometrium in clinic, this may not be easy as she is nulliparous and the gold standard is hysteroscopy because you can be sure that you are taking the biopsy from the correct part of the uterus. Ultrasound would be a useful investigation especially in relation to her ovaries (which will be difficult to feel because of her size) but a tissue diagnosis is needed here.

1.37 A 26-year-old woman attends for her first smear at the GP's surgery and mentions that she has experienced postcoital bleeding for the last 6 months. Whilst taking the smear, a friable 3 mm diameter red lesion is noted on her cervix, which bleeds profusely.

B. Colposcopy and cervical biopsy

As there is clinical suspicion of cancer in this case, a cervical biopsy is necessary whatever the result of the smear.

1.38 A 57-year-old woman goes to see her GP complaining of indigestion and abdominal distension. She has had a CA125 blood test done privately and the result is 60 iu/l.

I. Transvaginal ultrasound scan

The CA125 level is higher than normal and this suggests a closer look at the ovaries. Ultrasound is the cheapest and easiest method.

1.39 A worried 31-year-old refugee woman presents to the surgery a few weeks after arrival in the country saying that her younger sister has just died of cervical cancer back home. She wishes to be reassured that she does not have it too.

G. Liquid-based cervical cytology

Cervical cancer is not inherited or genetic in any way but the patient's anxiety is understandable. A smear should be adequate and she has should commence on the screening programme anyway.

1.40 A 32-year-old nulliparous woman presents with lower abdominal pain and severe dysmenorrhoea 3 years after radiotherapy treatment for cancer of the cervix. On examination her cervix looks normal but atrophic with radiotherapy changes and an USS shows that the cavity of the uterus is distended with blood.

C. Dilatation and curettage

This patient has a haematometria that is probably the result of radiotherapy. Although it is important to rule out recurrence of her original cancer, the situation needs treatment to let the blood out of the uterus and get rid of her pain. We do not do dilatation and curettage as a diagnostic procedure anymore (now that hysteroscopy is available and is more accurate), but in this case it is actually the correct procedure.

A	Discuss with on-call consultant
B	Discuss with on-call registrar (ST4, specialty trainee year 4)
C	Leave for consultant to deal with on his return
D	No action required
E	Phone GP
F	Phone patient
G	Post a prescription to patient
H	Recall urgently to gynaecology clinic next week
I	Refer to gynae-oncology MDT meeting
J	Routine gynaecology clinic follow-up
K	Write to GP
L	Write to patient

The rest of your clinical team are away and your consultant's secretary has asked you to go through some messages and results in his in-tray. For each of the following scenarios select the most appropriate course of action to ensure the best use of NHS time and resources, as well as considering the safest and most convenient solution for the patient.

Each option may be used once, more than once, or not at all.

1.41 A 28-year-old woman attended the antenatal clinic a few days ago for a growth scan at 28 weeks of gestation and gave a history of an offensive vaginal discharge for the last week. The result of the high vaginal swab is reported as showing clue cells on microscopy and profuse anaerobes on culture.

G Post a prescription to patient

The results of the high vaginal swab suggests bacterial vaginosis (BV) and because she is symptomatic she needs antibiotic treatment. In addition, we always treat BV in pregnancy as it can cause miscarriage and premature labour. The most efficient way of organising this is to provide a prescription directly to the patient. An alternative would be to write to her asking her to see her GP for a prescription but that would mean an extra visit to the GP and possibly a delay in starting treatment.

1.42 An 18-year-old woman attended the emergency gynaecology clinic 2 days ago with pelvic pain, discharge, and postcoital bleeding for the preceding fortnight. The endocervical swab result shows chlamydia trachomatis detected by PCR.

L Write to patient

The reason for writing to the patient rather than just issuing a prescription is that she needs to be informed of the result and referred to the genito-urinary (GU) medicine clinic for treatment, screening for other sexually transmitted infections including HIV, and contact tracing. Your letter would be able to explain all this. You would copy this to the GP but you wouldn't write to the GP asking him or her to do the referral to GU medicine as it is the gynaecology team's responsibility to action results on investigations they have done.

1.43 A GP has written a letter about a 30-year-old woman with a 2-year history of pelvic pain. She has been previously seen in the gynaecology clinic by your consultant and was advised to start the combined oral contraceptive pill. She is getting headaches so has discontinued the pill but is still getting pelvic pain.

J Routine gynaecology clinic follow-up

Because this woman is unable to tolerate the suggested management plan, she should be seen again in clinic to explore other options and possibly consider laparoscopy, but it is not an urgent situation.

1.44 A 23-year-old woman was seen in the gynaecology clinic 2 weeks ago with a 3-month history of pelvic pain throughout the cycle. Examination showed no abnormality, in particular no tenderness on vaginal examination, and the high vaginal and endocervical swabs were negative. In clinic, you gave her an advice leaflet about irritable bowel syndrome and organised an USS. The scan result shows a normal-sized anteverted uterus; both ovaries are clearly seen and are normal. There is no free fluid and there are no adnexal masses.

L Write to patient

It is a more efficient use of time and resources to write to the patient directly with results rather than bring them back to a gynaecology clinic just to tell them that everything is normal. There is good evidence that functional bowel pain is a significant cause of pelvic pain. If she continues to have pain it would be more appropriate for her to see her GP and have a trial of treatment with laxatives and antispasmodics before considering referral back to the gynaecology clinic for laparoscopy.

1.45 A 22-year-old woman was admitted as an emergency 1 week ago. She was found to have a torted ovarian cyst and had a laparoscopic oophorectomy. The rest of her pelvis was normal and she was given that information before discharge.

The histology report on the cyst shows a mature cystic teratoma (dermoid cyst).

L Write to patient

The patient needs to know the result and writing to her is the most efficient use of time and resources. Because this was laparoscopic surgery she doesn't need to be seen back in clinic for review of wound healing; this would only be necessary if she'd had a laparotomy. This is a mature dermoid cyst which is benign, so there is no need to involve the gynae-oncology multidisciplinary team.

A	Appendicitis
B	Complete mole
C	Ectopic pregnancy
D	Hyperemesis gravidarum
E	Incomplete miscarriage
F	Missed miscarriage
G	Partial hydatidiform mole
H	Threatened miscarriage
I	Urinary tract infection

These clinical scenarios describe pregnant women presenting with acute problems. In each case select the most likely diagnosis.

Each option may be used once, more than once, or not at all.

1.46 Having had a positive pregnancy test 2 weeks after her missed period, a 29-year-old primigravid woman is referred to have a scan because of vaginal bleeding. On arrival in the Early Pregnancy Unit the bleeding is noted to be heavy, and when you insert a speculum you find that the cervical os is open.

E. Incomplete miscarriage

The cervical os being open gives this diagnosis. It could also be an inevitable or complete miscarriage – a scan would differentiate – but we have not given you these options.

1.47 A 28-year-old woman has a transvaginal ultrasound scan on the Early Pregnancy Unit at 8 weeks of gestation because of vaginal bleeding. The uterus is larger than expected with a closed os. The scan shows an abnormal-looking intrauterine sac with a fetal pole but no heart pulsation detected. Her serum βhCG is 150 000 IU/ml.

G. Partial hydatidiform mole

The very high human chorionic gonadotrophin (hCG) levels suggest this diagnosis. Partial moles often present as miscarriage (unlike complete moles, which have a typical snowstorm appearance on scan).

1.48 A 28-year-old woman attends her GP's surgery asking for a pregnancy test after 14 weeks of amenorrhoea. She feels unwell and has been vomiting throughout the day. On examination she is tachycardic, sweaty, and has a tremor. Her uterus is easily palpable and the fundus is just below the umbilicus.

B. Complete mole

The combination of a uterus that is large for dates and symptoms of thyrotoxicosis suggest this diagnosis (hCG has an alpha subunit in common with thyroid stimulating hormone (TSH)). The diagnosis could also be hyperemesis with the pregnancy being more advanced than expected from the dates (which would account for the uterus reaching the umbilicus), but hyperemesis usually occurs in the first trimester.

1.49 Having reached 11 weeks of gestation, a 22-year-old woman is relieved when her morning sickness disappears. A week later she is devastated when her booking scan shows an irregular sac which is 10 weeks' size. A fetal pole is present but cardiac activity is absent.

F. Missed miscarriage

The diagnosis is missed miscarriage because she has had no bleeding. The woman is unaware that her pregnancy has failed and the diagnosis is often made in the scan department.

1.50 A GP refers a pregnant 19-year-old woman at 14 weeks of gestation because she has been vomiting for the last week. She has no diarrhoea but is clinically very dehydrated. Urine dip is positive for ketones, nitrites, and protein.

I. Urinary tract infection

The diagnosis could be hyperemesis gravidarum but the nitrites and protein as well as ketones in the urine suggest urinary tract infection (UTI) instead. It is also a bit unusual to start experiencing hyperemesis in the second trimester.

Curriculum Module 2

Answers

Single Best Answer Questions

2.1 A woman is about to have a caesarean section for placenta praevia and has been counselled about the risk of haemorrhage. She asks if there is a cell saver available for her operation.

Which of these statements is correct regarding the use of intraoperative cell savers in obstetrics?

A. Antibiotics should be given routinely if salvaged blood is transfused

B. Cell salvage is not recommended for rhesus negative mothers

C. Cell savers cannot be used in caesarean section because of the risk of amniotic fluid embolism

D. ***If the mother is rhesus negative she needs anti-D after reinfusion of salvaged blood**

E. The leucocyte-depletion filter will remove fetal blood cells

Cell salvage is recommended for patients where the anticipated blood loss is great enough to induce anaemia or anticipated to exceed 20 per cent of blood volume. The filters have been shown to remove some markers of amniotic fluid contamination such as squamous cells, and amniotic fluid embolism does not seem to be an issue in the studies conducted so far. However, the filters do not remove fetal red cells so there is a risk of sensitisation in rhesus negative mothers; hence the need for anti-D and a Kleihauer test 40 minutes after the procedure to ensure enough anti-D has been given.

Source: RCOG Green-top Guideline, No. 47, 'Blood Transfusion in Obstetrics' (2015).

2.2 One of the more serious complications of laparoscopy is bowel damage occurring at insertion of the laparoscope. Which of these patient characteristics makes this complication most likely?

A. BMI less than 20

B. BMI more than 40

C. Previous diagnostic laparoscopy

D. ***Previous caesarean section scar**

E. History of endometriosis

You might think that a Pfannenstiel incision is a long way from the umbilicus but the peritoneum is split right up to that level once the rectus sheath is opened at the start of the caesarean, so the bowel can stick to the back of the anterior abdominal wall at any level as the wound is healing. All of these characteristics (except perhaps previous laparoscopy) are risk factors for bowel damage but the caesarean is the most likely.

2.3 If a woman has been delivered by caesarean section in her first pregnancy, it is good practice to read the previous operation notes to see if there were any intraoperative complications.

In which of these indications for caesarean may the surgical details on the operation notes explain an underlying anatomical reason for the caesarean indication?

A. Cord prolapse
B. ***Breech presentation**
C. Failed forceps delivery
D. Fetal distress
E. Placenta praevia

One of the causes of breech presentation is uterine abnormality, for example, bicornuate uterus or septum, which would be noted by the surgeon when he or she was cleaning out the uterine cavity after removal of the placenta.

2.4 On the labour ward a woman needs an emergency caesarean section for cord prolapse but she cannot sign the consent form as she is illiterate.

Select the best course of action in the absence of her written consent:

A. Ask her husband to sign the consent form
B. Cancel the operation
C. Do the operation without consent in her best interest
D. Get permission through a court order on the telephone
E. ***Obtain verbal consent**

Written consent is the norm. If it is not possible to obtain written consent because of the extreme nature of the emergency, for example, cord prolapse, then verbal consent is acceptable. We must record the reasons for proceeding without written consent in the notes. Where a woman's capacity to consent is in doubt, legal advice is obtained if time allows in accordance with the Mental Capacity Act 2005, but that would not be the case in a cord prolapse situation. Relatives cannot consent on behalf of an adult patient who lacks capacity although it is good practice to involve the next of kin in any discussions.

2.5 Some elective gynaecological operations are more likely to result in primary haemorrhage, needing transfusion, than others.

Select the operation where cross-matched blood should be available rather than just 'group and save' being requested:

A. Adhesiolysis
B. Hysterectomy for dysfunctional uterine bleeding
C. ***Myomectomy**
D. Ovarian cystectomy
E. Posterior vaginal repair

Myomectomy is not done very often because most patients with fibroids are past childbearing age and have a hysterectomy (or other treatment such as embolization). During a myomectomy operation the blood loss can be torrential and sometimes the surgeon must carry on and do a hysterectomy to save the woman's life. Cross-matching at least two units is recommended

2.6 Elderly women, especially if they have cancer, are more at risk of wound dehiscence. Following a hysterectomy, postoperative dehiscence of an abdominal wound is more likely to occur if:

A.   The urinary catheter is left in too long

B.   The patient is mobilised too early

C.   *The patient develops a postoperative ileus

D.   The patient develops a vault haematoma

E.   The wound is transverse rather than vertical

Elderly, unfit patients with poor nutritional status, especially those with cancer, are at risk of wound breakdown. Poor healing can be expected if the wound gets infected or if the abdomen is distended because of ileus.

The Pfannenstiel incision we use for most gynaecological surgery is very robust and rarely comes apart, so we sew the rectus sheath up with dissolvable suture material whereas we must use more long-lasting stitches for vertical wounds as the rectus sheath in the midline has a relatively poor blood supply and healing takes longer than a transverse incision.

2.7 One of your patients is about to be admitted for a hysterectomy and has been counselled about the 'enhanced recovery pathway' at her pre-op checkup appointment. This care plan has been introduced for patients undergoing major gynaecological surgery to shorten their hospital stay, thereby reducing costs.

Which of these is part of this pathway?

A.   *Avoiding dehydration by limiting fluid restriction to 2 hours before surgery

B.   Cooling the patient during surgery

C.   Mechanical bowel preparation helps avoid bowel trauma and enhances recovery

D.   Preloading with a sachet of amino acid solution

E.   Routinely using drains to avoid pelvic haematoma formation

Maintaining the body temperature, rather than cooling, reduces complication rates.

The pathway advises avoiding bowel prep to speed up return of bowel function.

The solution used is a carbohydrate solution, not amino acid.

Surgeons are encouraged to avoid drains as they slow up mobilisation postoperatively.

Source: The Obstetrician and Gynaecologist, 'Enhanced Recovery in Gynaecology' 15 (4) (2013).

2.8 A patient who is due to have a pelvic floor repair mentions at the preoperative checkup that she is allergic to latex. Her surgery is scheduled for the middle of the operating list the following morning.

Her general health is good and she has no other allergies.

Select the most appropriate action:

A.   Add an 'alert' to the operating list

B.   Cancel the operation

C.   *Move her operation to the beginning of the list

D. Tell the theatre staff at the start of the list during the briefing

E. Reassure her that nonlatex gloves will be used

Latex allergies can be severe so we would not just use latex-free gloves, we would also make sure that the patient did not come into contact with latex parts of the operating table and stirrups. There must be a 20-minute gap between her operation and a previous operation where latex was used (to allow the air in the operating theatre to be changed in case there are any latex particles in it) so this would cause a significant delay in the list unless she was the first patient in the morning. It is too late to mention it during the 'World Health Organisation' checklist.

2.9 Which procedure requires perioperative antibiotic prophylaxis?

A. ***Caesarean section**

B. Forceps delivery

C. Laparoscopic removal of ectopic pregnancy

D. Oophorectomy for ovarian cyst

E. Perineal repair of second-degree tear

Any surgery that involves opening the vagina or operating on the vagina leads to an increased risk of infection, so that prophylactic antibiotics are indicated. The increased chance of infection in caesarean delivery is because the surgeon reaches down into the vagina to bring the baby's head back into the abdomen.

2.10 During an abdominal hysterectomy operation, the risk of ureteric injury is higher if:

A. Ovaries are being conserved

B. Patient is postmenopausal

C. She is immunosuppressed

D. ***The patient has a duplex kidney**

E. There is endometriosis involving the Pouch of Douglas

The chance of injuring a ureter is increased if there is abnormal anatomy (the duplex kidney may have two ureters) or adhesions due to endometriosis. In this case the endometriosis is nowhere near the ureters. If the ovaries are not being dissected off the pelvic side wall and removed, the risk of ureteric injury is less.

2.11 You are about to sign a consent form with a patient who is having a caesarean section. After you have listed the complications for her, she asks you which is the most common:

A. Wound dehiscence

B. Subsequent subfertility

C. Pseudo-obstruction of the bowel

D. ***Excess blood loss during surgery**

E. Fetal laceration

These complications of caesarean section occur relatively rarely except the excess blood loss, which is almost inevitable. We teach our trainees how to minimise blood loss at caesarean, but patients usually lose far more than those who have a vaginal delivery.

2.12 In the antenatal clinic you see a primigravid woman who has been referred by her community midwife at 37 weeks because the fetus is lying transversely. You organise an USS that shows that the reason for the abnormal lie is an 8 cm diameter ovarian cyst filling her pelvis. Your consultant tells

you to arrange a caesarean section and the woman asks you about the management of the cyst. Select the most appropriate advice in this clinical situation:

A. It will be dealt with later as the ovaries are not accessible during a caesarean

B. Spontaneous resolution of the cyst is likely after delivery

C. Removing the cyst at the time of caesarean will require a general anaesthetic

D. Caesarean and removal of the cyst should take place now in case the cyst torts

E. *Ovarian cystectomy during a caesarean at 39 weeks is appropriate

You will have seen the surgeon checking the ovaries routinely at the end of a caesarean operation before closing the abdomen, so the ovaries are obviously accessible. Spontaneous resolution is unlikely as this cyst cannot be an ovulatory cyst; otherwise it would have disappeared months ago whilst she has been pregnant. It does need to come out at the time of the caesarean, which is possible after the baby is delivered and the uterine incision closed. It can be done under spinal anaesthetic as it shouldn't increase the operating time by very much so it is unlikely that the spinal will wear off before the cystectomy has been done. In terms of the timing of the caesarean, the knowledge that is being tested here is that, if the baby is delivered at 37 weeks, there is a risk of transient tachypnoea of the newborn and the paediatricians prefer us to delay elective deliveries until 39 weeks of gestation.

2.13 You have seen a woman in preoperative assessment clinic who is due to undergo hysterectomy for prolapse in a few weeks' time. Which one of these is the most important factor to warn the anaesthetist about from her case notes?

A. She lives alone and has no postoperative social arrangements for care

B. Her mother had a DVT during chemotherapy many years ago

C. She has hypertension that is adequately treated with bendroflumethiazide

D. She is allergic to penicillin

E. *There is a family history of suxamethonium apnoea

The anaesthetist will want her to have a test to see if she has suxamethonium apnoea too. Although all the other factors are relevant to her hospital admission they are not so important to the anaesthetic team.

2.14 You are filling out a thromboprophylaxis risk form in the preoperative assessment clinic for a woman about to undergo a pelvic floor repair. Which of the following does not contribute to her risk score for venous thromboembolism?

A. The woman has a BMI of 44

B. The woman has inflammatory bowel disease

C. *The woman has essential hypertension

D. The woman has protein S deficiency

E. The woman has a history of recent breast cancer

If you have ever filled out a thromboprophylaxis risk form in a preoperative clinic you will recognise most of these risk factors.

2.15 A 45-year-old woman has been put on the waiting list for endometrial abla-tion to treat her menorrhagia. She visits the GP surgery to ask for further information as she wasn't given adequate time to discuss the procedure in the gynaecology clinic.

Which one of the following statements about endometrial ablation is correct?

A.   Endometrial ablation is always done under general anaesthetic
B.   Endometrial sampling is not required prior to the procedure
C.   It cannot be undertaken in the presence of a caesarean scar
D.   *She should continue using contraception afterwards
E.   The operation has a 90 per cent chance of producing amenorrhoea

This operation is not contraceptive and there have been reported pregnancies fol-lowing the procedure. The scarring in the uterine cavity means that they often miscarry but there have been some reports of pregnancies going to term. We do worry a bit about caesarean scars and may arrange a scan to look at the thickness of the myometrium in the lower part of the uterus, but it is not a contraindication. Some of the newer methods of ablation can be done under local anaesthetic.

2.16 A woman attends A&E due to heavy vaginal bleeding a week after having a LLETZ procedure for CIN 3. Her pulse and blood pressure are normal and her haemoglobin is 120 g/L

On speculum examination there is active bleeding from the cervix. What is the most appropriate initial management in this case?

A.   Arrange the operating theatre immediately for suturing of the cervix
B.   *Pack the vagina and give broad spectrum antibiotics
C.   Prescribe oral norethisterone and allow home
D.   Prescribe tranexamic acid and allow home
E.   Take a swab and commence broad spectrum oral antibiotics

As she is actively bleeding you must do something about this situation and can-not just send her home. Secondary bleeding like this is usually due to infection so she needs some antibiotics. Packing the vagina is usually enough to stop the bleeding but she may need to go to theatre if that does not work.

2.17 You would have concerns about the legitimacy of one of these patients signing their consent form for surgery. Which patient?

A.   A girl aged 15 years requesting termination of pregnancy
B.   An elderly woman who has had a stroke
C.   A woman requesting sterilisation whose husband did not agree
D.   A Jehovah's Witness who needs a caesarean for placenta praevia
E.   *A non-English-speaking woman whose husband is translating for her

A teenager who seems competent to understand what she is agreeing to (so-called Gillick or Fraser competent) is not a worry. The only problem here is the woman whose husband is the only way of communicating with her – he may have a vested interest and may not convey to her exactly what you tell him. In these circum-stances, an independent interpreter is recommended.

2.18 An 86-year-old woman presents to the gynaecology outpatient clinic with postmenopausal bleeding. Having examined her, the consultant decides that hysteroscopy and cervical biopsy are necessary but she is currently taking warfarin on account of an artificial heart valve. Select the most appropriate option regarding her anticoagulation:

A.   *Change to heparin and omit dose on morning of surgery
B.   Continue with current dose of warfarin
C.   Omit anticoagulation on morning of surgery
D.   Omit warfarin for 3 days before surgery and check INR
E.   Postpone surgery until anticoagulant therapy completed

This woman's anticoagulation therapy will not 'complete' because she will be on it for life, so option E is irrelevant. It is not advisable to continue with surgery whilst she is fully anticoagulated as she is likely to bleed excessively, so a method of stopping it temporarily must be found. The best option is to switch to heparin, which can be stopped and restarted more easily, with the possibility of staying on heparin until the histology report is available and you know whether she is going to need major surgery such as a hysterectomy for cancer in the near future.

2.19 You are asked to review a woman on the Day Case Unit who had a laparoscopic sterilisation yesterday. She has had four children between the ages of 6 months and 4 years, all delivered by caesarean section using a Pfannenstiel incision. The nurses are concerned because she has abdominal pain and she is still not well enough to go home, although your consultant saw her last night after the operating list had finished and discharged her.

When you examine her you notice some watery discharge from her suprapubic incision, which is soaking through the dressing.

Which one of the following statements applies to this case?

A.   Bowel damage is unlikely because her previous incision was suprapubic
B.   She is probably evading being discharged because the children exhaust her
C.   She should be sent home because your consultant discharged her
D.   *There could be a hole in her bladder
E.   Unrecognised laparoscopic bowel injury is a likely diagnosis

Laparoscopy carries a risk of serious complications of about 2 in 1,000 and it is important for GPs to be able to recognise them. If you have assisted in theatre, you will know that a Pfannenstiel incision involves opening the peritoneum as far as the umbilicus, so it possible to have bowel stuck to the back of the scar all the way up the anterior abdominal wall, even if the skin incision is suprapubic. As a caesarean incision heals, it is not unusual for the bladder to become adherent – to the front of the uterus and to the back of the abdominal incision – so it is possible that the second port for the sterilisation has gone through the bladder. It could be urine leaking out of the wound. We know that bowel damage at laparoscopy is not always recognised at the time of injury and that the presentation is often delayed so that the patient has returned home by the time she develops symptoms of peritonitis.

Source: RCOG Green-top Guideline, No. 49, 'Preventing Entry-Related Gynaecological Laparoscopic Injuries'. This guideline was published in 2008 and has been updated and transferred to the British Society of Gynaecological Endoscopy (BSGE) website.

2.20 An asthmatic woman is breathless on return to the Day Case Unit from the operating theatre recovery room and you are asked for advice. She has had an uncomplicated evacuation of uterus performed, but the clinical notes mention that she did have a coughing fit as she was being anaesthetised. Select the most appropriate immediate course of action in this situation:

A. Send her for an urgent chest x-ray

B. Organise a peak flow estimation

C. Prescribe nebulised salbutamol

D. Ask the anaesthetist to review her at the end of the list

E. ***Check her airway and give her oxygen by face mask**

These actions are appropriate but the first thing to do is ABC – check her airway and give oxygen. You are not sure at this stage whether she is having an exacerbation of her asthma, has a pneumothorax, or has aspirated.

Extended Matching Questions

A	CA125
B	Chest x-ray
C	Clotting screen
D	CT scan of abdomen and pelvis
E	Electrocardiogram
F	Endocervical chlamydia swab
G	Ferritin
H	Haemoglobin
I	High vaginal swab
J	Plain abdominal x-ray
K	Pregnancy test
L	Thrombophilia screen
M	Ultrasound guided biopsy
N	USS of the pelvis

These clinical scenarios describe women who are on the waiting list for various gynaecological operations. Select the single most appropriate preoperative investigation for each case.

Each option may be used once, more than once, or not at all.

2.21 A 31-year-old woman requesting fertility investigations is to be admitted to the Day Case Unit on day 8 of her next menstrual cycle for a laparoscopy and dye test to check tubal patency because she has a history of pelvic inflammatory disease.

F Endocervical chlamydia swab

Although most patients undergoing minor gynaecological procedures will have haemoglobin estimation this is not necessary unless they have heavy periods. For this patient it is more important to check that she does not have an undiagnosed chlamydia infection as dye laparoscopy may result in a further episode of acute pelvic inflammatory disease. Another distracter here is pregnancy test but she is day 8 of the cycle so this is not relevant.

2.22 To investigate her severe long-standing menorrhagia a 49-year-old woman is going to undergo hysteroscopy and endometrial biopsy and she has chosen to have it done under general anaesthetic.

H Haemoglobin

This woman is likely to have iron deficiency anaemia and hopefully the GP will have already done the haemoglobin before referring her for a gynaecological opinion. The distracters are ferritin level (which you would do if she was anaemic) and USS of the pelvis.

2.23 A woman aged 42 years has an USS revealing a left ovarian cyst measuring 9 cm with solid elements in it. The right ovary seems normal on the scan and there is no ascites. Your consultant is trying to decide whether to remove the uterus and other ovary as well as the diseased ovary.

A CA125

The main issue here is whether the cyst is likely to be malignant or not. If there is any suspicion of malignancy the correct operation is total hysterectomy, bilateral salpingo-oophorectomy, and omentectomy for staging of the disease. A CT scan might give some idea of omental or other abdominal spread of tumour but the CA125 blood level is the most useful piece of information when deciding on the extent of surgery to be performed. A normal chest x-ray would exclude stage 4 disease if there are no pleural effusions, but not as useful as the CA125.

2.24 A 32-year-old multiparous woman is admitted as a day case for laparoscopic sterilisation. She has been using a copper coil for contraception but you cannot see the strings and she thinks it was extruded from the uterus during an unusually heavy period 4 weeks ago.

K Pregnancy test

You might want to do a haemoglobin level in view of the recent heavy period but the main worry here is that she has not had contraceptive protection for the last few weeks giving her a chance to conceive prior to being sterilised. Although she has not actually missed her period yet, pregnancy tests are now sensitive enough to pick up measurable levels of hCG by a week after implantation. If you are worried about where the coil is you might want an USS of the pelvis or even a plain x-ray to locate it but the pregnancy test comes first.

2.25 A 40-year-old woman is going to have a hysterectomy for endometriosis. Scan reveals bilateral chocolate cysts on the ovaries. She has not had any surgery before but her mother had a DVT following hysterectomy at the same age.

L Thrombophilia screen

If this woman has inherited a thrombophilia she may need anticoagulation to cover the hysterectomy.

A	Chest x-ray
B	CT scan of abdomen and pelvis
C	Electrocardiogram (ECG)
D	Haemoglobin
E	High vaginal swab
F	Intravenous Pyelogram (IVP) x-ray
G	Plain abdominal x-ray
H	Serum calcium
I	USS of kidneys
J	Urea and electrolytes (U&E)
K	Urine culture

These clinical scenarios describe women developing complications after gynaecological operations. Select the most appropriate investigation for each case.
  Each option may be used once, more than once, or not at all.

2.26 Three days after a hysterectomy for endometrial cancer, a 60-year-old woman still has a distended abdomen with no bowel sounds. Which investigation will help you most with planning her management?

J Urea and electrolytes

As she has no bowel sounds, the diagnosis is paralytic ileus. You do not really need an abdominal x-ray to diagnose this – just use your stethoscope – but it can be associated with a low potassium level therefore the U&E is more use than an x-ray in the management of this patient because it will help you decide which intravenous fluids to prescribe.

2.27 An obese 58-year-old woman who normally smokes twenty cigarettes a day develops severe left-sided chest pain 2 days after a prolapse operation. She is tachycardic and tachypnoeic. On examination you find an inspiratory wheeze but normal air entry all over the chest. Which investigation would you carry out initially?

C Electrocardiogram

You would not want to send her down to the x-ray department for a chest x-ray until you have excluded acute myocardial infarction with an ECG.

2.28 Having undergone hysteroscopy and insertion of a Levonorgestrel intrauterine system (Mirena®) for menorrhagia under general anaesthetic, a 42-year-old woman was not well enough to be discharged home and has stayed in hospital overnight because of severe lower abdominal pain. The next morning, she is still in pain and has a temperature of 38°C. You cannot locate the coil strings on speculum examination.

G Plain abdominal x-ray

The suspicion is that the intrauterine system (IUS) has perforated the fundus of the uterus. You should be able to locate it on an abdominal film (although an ultrasound of the uterus would also be useful but we haven't given you this option).

2.29 On the fourth day following a difficult hysterectomy and bilateral salpingo-oophorectomy operation for endometriosis a 38-year-old woman has a swinging pyrexia and unilateral loin pain. She is still nauseous and seems to have a persistent ileus.

I USS of kidneys

Although this clinical scenario sounds like pyelonephritis and therefore MSU would be indicated, there is possibly a much more sinister cause of her symptoms that must not be overlooked. UTI does not usually cause ileus. The persistent ileus could be due to urine in the peritoneal cavity as a result of ureteric damage during surgery and the consequences of missing that diagnosis are potentially much more serious, with loss of renal function on the affected side. A normal ultrasound of the kidneys excludes ureteric damage and is a better investigation than IVP as it does not involve radiation.

2.30 Six days after leaving hospital following a vaginal hysterectomy operation, an anaemic woman is readmitted with further vaginal discharge and pain. She was sent home on iron tablets and analgesics. On readmission she is pyrexial and bimanual pelvic examination reveals a palpable tender mass at the vault with offensive brown blood in the vagina.

E High vaginal swab

Although a haemoglobin level would be routine here, you already know that she is anaemic and is being treated for it. The diagnosis is vault haematoma that is likely to be infected. You will be prescribing antibiotics for this patient anyway but the point of a high vaginal swab is to check that the treatment is correct depending on the sensitivities. If you can feel a palpable haematoma, imaging is superfluous to the diagnosis.

A	A guardian with power of attorney should sign the consent form
B	Consent from the patient is valid
C	Defer the operation until a court order can be obtained
D	Defer the operation until an independent interpreter is available
E	Defer the operation until the woman is fully recovered
F	Operate without consent in the patient's best interest
G	The consent already given is no longer valid
H	The woman has a right to refuse consent

I	The woman should not be asked to participate in the research
J	Verbal consent from the patient is adequate
K	Written consent could be obtained from the patient's husband

These clinical scenarios describe women in different situations where consent may be an issue. Select the most appropriate advice for each case.

Each option may be used once, more than once, or not at all.

2.31 A 51-year-old woman with severe learning difficulties is brought into A&E as an emergency with prolonged heavy bleeding. On admission her haemoglobin is 93 g/l. She needs a hysteroscopy to investigate the problem but cannot understand what is being proposed.

A. A guardian with power of attorney should sign the consent form

It is clearly in the best interests of this patient for her to have the investigation done especially as the bleeding has made her anaemic. The best option is for her family to be involved in the decision. In the absence of family, it is likely that she will have a legal guardian who could sign the consent form for her. In fact, the 'consent form' is form 4, which is a statement of why the procedure is in her best interests and ideally the legal guardian would sign in agreement to the procedure.

2.32 On the labour ward a primigravid woman has reluctantly had a fetal blood sample done at 4 cm dilatation and the result shows that the baby is hypoxic. She has a needle phobia and adamantly refuses caesarean section to deliver the baby quickly. Both the obstetric consultant and the paediatrician have explained the possible consequences to her.

H. The woman has a right to refuse consent

Although the consequences of this woman's decision could have profound effects on her baby's health, the baby has no rights in law until it is born. It is her right to refuse consent, and the responsibility of the health professionals involved is to ensure that her decision is fully informed. You might need to take into account the effects of any drugs she might have had for pain relief in labour and take care to document fully everything that is explained to her. Her husband cannot give consent on her behalf.

2.33 A Jehovah's Witness has a hysterectomy operation for endometrial cancer. She specifically states that she will not accept blood transfusion and signs a disclaimer form preoperatively. In the recovery room it becomes apparent that she has internal bleeding and the consultant decides to take her back to theatre. She has had a great deal of opiates to control her pain and is very drowsy.

F. Operate without consent in the patient's best interest

The blood transfusion issue is not relevant to consent in this situation but the longer the return to theatre is delayed, the more likely she is to die. The surgeon can take her back to theatre urgently to stop the bleeding without further consent especially as she will not accept blood transfusion. Her husband cannot give consent on her behalf.

2.34 On the labour ward a new research project is underway comparing two different drugs to treat postpartum haemorrhage. You are called in to put a drip up for a woman who has lost 400 ml of blood already and the blood loss seems to be ongoing. Although it has not been discussed previously with the patient, the midwife mentions the possibility of the patient being asked to participate in the research project.

I. The woman should not be asked to participate in the research

It is not appropriate to take consent for participation in a research project in an emergency situation. There is no time available for the woman to consider the options and either participate or withdraw consent if she wants to and these things are best discussed earlier in pregnancy.

2. 35 A 15-year-old schoolgirl presents to clinic requesting surgical termination of pregnancy accompanied by her 15-year-old boyfriend. She will not tell her parents about the pregnancy and after much discussion she is thought to be able to understand the risks of the procedure.

B. Consent from the patient is valid

If the teenager is deemed to be competent to understand the implications of her decision (so-called Fraser competence), then she can give consent for the procedure. It is always best if she does tell her parents (especially if she develops a complication) and we would always encourage her to think about doing that.

A	Cancel the operation as it is not the correct procedure for this patient
B	Go ahead with the operation as planned
C	Postpone the operation and arrange counselling
D	Postpone the operation and arrange review in genito-urinary medicine clinic
E	Postpone the operation and arrange routine gynaecology clinic review
F	Postpone the operation and arrange urgent gynaecology clinic review
G	Postpone the operation and organise an USS
H	Postpone the operation until you can arrange further tests
I	Refer her urgently to her GP for a prescription
J	Suggest that the patient has a spinal anaesthetic

The patients that you are seeing in the preoperative clinic are about to undergo gynaecological operations and unfortunately your consultant is not immediately available for advice.

Select the most appropriate management plan for each clinical scenario.

Each option may be used once, more than once, or not at all.

2.36 The waiting list clerk has arranged for a 49-year-old woman to fill a cancelled slot on the operating list at short notice. She is due to have an abdominal hysterectomy in 3 days' time and you are doing her preoperative check. She had a hysteroscopy done under local anaesthetic for irregular heavy bleeding recently but the histology on the endometrium from that operation is not yet available.

F Postpone the operation and arrange urgent gynaecology clinic review

The original symptoms may be caused by endometrial cancer, so irregular peri-menopausal bleeding should be dealt with urgently (in the same way as post-menopausal bleeding). You need to check the histology before she has her uterus removed as hysterectomy for endometrial cancer is a different operation from that for benign disease (e.g., the surgeon would take peritoneal washings and remove the ovaries as well).

2.37 A 37-year-old woman presented to clinic with left iliac fossa pain radiating down her left leg several weeks ago and USS revealed a 7 cm simple left ovarian cyst. She was put on the waiting list for an ovarian cystectomy but her symptoms have now disappeared.

G Postpone the operation and organise an USS

It is possible that this was an ovulatory cyst that may now have resolved. An ultrasound will resolve the issue.

2.38 A healthy 62-year-old woman is due to be admitted for a prolapse repair. She mentions a family history of 'difficulty waking up' after anaesthetics but is not sure of the clinical details.

H Postpone the operation until you can arrange further tests

This patient may have inherited suxamethonium apnoea and it is possible to test for this. Even though she wants a spinal anaesthetic, this may not give enough analgesia on the day of surgery and the anaesthetist will want to know that it is safe to give her a general anaesthetic.

2.39 A 33-year-old woman is to be admitted for endometrial ablation to treat her menorrhagia. She has turned down the option of a Mirena® IUS because she wishes to have another baby within the next couple of years.

A Cancel the operation as it is not the correct procedure for this patient

This patient is obviously unaware that endometrial ablation is not a suitable operation if pregnancy is desired in the future. The operation is designed to remove the endometrial layers right down to the basal layer that regenerates each cycle. Pregnancy has been reported after this operation but it is not usually successful and we often recommend that patients considering this are sterilised concurrently.

2.40 When she was seen in the fertility clinic a couple of weeks ago, a 29-year-old woman had a speculum examination during which some routine swabs were taken. You look up the results before signing her consent form for a laparoscopy and dye test only to discover that the chlamydia swab is positive.

D Postpone the operation and arrange review in genito-urinary medicine clinic

It is inadvisable to proceed with her surgery until the chlamydia infection has been adequately treated and contact tracing has been done – which is the main reason for involving the genito-urinary medicine clinic. They are very good at taking a sexual history and following up contacts.

A	Acute primary haemorrhage
B	Chest infection
C	Deep vein thrombosis (DVT)
D	Haemolysis
E	Intestinal obstruction
F	Pelvic haematoma
G	Pulmonary embolus (PE)
H	Secondary haemorrhage due to vault infection
I	Ureteric injury
J	Urinary tract infection
K	Urinary retention
L	Vault granulations
M	Vault dehiscence

Each of these clinical scenarios describes a woman presenting with complications after hysterectomy; for each patient pick the most likely diagnosis based on the clinical information given.

Each option may be used once, more than once, or not at all.

2.41 You are called to see a morbidly obese 40-year-old woman who had a hysterectomy for endometrial cancer 3 days ago. She has gradually become more breathless over the previous 24 hours and now seems a little confused. She is hypoxic and expresses discomfort when you ask for deep breaths to auscultate her chest but there is normal air entry. Her temperature is normal and you do not see any abnormality on her chest x-ray.

G Pulmonary embolus

The hypoxia and chest pain on inspiration suggest either a chest infection, pulmonary embolism, or pneumothorax. She has at least three risk factors for thromboembolism.

The pain on deep inspiration and the normal chest x-ray are the reason the answer is PE rather than infection.

2.42 Three days after a hysterectomy for endometriosis, a 35-year-old woman is found to have a mild pyrexia and a tachycardia of 100 bpm. There is a moderate amount of old blood coming from the vagina and her haemoglobin has dropped from 127 g/l preoperatively to 82 g/l now. The estimated blood loss at operation was described as 250 ml.

F Pelvic haematoma

Causes of pyrexia following a hysterectomy include wound infection, vault infection, urinary tract infection, chest infection, ureteric obstruction, and thromboembolism. The drop in haemoglobin without a matching obvious massive vaginal loss suggests that this woman has a pelvic haematoma that is just starting to discharge down the vagina. The main distracter is secondary haemorrhage but that usually presents 7 to 10 days after the operation (and is due to infection involving the vaginal vault). Primary haemorrhage refers to blood loss during the operation.

2.43 A 30-year-old woman had a hysterectomy and left salpingo-oophorectomy for chronic pelvic inflammatory disease. The surgery was described as difficult due to dense adhesions between the hydrosalpinx and the left side of the pelvis. Blood loss during the operation is documented as 900 ml. Two days later she is pyrexial, has a distended abdomen with no bowel sounds, and is complaining of left loin pain.

I   Ureteric injury

The prolonged ileus is a clue because this can occur as a result of urine leaking into the abdomen and it can't be bowel obstruction because she has no bowel sounds.

Ureteric damage is more likely in the presence of adhesions especially if there is heavy bleeding obscuring the view of anatomical structures and the loin pain gives it away.

2.44 A woman who had a hysterectomy 10 weeks ago comes to your surgery because she has just started to bleed vaginally again. She has not seen any blood since a week after her hysterectomy but has not been examined following the operation as she did not go to the hospital for her postoperative checkup.

L   Vault granulations

It is so long since this woman's surgery that it cannot possibly be secondary haemorrhage due to vault infection as the vault will have healed up by now. Vault dehiscence is extremely rare and usually presents early as a result of a haematoma discharging down the vagina. The most likely finding on speculum examination will be granulation tissue, which can be treated by the application of silver nitrate.

As more postoperative care is moved out to primary care in the future, many GPs will be involved in doing the follow-up for hysterectomy patients. Excessive granulation tissue in association with watery discharge should alert you to the possibility of a fistula but this would have presented earlier than 10 weeks. Vault dehiscence is very rare and presents within the first week or so as the tissue breaks down.

2.45 On her fluid balance chart on the first postoperative day, you notice that a woman has apparently not passed urine since she returned from theatre despite having received more than 2 litres of fluid intravenously. She has a pelvic drain in situ which contains 400 mls. The nurses report that she asked for a bedpan twice during the night.

K   Urinary retention

This woman is most likely to be in retention and the next step is to catheterise her. If there is no urine there, you need to consider whether she is dehydrated, has bled into her abdomen, or (rarely) has a bilateral ureteric injury. She may have sustained a primary haemorrhage and be hypovolaemic but the most likely cause is retention. She needs a urinary catheter and a careful fluid balance chart until you have sorted out the problem.

A	Advise alternative method of contraception 4 weeks before surgery
B	Continue using current contraceptive method
C	Prescribe full therapeutic anticoagulation therapy
D	Prescribe local vaginal estrogen instead of systemic HRT
E	Switch HRT to transdermal method before surgery
F	Stop HRT 4 weeks before surgery
G	Stop HRT 12 weeks before surgery
H	Stopping HRT is not necessary
I	Stop contraceptive method 4 weeks before surgery

These clinical scenarios relate to women seeking advice relating to surgery and the risks of thromboembolism. In each case you should decide on the best course of action regarding her hormonal medication and select the most appropriate advice.

Each option may be used once, more than once, or not at all.

2.46 A 26-year-old woman is on the waiting list for scoliosis surgery and seeks advice about whether she should continue taking her COC.

A Advise alternative method of contraception 4 weeks before surgery

Scoliosis surgery will result in a prolonged period of immobility postoperatively. Combined hormonal contraception should be discontinued and another estrogen-free method used at least 4 weeks prior to surgery. You would not want to just stop the pill and not use another method as in option I because she may start her postoperative convalescence with an early pregnancy.

Source: RCOG Green-top Guideline, No. 40, 'Venous Thromboembolism and Hormonal Contraception'. Published 2010 and has been archived. Information still available on the Faculty of Sexual and Reproductive Healthcare website (statement on venous thromboembolism and hormonal contraception).

2.47 A 26-year-old woman is being admitted to hospital for scoliosis surgery in 6 weeks' time and seeks advice about whether she should have her next dose of Depo-Provera®, which is now due.

B Continue using current contraceptive method

POPs, injectables, implants, and Mirena® do not seem to be associated with an increased risk of venous thromboembolism.

Source: RCOG Green-top Guideline, No. 40, 'Venous Thromboembolism and Hormonal Contraception'. Published 2010 and has been archived. Information still available on the Faculty of Sexual and Reproductive Healthcare website (statement on venous thromboembolism and hormonal contraception).

2.48 A 26-year-old woman is on the waiting list for diagnostic laparoscopy to diagnose her pelvic pain. She is currently taking Dianette® for contraception and in the hope that it will improve her acne.

B Continue using current contraceptive method

Diagnostic laparoscopy is minor surgery not associated with prolonged immobility so she does not need to stop her contraceptive pill.

Source: RCOG Green-top Guideline, No. 40, 'Venous Thromboembolism and Hormonal Contraception'. Published 2010 and has been archived. Information still available on the Faculty of Sexual and Reproductive Healthcare website (statement on venous thromboembolism and hormonal contraception).

2.49 A fit 50-year-old woman started on systemic HRT (sequential tablet formulation) 6 months ago because of severe vasomotor and vaginal dryness symptoms. She has felt much better on it but is now on the waiting list for a posterior vaginal repair for prolapse. Apart from the surgery, you do not identify any risk factors for thromboembolism in her medical notes.

F Stop HRT 4 weeks before surgery

Each woman requires an individual assessment of the risks and benefits of stopping HRT before elective surgery. Although concurrent use of HRT must increase the risk of postoperative venous thromboembolism the risk is likely to be small and, in any case, many women having surgery will also have thromboprophylaxis. The operation that this woman is having is relatively short in terms of operative time but may be associated with more immobilisation than her normal lifestyle for a couple of weeks postoperatively. She is not likely to be prescribed thromboprophylaxis as she is otherwise low risk, so she should follow the guidance in the British National Formulary and stop her HRT 4 weeks prior to surgery.

Source: RCOG Green-top Guideline, No. 19, 'Venous Thromboembolism and Hormone Replacement Therapy'. This guideline was published in 2011 and has been archived but there is a guideline on the Faculty of Sexual and Reproductive Healthcare website.

2.50 A 45-year-old woman is taking tibolone (Livial®) HRT having had a complete pelvic clearance for endometriosis 6 months previously. She is about to undergo carpal tunnel surgery and seeks advice about her tibolone medication.

H Stopping HRT is not necessary

Carpal tunnel surgery is relatively minor, often done under local anaesthetic and does not usually involve a period of immobilisation. There is no need to worry about her HRT.

Source: RCOG Green-top Guideline, No. 19, 'Venous Thromboembolism and Hormone Replacement Therapy'. This guideline was published in 2011 and has been archived but there is a guideline on the Faculty of Sexual and Reproductive Healthcare website.

Curriculum Module 3

Answers

Single Best Answer Questions

3.1 A woman went into hospital at 29 weeks of gestation with fresh vaginal bleeding. An emergency USS confirmed that the placenta was not low lying and she was discharged home yesterday.

She is due to fly to Majorca in a week's time and attends surgery for advice about her holiday.

Select the most appropriate advice:

A.   Advise against travelling at all whilst pregnant
B.   Advise against travel after 32 weeks of gestation
C.   ***Defer the holiday for several weeks**
D.   Have another scan before leaving on holiday
E.   Make sure that she has adequate travel insurance to cover pregnancy complications

Examples of medical conditions that may contraindicate commercial air travel include recent haemorrhage, severe anaemia, serious cardiac or respiratory disease, recent sickling crisis, recent gastrointestinal surgery, and a fracture. In this case the main worry is that she may bleed again or go into labour with no facilities on the flight to help with delivery.

Source: Scientific Impact Paper, No. 1, 'Air Travel and Pregnancy' (May 2013); www.rcog.org.uk.

3.2 A woman books for antenatal care at 12 weeks of gestation in her second pregnancy. In the last pregnancy she developed gestational diabetes that was managed with insulin. The community midwife asks you whether she needs a GTT arranging.

Select the most appropriate management:

A.   ***Early GTT repeated at 28 weeks**
B.   GTT at 28 weeks
C.   HbA1C instead of GTT
D.   Random glucose at this booking appointment
E.   Refer straight to diabetic antenatal clinic

In a woman who has had gestational diabetes before, the options are to start an early self-monitoring blood glucose regime (but we haven't given you this option) or to have an early GTT done, repeated at 24–28 weeks.

The guidance states 'do not use fasting plasma glucose, random blood glucose, HbA1C, glucose challenge test or urinalysis for glucose to assess risk of developing gestational diabetes'.

We do measure HbA1C at the beginning of pregnancy to assess the risk for the pregnancy; but only in women with preexisting diabetes, not previous gestational diabetes.

Source: NICE Guideline, No. NG3, 'Diabetes in Pregnancy; Management from Preconception to the Postnatal Period' (2015).

3.3 A woman has been on antidepressants for years and attends your surgery for advice now that she is pregnant for the first time.

Which of the following statements is correct advice regarding her antidepressant medication during pregnancy and the puerperium?

A. Long-acting selective serotonin reuptake inhibitors (SSRIs) have no adverse neonatal effects

B. Breast-feeding is contraindicated when taking any antidepressants

C. ***Consider gradual reduction of the antidepressant during the third trimester**

D. Stop the antidepressant when the pregnancy reaches 37 weeks of gestation

E. Tricyclic antidepressants do not affect the baby

All antidepressants can cause neonatal withdrawal syndrome but long-acting SSRIs are the worst. Gradual withdrawal is advised, rather than stopping her medication abruptly.

Source: NICE Guideline, 'Antenatal and Postnatal Mental Health: clinical management and service guidance' (updated 2015) and Scottish Intercollegiate Guidelines Network (SIGN) Guideline, No. 127, 'Management of perinatal mood disorders' (2012).

3.4 A care worker is just about to start her first job in an old people's home and is planning a pregnancy next year. She asks occupational health about the possibility of catching chickenpox from a patient with shingles, which seems to be common amongst the elderly residents.

Select the correct information for occupational health to give her:

A. All pregnant women should avoid any contact with chickenpox and shingles

B. Chickenpox cannot be caught from an individual with reactivated zoster (shingles)

C. ***More than 90 per cent of individuals in the United Kingdom are seropositive for IgG varicella antibodies**

D. Pregnant women are routinely tested for immunity to chickenpox at booking

E. Vaccination is available, which can be given during pregnancy

Universal serological testing for previous chickenpox infection (IgG antibodies) is not recommended in pregnancy but women with no history of chickenpox infection can be tested and offered prepregnancy or postpartum vaccination. Most women in the United Kingdom and Europe are already immune so the advice about every pregnant woman avoiding people with chickenpox is unnecessary.

Source: RCOG Green-top Guideline, No. 13, 'Chickenpox in Pregnancy' (2015).

3.5 In the surgery you see a woman in her first pregnancy who is suffering from hyperemesis. You do not think that she needs admitting to hospital and prescribe an antiemetic. Her teeth are in poor condition.

Select the main reason for suggesting that she makes an appointment with a dentist:

A. Hyperemesis can result in damage to maternal teeth
B. ***Periodontitis is a risk factor for low birth weight**
C. Pregnant women are entitled to free dental care
D. The immune response to plaque bacteria is altered in pregnancy
E. There is an association between pregnancy and gingival hyperplasia

All the preceding are true. Pregnant women are more prone to dental caries, which is thought to be associated with premature delivery and low birth weight and is the main reason for allowing pregnant women access to free dental care.

They are entitled to free dental care and free prescriptions but this is not just during pregnancy – it continues until the baby is 1 year old.

Frequent exposure to gastric acid erodes dental enamel.

Gingival hyperplasia can sometimes be severe in pregnancy and there are pictures in textbooks if you don't know what this looks like.

Source: The Obstetrician and Gynaecologist, 'Dental Manifestations of Pregnancy' (2007).

3.6 A woman who was diagnosed with epilepsy many years ago when she was a schoolgirl consults her GP because she is thinking of starting a family. She is taking sodium valproate and has not had a fit for more than a year.

Select the best advice regarding her medication:

A. It is better to have a fit than to take antiepileptic medication
B. ***Monotherapy with one drug is the preferred option in pregnancy**
C. She should be advised to take 0.5 mg folic acid daily when she gets pregnant
D. Sodium valproate should be continued as it is associated with the least risk of abnormality
E. The increased risk of congenital abnormality will be avoided if she stops taking valproate

Antiepileptic drugs are associated with an increased risk of congenital abnormalities and neurodevelopmental delay, but the outlook is worse if the woman stops taking them and has frequent fits as a consequence. Sodium valproate is particularly worrying in terms of the risk of congenital abnormality.

Polytherapy carries the highest risk.

Women and girls with epilepsy should be encouraged to take 5 mg folic acid daily in case pregnancy ensues.

Sudden unexpected death in epilepsy remains a major cause of death in pregnant women

Source: RCOG Green-top guideline no. 68 'Epilepsy in Pregnancy' (2016).

MBRRACE-UK (Mothers and Babies: Reducing Risk through Audits and Confidential Enquiries across the UK) 2015 report: 'Surveillance of Maternal Deaths in the UK 2011–13 and Lessons Learned to Inform Maternity Care from the UK and Ireland Confidential Enquiries into Maternal Deaths and Morbidity 2009–13'; accessible through RCOG website or at www.npeu.ox.ac.uk.

3.7 A newly pregnant morbidly obese woman in your surgery asks for information about 'the new screening test that can be done looking for the baby's genetic material in her blood'.

Which of the following statements is correct information about noninvasive testing using maternal plasma DNA?

A. A monochorionic twin pregnancy cannot be tested as the results will be inaccurate

B. It is only used to detect chromosomal abnormalities

C. She does not need to have a scan before the test

D. The test can only be performed in the first trimester

E. ***The test will be less accurate because of her obesity**

If a twin pregnancy is monochorionic, both the fetuses will have the same DNA and the test is accurate. It is dichorionic twins where there is a problem.

The reason that the test is less accurate in obese women is that there is a lower percentage of fetal DNA in the maternal circulation.

It is used to determine fetal sex in X-linked diseases and the fetal blood group in pregnancies affected by red cell antibodies, for example, rhesus.

It is not advisable to have the test before 10 weeks, so dating the pregnancy with a scan avoids false negative results.

The trisomies commonly tested for with this are 21, 13, and 18.

Source: RCOG Scientific Impact Paper, No. 15, 'Non-invasive Prenatal Testing for Chromosomal Abnormality Using Maternal Plasma DNA' (March 2014).

3.8 A community midwife is concerned about one of the pregnant women on her caseload because she has noted bruises of different ages on the woman's body whilst auscultating the fetal heart during a home visit.

Which of the following situations should also raise concerns about domestic violence?

A. All her older children are brought to antenatal appointments even during school terms

B. Her whole family including her parents come to antenatal appointments

C. Partner is always present at antenatal appointments

D. ***Poor attendance at antenatal clinic appointments**

E. Woman's previous children are all fathered by different men

Features that make you suspect domestic violence are injuries to the abdomen, genitals, and breasts; explanation of injury does not fit; woman trivialises injuries or does not seek medical help for them; late booking for antenatal care or frequent DNAs; partner controls woman during appointments and answers questions on her behalf; woman presents frequently with trivial or undiagnosable symptoms; and woman is reluctant to be discharged from hospital.

3.9 A multiparous woman with an uncomplicated pregnancy of 24 weeks' gestation is about to go on a long-haul flight. She has a BMI of 42, no medical problems, and is a nonsmoker.

Select the best advice regarding thromboembolism prevention in her case:

A. Aspirin 75 mg oral tablets

B. Graduated compression stockings

C. Hydration and mobilization during flight

D. ***Low molecular weight heparin injections**

E. No special measures needed

Prolonged air travel results in a threefold increase in the risk of VTE but wearing graduated compression stockings results in 16.2 fewer DVTs per 10,000 people (although these results are from a nonpregnant population). It is suggested that all pregnant women wear compression stockings but this woman is multiparous and has a BMI of 42, both of which increase her risks. If she needs formal thromboprophylaxis because she has other risk factors, low molecular weight heparin is more effective than aspirin.

Source: Scientific Impact Paper, No. 1, 'Air Travel and Pregnancy' (May 2013); www.rcog.org.uk.

3.10 A pregnant woman from your GP practice with insulin-dependent diabetes is referred to the hospital diabetic obstetric clinic for antenatal care.

How often should she be scanned for growth and amniotic fluid volume?

A. Fortnightly from 24 weeks of gestation

B. Fortnightly from 28 weeks until term

C. ***Monthly from 28 weeks of gestation until 36 weeks**

D. Monthly from 28 weeks until term

E. No growth scans necessary unless the symphysial-fundal height measures 'small for dates'

There is a chart on this guideline that gives details of what should be done at every antenatal visit, including screening the mother for complications such as retinopathy and nephropathy.

Source: NICE Guideline, No. NG3, 'Diabetes in Pregnancy; Management from Preconception to the Postnatal Period' (2015).

3.11 Intrahepatic cholestasis of pregnancy is an uncommon but serious complication. Which of the following statements about this condition is correct?

A. Antenatal administration of vitamin K to the mother reduces the itching

B. ***Meconium in the liquor during labour is to be expected**

C. The condition only occurs in primigravid women

D. The problem affects the mother's health, but the baby is not at risk

E. The recurrence risk in a subsequent pregnancy is 5 per cent

Although meconium liquor can occur in pregnancies affected by cholestasis, it should not be ignored because it is sometimes an indication of fetal hypoxia.

The recurrence risk is quoted as between 45 and 90 per cent in the next pregnancy.

Source: RCOG Green-top Guideline, No. 43, 'Obstetric Cholestasis'. Published 2011.

3.12 Which of the following statements concerning HIV in pregnancy is true?

A. In HIV-positive mothers on antiretroviral treatment breast-feeding is safe
B. ***Infants born to women who are HIV positive should be treated with antiretroviral therapy from birth**
C. Interventions can reduce the risk of vertical HIV transmission from 30 per cent to zero
D. Use of short-term steroids to promote fetal lung maturation is inadvisable
E. Women who do not require treatment for their own health do not need to take antiretroviral therapy during pregnancy

To reduce the chance of passing on HIV to the baby, the mother should take antiretroviral drugs during pregnancy, be delivered by caesarean section (unless her viral load is very low), and avoid breast-feeding. The incidence of vertical transmission does not reach zero even with these measures.

The baby should get antiretroviral therapy until it is possible to check HIV status at 3 months of age.

Source: British HIV Association Guideline for the management of HIV infection in pregnant women. Published 2012, reviewed 2014. www.bhiva.org

3.13 A refugee woman from Ethiopia books for antenatal care in her first pregnancy and discloses to the midwife that she has undergone FGM in the past. Which of these statements about FGM is true?

A. ***FGM can be surgically 'undone' before delivery**
B. If her baby is female, she may be at risk of FGM as a teenager in the future
C. She must be delivered by elective caesarean section
D. Usually involves complete closure of the vaginal introitus except for a tiny hole
E. UK law states that the suturing can legally be restored after delivery

If you suspect that a woman has undergone FGM, she should be referred to a clinic with experience of dealing with this as it is entirely possible to 'undo' the introitus so that she can have a vaginal delivery without too much trauma. In the United Kingdom it is illegal to resuture the vaginal introitus so that it is closed again. There may be child protection issues; there is often intense cultural pressure to inflict the same procedure on young girls, but the surgery is normally carried out well before puberty. There are several different types of FGM resulting in varying degrees of closure of the introitus.

3.14 You see a pregnant woman in your surgery who has just been to the hospital for a dating scan at 11 weeks of gestation that reveals that she has monochorionic twins in separate sacs.

Which of the following statements is true about this type of twin pregnancy?

A. ***Delivery should be planned for 36 weeks if she has not laboured**
B. Monochorionic twins are at lower risk of twin-twin transfusion syndrome than dichorionic twins
C. Regular growth scans will be offered from 32 weeks of gestation
D. She should be delivered by caesarean section as there is a risk of cord entanglement
E. She will not be able to have any sort of screening for Down syndrome

Monochorionic twins are at risk of twin-twin transfusion syndrome rather than dichorionic and, because of this, her growth scans will start earlier at 24 weeks. There is a risk of cord entanglement but these twins are in separate sacs and this is not a reason for caesarean delivery. There is a risk of stillbirth if the pregnancy goes to term so we would normally deliver by 36 weeks. She could have nuchal translucency scans to screen for Down syndrome but there is an ethical dilemma regarding the results – what if one of the twins has a thickened nuchal fold and the other one doesn't? The subsequent diagnostic test is also problematic if required.

Source: RCOG Green-top Guideline, No. 51, 'Management of Monochorionic Twin Pregnancy'. Published 2016.

3.15 You are consulted by a primigravid woman at 24 weeks of gestation who has an unbearable headache. She has a history of severe migraines that she has consulted you about before several times. You do a thorough examination and find epigastric tenderness. Testing her urine reveals proteinuria +++.

Which one of the following statements about her situation is correct?

A. Fundal height is irrelevant as poor growth will not be apparent at this early gestation

B. If her blood pressure is 125/80 mmHg the diagnosis cannot be pre-eclampsia

C. Prescribing antibiotics without awaiting the results of an MSU is not advisable

D. *She needs assessment by an obstetrician urgently

E. The diagnosis cannot be pre-eclampsia because of the early gestation

In general practice you might be consulted about symptoms by patients who have pre-eclampsia, so it is important to recognise the symptom cluster of unremitting frontal headache, visual disturbance, and epigastric pain, sometimes with nausea and vomiting. The measured BP should be compared with the booking blood pressure to quantify the rise, although very occasionally patients can develop eclampsia with normal blood pressure so the presence of proteinuria with the preceding symptoms should prompt referral to the obstetric unit for assessment. Occasionally pre-eclampsia happens at a very early gestation.

3.16 Consultant referral is necessary so that antenatal serial growth scans can be arranged to check on fetal growth if the pregnancy is affected by which of the following conditions in the mother:

A. History of polycystic ovarian syndrome

B. 'Slapped cheek' syndrome

C. Previous delivery by caesarean section

D. *Recurrent unexplained antepartum haemorrhage

E. Vitamin B12 deficiency

Polycystic ovarian syndrome increases the risk of miscarriage and diabetes but not intrauterine growth restriction (IUGR). The other conditions are good reasons for referring for consultant care but for reasons other than the potential for poor fetal growth.

'Slapped cheek' syndrome is due to parvovirus infection, which can cause severe fetal anaemia and intrauterine fetal death but not usually growth restriction.

There is no known association between any maternal vitamin deficiency and growth problems.

Source: RCOG Green-top Guideline, No. 31, 'The Investigation and Management of the Small-for-Gestational-Age Fetus'. Published 2013.

3.17 A 14-year-old schoolgirl is brought to your surgery by her mother having been sent home with a note from the school nurse suggesting that she might be pregnant. On examination it is obvious that her abdominal swelling is due to a pregnancy of about 36 weeks of gestation; fetal movements can be clearly seen and the fetal heart auscultated.

Which of the following is true regarding this teenage pregnancy?

A. Her due date can be accurately predicted when she has a scan at the hospital

B. She is no more likely to deliver a small-for-dates infant than mothers aged 20–30

C. ***She should be offered chlamydia screening**

D. There is no point in discussing contraception

E. You should involve the police because her pregnancy must be the result of rape

There is a higher incidence of sexually transmitted infections in teenage mothers.

Teenagers who get pregnant are far more likely than older mothers to have infections such as chlamydia and some antenatal clinics routinely screen teenagers for STIs. Although it may seem like 'shutting the stable door after the horse has bolted' a discussion about future contraception is advisable during antenatal clinic appointments so that a method can be prescribed as soon as she delivers; otherwise a proportion of these teenagers will be back in antenatal clinic sooner than everyone would like.

Having sexual intercourse with anyone under the age of 16 years is illegal but in practice it does not seem appropriate to refer pregnant teenagers to the police; we want them to engage with services, not conceal their pregnancies until delivery. There is a caveat here – if her partner is much older than her or there is any suspicion of incest, there may be child protection issues and you should take advice from your local Child Protection Lead and Social Services in that case.

Teenage mothers are more at risk of IUGR and should have growth scans. As she is booking late, the dating of the pregnancy from ultrasound will be hopelessly inaccurate so she will need a growth scan 2 weeks later anyway to check that the baby is growing along the same centile as her first scan.

3.18 A 34-year-old woman who has had two uncomplicated pregnancies previously expresses a wish to have a home birth this time. At her 28-week checkup with the midwife she mentions that she has had a couple of minor episodes of vaginal bleeding following intercourse during the previous few weeks. Her blood group is A rhesus negative.

Which one of the following statements about her care is appropriate?

A. A normal 20-week anomaly scan will exclude placenta praevia as a cause

B. Bleeding is unlikely to be caused by cervical cancer if her recent smear is normal

C. Kleihauer testing will help diagnose placental abruption

D. She could still have a home birth if the placenta is not low

E. ***She should be referred to consultant-led antenatal care for growth scans**

She needs an USS to rule out placenta praevia, which is sometimes missed on the anomaly scan. Undiagnosed recurrent antepartum haemorrhage is associated with growth restriction and cerebral palsy so her antenatal care should be transferred to an obstetric consultant for growth scans. We would not advise home birth because of the increased risk of fetal distress in labour. The Kleihauer test is performed to discover how much anti-D a rhesus negative mother needs after a potential sensitising event, not to diagnose abruption.

3.19 You see a primigravid woman in clinic who has just had a 20-week detailed (anomaly) scan that reveals a low-lying placenta. Her haemoglobin was 107 gm/L at booking and she takes ferrous sulphate 200 mg daily.

Which is the most appropriate advice for her?

A. Admission to hospital will be necessary later in the pregnancy

B. ***Avoid sexual intercourse**

C. Delivery will be by caesarean section at 37 weeks

D. Increase the dose of oral iron to three times daily

E. Take folic acid 5 mg daily

Although the placenta is low lying at this gestation it may not be on a subsequent USS, so she could still have a vaginal delivery if the placenta is no longer low at term. There is no point in arranging the repeat scan before 32 weeks of gestation because the lower segment of the uterus does not start to form until then.

It is worth avoiding anaemia but she does not necessarily need increased iron or folic acid. Even if the placenta does turn out to be low lying later on, it is no longer considered mandatory to admit women with a low-lying placenta in the third trimester. If there has been no bleeding and the placenta doesn't cover the os she can remain at home until near term, particularly if she lives close to the hospital.

Not having intercourse is sensible advice to avoid causing vaginal bleeding (and the release of prostaglandin in the vagina will make the uterus contract).

3.20 You are looking after a 'grand multip' pregnant with her fifth baby who has had four normal births before.

Which pregnancy complication is she most at risk of?

A. Anaemia

B. Hypertension

C. Low-lying placenta

D. Placenta accreta

E. ***Postpartum haemorrhage**

It is the poor contractility of the myometrium that makes a 'grand multip' more at risk of postpartum haemorrhage. This was the cause of death of Mumtaz Mahal who died of haemorrhage giving birth to her thirteenth child (resulting in the construction of the incredible Taj Mahal).

Hypertension is more common in older mothers but a grand multip is not necessarily older. Placenta accreta is more common after several caesarean sections but not after vaginal births.

Extended Matching Questions

A	Alpha-fetoprotein level
B	Amniocentesis
C	Chorionic villus sampling
D	Combined nuchal translucency scan and serum screening
E	Cordocentesis
F	Detailed ultrasound scan
G	Karyotype both parents for balanced (Robertsonian) translocation
H	Nuchal translucency scan
I	Serum screening with hCG/alpha-fetoprotein/oestriol levels
J	Third trimester growth scan
K	3-D ultrasound scan

These clinical scenarios relate to prenatal screening and diagnostic tests. For each woman select the most appropriate investigation.

Each option may be used once, more than once, or not at all.

3.21 The wife of a prominent politician is referred to a private obstetric clinic at 10 weeks of gestation because she has conceived unexpectedly many years after the birth of her last child and is now aged 42. She wishes to be absolutely reassured that the baby does not have Down syndrome as soon as possible because she feels that it would hamper her contribution to her husband's career.

C Chorionic villus sampling

If she wishes to have a quick definitive answer from a diagnostic test rather than a screening test, then chorionic villus sampling (CVS) is the best option despite the increased miscarriage risk. The current NHS screening programme would not provide a diagnostic CVS or amniocentesis on grounds of maternal age.

3.22 A patient with a history of a previous pregnancy affected by neural tube defect wishes to have the most sensitive test in this current pregnancy.

F Detailed USS

Although the alpha-fetoprotein level would give some idea of the likelihood of neural tube defect (NTD) it is not diagnostic and misses some cases, especially closed NTDs; therefore detailed ultrasound is the best option. Very few cases of NTD are missed on ultrasound these days because the scan machines have much-improved resolution.

3.23 A 36-year-old woman has conceived after many years of infertility. She wishes to have a screening test for Down syndrome with the least false positive rate.

H Nuchal translucency and serum screening

This patient is seeking a screening test rather than a diagnostic test with a risk of miscarriage attached, and this combination gives the most accurate option. If the result is in the high-risk category she must decide whether to risk miscarriage by opting for a diagnostic test.

3.24 A couple who know that they are both carriers of cystic fibrosis present at 9 weeks' gestation requesting prenatal diagnosis.

C Chorionic villus sampling

It is possible to exclude this condition now at an early gestation by offering CVS.

3.25 A 40-year-old woman who has reached 15 weeks of gestation having had three previous first-trimester miscarriages wishes to have a diagnostic test for Down syndrome because her partner has a balanced Robertsonian translocation.

B Amniocentesis

If this patient wishes to have a diagnostic test she must accept the risk of miscarriage and have an amniocentesis. Serum screening and detailed scan might suggest a problem but are not diagnostic. The balanced translocation increases the risk of trisomy, and we probably know about it because of investigation of recurrent miscarriage in this couple.

A	Abruptio placentae
B	Appendicitis
C	Constipation
D	Pancreatitis
E	Pre-eclampsia
F	Red degeneration of a uterine fibroid
G	Torsion of an ovarian cyst
H	Ureteric calculus
I	Urinary tract infection
J	Uterine rupture

These clinical scenarios relate to the emergency presentation of a pregnant woman with abdominal pain. For each woman select the most likely diagnosis for her pain.

Each option may be used once, more than once, or not at all.

3.26 Two years after a myomectomy operation, a 42-year-old woman has conceived following IVF treatment. At 32 weeks of gestation she is admitted to the obstetric unit with increasing pain in her abdomen for 3 days, which only responds to opiate analgesia. Apart from nausea she has no systemic symptoms. On examination she is apyrexial and normotensive but has a tachycardia. There is localised tenderness only at the fundus of the uterus.

F   Red degeneration of a uterine fibroid

Apart from a tachycardia her observations are normal and the tenderness is over the uterus. This makes appendicitis, urinary tract infection, and pancreatitis less likely. If the cause of the pain was uterine rupture or abruptio placenta it would not have been going on for several days and she would be much more unwell. As she has had a myomectomy previously she may well have another fibroid. Red degeneration happens when a fibroid grows so rapidly that it outgrows its vascular supply and the middle of the fibroid becomes necrotic. This is not uncommon during pregnancy and the pain can be severe.

3.27 An 18-year-old primigravid woman presents in A&E at 16 weeks of gestation with lower abdominal pain and vomiting. She has foetor oris and a temperature of 37.8°C.

B   Appendicitis

The gastrointestinal upset and foetor oris suggests appendicitis rather than urinary tract infection. Appendicitis can be a difficult diagnosis to make in pregnancy.

3.28 At 32 weeks of gestation a woman pregnant with her second baby is admitted by an ambulance having collapsed in a supermarket due to sudden onset of severe abdominal pain. Her observations are stable apart from a maternal tachycardia. The uterus is tender and unfortunately no fetal heartbeat is detectable.

A   Abruptio placentae

The uterus is described as 'woody hard' if abruption occurs. If there is no vaginal bleeding the diagnosis is concealed abruption.

3.29 At 17 weeks of gestation a 38-year-old primigravid woman is rushed in to A&E with severe unilateral colicky loin pain. She was writhing about on the bed but the pain has now subsided following a dose of morphine. Urinalysis reveals haematuria and her temperature is normal.

H   Ureteric calculus

The history of the pain and lack of pyrexia suggest that this is more likely to be ureteric calculus than urinary tract infection (although colic is uncommon in pregnancy because high progesterone levels relax the smooth muscle of the ureters). Torsion of an ovarian cyst would not produce haematuria.

3.30 A primigravid woman on holiday in London attends an NHS 'walk-in' centre with severe epigastric pain and headache. Her pregnancy has been uncomplicated so far and she is now 30 weeks of gestation. On admission, urinalysis reveals that there is a great deal of protein in her urine.

E   Pre-eclampsia

This could be a urinary tract infection but the symptoms are more suggestive of pre-eclampsia, even at this early gestation. Taking her blood pressure should be the next move.

A	Aim for vaginal delivery but with a shortened second stage
B	Await spontaneous labour and aim for vaginal delivery
C	Classical caesarean section
D	Elective caesarean section at 39 weeks of gestation
E	Elective caesarean section at 39 weeks of gestation and sterilisation
F	Elective caesarean section at 40 weeks of gestation
G	Emergency caesarean section
H	Induction of labour at 38 weeks of gestation and aim for vaginal delivery
I	Offer external cephalic version and await spontaneous labour
J	Offer external cephalic version and if successful induce labour

These scenarios relate to a woman with a complicated pregnancy or underlying medical condition. How would you counsel her regarding delivery?

Each option may be used once, more than once, or not at all.

3.31 Having been delivered by caesarean section in her two previous pregnancies a 30-year-old woman books for antenatal care at 17 weeks of gestation.

D Elective caesarean section at 39 weeks of gestation

It is usual to offer caesarean delivery if the patient has had two previous sections because of the increased risk of scar rupture. In terms of timing, we normally choose 39 weeks of gestation because babies rarely develop transient tachypnoea of the newborn if delivery is deferred until then.

3.32 Having had a myomectomy operation a few years ago, a 39-year-old woman is followed up carefully in antenatal clinic because she has several more fibroids in the uterus. Serial scans show that the baby is well grown but at 37 weeks the ultrasonographer notes that the fibroid in the lower segment has grown to 8 cm diameter and the baby is lying transversely above it.

C Classical caesarean section

Myomectomy does not necessarily mean that she must have a caesarean section and vaginal delivery is feasible. However, a fibroid occupying the lower segment of the uterus – especially one that is nearly as large as the baby's head – is likely to obstruct labour. It would also make a lower segment caesarean tricky so that the best option would be to open the uterus longitudinally above the fibroid with a classical incision. We very rarely perform classical caesarean sections and there are implications for her next pregnancy, so if you know that your patient has had one before, you should take pains to point that out in your next referral letter.

3.33 A woman with HIV attends antenatal clinic at 36 weeks of gestation. She is on antiretroviral medication and her viral load is extremely low at < 50 copies per ml.

B Await spontaneous labour and aim for vaginal delivery

HIV-positive patients are normally delivered by caesarean to reduce the chance of vertical transmission. However, if her viral load is extremely low (as in this case) we know that the mode of delivery makes no difference to the baby. There are rules to follow that include avoiding prolonged labour and leaving the membranes intact as long as possible; therefore avoiding induction of labour is a good idea.

3.34 A primigravid woman is referred to hospital antenatal clinic at 37 weeks of gestation because the presentation is found to be breech. Scan confirms that the baby is of average size and the presentation is flexed breech.

I Offer external cephalic version and await spontaneous labour

There are several 'distractors' in this question. If the presentation remains breech, this woman is likely to be offered elective caesarean; therefore the best option is to try and turn the baby. It is unnecessary to induce labour if external cephalic version is successful, as spontaneous labour is more efficient than induced.

3.35 Just prior to conceiving, a 34-year-old woman was treated for a cerebral aneurysm, which was successfully clipped leaving no neurological deficit. Her craniotomy wound has healed well and she is now 36 weeks of gestation in her first pregnancy.

A Aim for vaginal delivery but with a shortened second stage

A history of previous intracranial problems such as bleeding, detached retina, and treated aneurysm make it inadvisable for a woman to be performing the Valsalva manoeuvre every couple of minutes for an hour in labour so we would plan to have an elective assisted delivery to shorten the second stage. We don't need to consider caesarean delivery because she has had her aneurysm successfully treated.

A	Admit immediately to a psychiatric 'mother and baby' unit
B	Advise that depression is common and resolves after delivery
C	Advise that she should stop medication as it can harm the baby
D	Arrange specialist counselling
E	Ask a psychiatric liaison worker to visit at home
F	Continue medication and seek psychiatric advice
G	Recommence psychiatric medication immediately
H	Refer to her previous psychiatrist
I	Routine opinion from a specialist obstetric psychiatric clinic
J	Suggest that she considers short-term use of sleeping tablets
K	Suggest that she takes an antidepressant
L	Urgent opinion from a specialist obstetric psychiatric clinic

These scenarios relate to psychiatric problems in pregnant women. In each case decide the most appropriate course of action.

Each option may be used once, more than once, or not at all.

3.36 Having been diagnosed with schizophrenia at university many years ago, a 34-year-old woman books for antenatal care very late as she had not realised that she was pregnant until the third trimester. She has been off medication for many years and has been psychiatrically well since.

L Urgent opinion from a specialist obstetric psychiatric clinic

The chance of this woman developing a puerperal psychosis after delivery is very high (around 30 per cent) and she needs surveillance postpartum with easy recourse to urgent specialist obstetric psychiatric advice if she becomes ill. Ordinary psychiatrists sometimes do not appreciate the urgency of the problem and something drastic can happen before psychiatric admission can be organised. As she is near term, this needs urgent action. This message came over very clearly from the 2000–2002 maternal mortality reports (when maternal suicide was the leading cause of maternal death in the United Kingdom).

3.37 A primigravid woman at 28 weeks of gestation consults you in surgery about feeling very low in mood and having trouble sleeping following the death of her mother. She denies thoughts of self-harm.

D Arrange specialist counselling

Although this woman does sound depressed, it is a reactive depression and likely to respond to simple measures. The use of antidepressants in pregnancy is reasonable if the benefits outweigh the risks, but there is limited information about the safety of many drugs regarding the fetus, so it is better if she can cope with nondrug therapy.

3.38 A young woman with bipolar disorder has been well controlled on lithium for a few years and seeks preconceptual counselling. She is planning pregnancy soon and has no other medical problems.

F Continue medication and seek psychiatric advice

Patients on lithium to stabilise their mood can become quite unwell if they stop it abruptly and in this situation the risks of stopping the lithium outweigh the benefits. She needs advice from her psychiatrist to decide if it is advisable to come off her medication to reduce the chances of damaging the fetus especially in the first trimester. It is good that she has come for preconceptual counselling as it gives an opportunity to organise withdrawal before pregnancy if she is well enough.

3.39 The midwife caring for one of your patients contacts you with concerns about a 42-year-old first-time mother who has refused to allow her access to the house for the previous 3 days. The husband reveals on the telephone that his wife has not slept since the baby was born and is making bizarre comments about the health of the baby. Her psychiatric liaison worker has left a written care plan in her obstetric notes.

A Admit immediately to a psychiatric 'mother and baby' unit

This woman appears to have developed postpartum psychosis and needs inpatient assessment done by an experienced team. If she goes into a specialised unit she can take the baby with her, which is better for bonding as she improves in the long run. If there is a written care plan it is likely that she has previous history and the plan should be accessible to everyone looking after her.

3.40 A woman books for antenatal care at 10 weeks in her second pregnancy. She gives a history of postnatal depression that involved several months of in-patient care following her previous delivery. She is currently well and not on any medication.

I Routine opinion from a specialist obstetric psychiatric clinic

This woman has booked early, which provides the obstetric and psychiatric medical team a great deal of time to look into her history and assess the risk for this pregnancy. The fact that she was looked after as an in-patient previously increases the likelihood of it having been a psychosis rather than an ordinary depression, but this can be investigated to confirm the previous diagnosis to work out her recurrence risk. 'Postnatal depression' is an acceptable diagnosis to many patients, so any sort of mental illness may be referred to as depression (when it was actually a psychosis).

A	Abdominal USS
B	Computed Tomogram scan
C	Doppler measurement of cerebral artery flow
D	Electronic cardiotocograph fetal monitoring
E	Fetal growth scan in 2 weeks
F	Speculum examination of the cervix with fibronectin swab
G	Speculum examination of the cervix with microbiology swabs
H	Transvaginal ultrasound scan
I	USS with umbilical artery Doppler measurement
J	Vaginal examination in theatre with the operating team standing by

These clinical scenarios relate to women in the third trimester of pregnancy, presenting with vaginal bleeding. In each case, choose the most appropriate initial investigation.

Each option may be used once, more than once, or not at all.

3.41 A woman attends the labour ward at 35 weeks of gestation on account of a small amount of vaginal bleeding, which has now stopped. Initially there was some minor abdominal pain, but this has settled and there is no uterine activity. There have been reduced fetal movements since the episode of bleeding. On examination the size of the uterus is compatible with dates.

D Electronic cardiotocograph fetal monitoring

Although the diagnosis here could be placenta praevia, therefore an ultrasound is a good idea; it is important to check that the baby is healthy before she goes to scan because another potential diagnosis is placental abruption. At some stage she will also need a speculum examination to exclude a cervical cause of the bleeding – such as chlamydial infection – but this should not be done until after the scan excludes placenta praevia.

3.42 A primigravid 37-year-old woman presents with a heavy vaginal bleed at 39 weeks of gestation. The uterus is nontender and the baby is well grown but appears to be lying transversely. There are no contractions and the condition of both the mother and the baby is stable.

A Abdominal USS

Transverse lie is extremely unusual in a primigravid patient and this makes the diagnosis of placenta praevia very likely – so she needs an abdominal scan. If she were contracting (so you haven't much time to make the diagnosis) we would consider examining her in theatre, in case doing that makes her bleed torrentially from a low-lying placenta.

3.43 A primigravid patient is seen in the antenatal assessment unit because of recurrent episodes of antepartum haemorrhage over the previous few weeks. The uterine fundus measures 'small-for-dates' at 37 weeks of gestation. An USS confirms that the baby's abdominal circumference is on the tenth centile of the growth chart and the liquor volume is less than expected.

D Electronic cardiotocograph fetal monitoring

Recurrent antepartum haemorrhage is sometimes associated with intrauterine growth restriction. Although a Doppler is indicated here and another growth scan in 2 weeks' time, it is important to check that the baby is healthy now before planning future management.

3.44 Having booked late for antenatal care because she tried to conceal her pregnancy, a 15-year-old primigravid woman comes in to labour ward late one evening with a small amount of postcoital bleeding at term. The baby is moving normally and the uterus is nontender.

G Speculum examination of the cervix with microbiology swabs

The lack of uterine tenderness rules out abruption as a diagnosis and it is likely that she has had a scan (which would have picked up placenta praevia) even though she booked late. The rate of chlamydial carriage in teenagers is very high and this infection is the most likely cause of her postcoital bleeding.

3.45 The emergency ambulance brings a 23-year-old woman to hospital at 34 weeks in her second pregnancy because she experienced sudden onset of abdominal pain and vaginal bleeding an hour ago. On examination the uterus is very tender and feels hard.

D Electronic cardiotocograph fetal monitoring

The diagnosis here is likely to be placental abruption so the first priority is to check that the baby is healthy.

A	Candida albicans
B	Chlamydia trachomatis
C	Escherichia coli
D	Gardnerella vaginalis
E	Gonococcus

F	Group B streptococcus
G	Listeria monocytogenes
H	Parvovirus B19
I	Rubella
J	Streptococcus faecalis
K	Toxoplasma gondii

These clinical scenarios relate to women with infectious diseases in pregnancy. For each case select the single most likely infecting organism.

Each option may be used once, more than once, or not at all.

3.46 A woman presents in the surgery at 22 weeks of gestation complaining of increasing abdominal discomfort and on examination the uterus is tense and large for dates. She gives a history of a mild flu-like illness 2 weeks previously. The community midwife refers her to hospital for an USS, which shows polyhydramnios and fetal hydrops.

G Listeria monocytogenes

Rubella, toxoplasma, and listeria all cause a mild flu-like illness in pregnancy and all three organisms can cross the placenta and infect the fetus. Listeria monocytogenes causes suppression of fetal bone marrow and leads to severe fetal anaemia that causes the classical picture of hydrops fetalis. The knowledge of how to diagnose and treat hydrops fetalis is clearly not part of the DRCOG syllabus. However, the core knowledge being tested is the risk that listeria poses to the pregnant woman and the dietary advice given to all pregnant women to avoid unpasteurised foods.

3.47 A primigravid woman presents at 34 weeks of gestation with a history of feeling increasingly unwell, rigours, and right-upper-quadrant pain. On examination she is flushed, has a tachycardia of 100 bpm, and has a temperature of 38°C. She is tender in the right renal angle.

C Escherichia coli

This should be a familiar clinical example; the woman clearly has a urinary tract infection and the high pyrexia suggests pyelonephritis. You know that E. coli is the commonest cause of UTI in women. It is tempting to think that the answer is too obvious and look for complexity where there is none, so-called overthinking the question. Not all questions will have complex answers; pyelonephritis is a risk for premature labour and, therefore, this is important core knowledge to be tested.

3.48 A 17-year-old woman presents at 30 weeks of gestation in her first pregnancy with a history of recurrent postcoital bleeding. Her booking scan at 20 weeks showed a normally sited placenta. Speculum examination reveals a florid ectropion with contact bleeding on taking swabs.

B Chlamydia trachomatis

There are two possible answers to this question, Chlamydia trachomatis and Gonococcus. Both may cause postcoital bleeding (PCB) but Chlamydia is significantly more common, especially in younger women. Candida albicans causes vaginal irritation and discharge but rarely causes PCB. The fact that the scenario makes no mention of any symptoms other than PCB should allow you to discount Candida as the correct answer.

3.49 In antenatal clinic at 17 weeks of gestation a primigravid woman complains of vaginal discharge and soreness. On speculum examination there is a thick, white discharge adherent to the vaginal walls.

A   Candida albicans

The nature of the discharge and the symptoms suggest thrush infection, which is exceedingly common in pregnancy.

3.50 A 28-year-old primary school teacher is pregnant for the first time. Several children in her class have 'slapped cheek syndrome' at the start of term and when she comes to hospital for her routine anomaly scan her baby is found to be hydropic.

H   Parvovirus B19

Children with slapped cheek syndrome due to parvovirus do not feel ill and are therefore sent to school where the parvovirus poses a risk to the pregnancy. It causes fetal anaemia, which is why the baby looks hydropic on the scan – high output cardiac failure.

Curriculum Module 4

Answers

Single Best Answer Questions

4.1 In antenatal clinic a woman who was delivered by caesarean section in her last pregnancy is discussing the prospect of vaginal birth after caesarean section (VBAC) for her current pregnancy.

In the last pregnancy she had a very slow first stage of labour and got stuck at 9 cm dilatation. The baby was in the occipito-posterior (OP) position but there was no evidence of cephalo-pelvic disproportion.

What is her chance of achieving a vaginal birth this time?

A.   30 per cent
B.   40 per cent
C.   50 per cent
D.   60 per cent
E.   *70 per cent

The chances of a successful VBAC vary according to the reasons for the caesarean last time and depending on how many centimetres dilatation the cervix reached during the previous labour, but a figure of 70 per cent overall is generally quoted to patients.

The RCOG Green-top Guideline states 'Women considering their options for birth after a single previous caesarean should be informed that, overall, the chances of successful planned VBAC are 72–76%'.

Source: RCOG Green-top Guideline, No. 45, 'Birth after Previous Caesarean Birth'. Published 2015.

4.2 A woman who is considering a VBAC is discussing her birth plan with her community midwife.

Which of these factors increases the chances of rupture of the uterine scar during labour?

A.   Fetal distress in the previous labour
B.   Having a water birth in this labour
C.   Maternal BMI >30
D.   Onset of spontaneous labour after the due date in this pregnancy
E.   *Previous labour complicated by chorioamnionitis

Water birth does not compromise the scar, but one of the signs of scar rupture is fetal distress, and it is recommended that patients undergoing VBAC should have continuous fetal monitoring as well as IV access. It is also difficult to assess maternal condition in terms of scar tenderness if she is in a birthing pool.

High BMI compromises the chances of a successful VBAC, but this is due to poor contractility of the uterus rather than increased risk of scar rupture.

The risk of uterine rupture is increased if the previous section was complicated by infection because it compromises the healing of the uterine scar. There is limited evidence from a case-control study that women who experienced both intrapartum and postpartum fever in their prior caesarean birth were at increased risk of uterine rupture in their subsequent planned VBAC labour (OR 4.02, 95 per cent CI 1.04–15.5).

Source: RCOG Green-top Guideline, No. 45, 'Birth after Previous Caesarean Birth'. Published 2015.

4.3 Which of the following obstetric conditions or situations predisposes to cord prolapse during labour?

A. ***Breech presentation**

B. Maternal diabetes

C. Oligohydramnios

D. Placenta praevia

E. Waterbirth

Cord prolapse is an obstetric emergency necessitating immediate delivery and is more likely where the presenting part is either not in the pelvis (e.g., with a transverse lie) or does not fit it well (e.g., with a high head that is 5/5 palpable or a breech presentation as the breech may be smaller than the head especially before 37 weeks).

4.4 Induction of labour is clinically indicated in which of the following conditions?

A. Maternal urinary tract infection

B. Pathological CTG tracing

C. ***Pregnancy-induced hypertension**

D. Symphysis pubis dysfunction

E. Undiagnosed antepartum haemorrhage

Urinary tract infection is not an indication for induction, and active infection in the pelvis during labour may increase the chances of septic complications.

A pathological CTG tracing usually indicates the need for immediate delivery (or fetal blood sampling, which is not likely to be possible if labour has not yet started).

There is no evidence that inducing labour is beneficial to patients with symphysis pubis dysfunction although they usually request induction (or even caesarean).

Although antepartum haemorrhage is an indication for induction of labour it is important to exclude placenta praevia before planning induction.

4.5 Which of the following is a contraindication to a home delivery?

A. A woman with a BMI of 37 who has had two normal births before

B. ***Grand multiparity**

C. Poor rapport with community midwife

D. Spontaneous labour occurring 10 days postdates

E. Second labour after previous forceps delivery

Women with a significantly raised BMI, that is, over 35, should be advised against home birth due to increased risk of complications such as shoulder dystocia. Although this woman's BMI is raised she could opt for home birth if she wishes in accordance with national guidance. Although it is not ideal for a woman who did not manage a normal delivery last time or does not get on well with her midwife to plan a home birth she is still likely to be able to deliver without medical intervention.

A grand multip is more likely to have a postpartum haemorrhage and therefore should be advised to plan delivery in a consultant-led unit.

4.6 **Which of the following pregnant women should be counselled against planning to labour in a birthing pool in hospital?**

A. A primigravid woman whose baby is in the occipito-posterior position at the start of labour

B. A multiparous woman whose pregnancy is complicated by mild rhesus disease

C. ***A woman with a BMI of 45 and an otherwise uncomplicated pregnancy**

D. A woman with an otherwise uncomplicated pregnancy who has had a successful external cephalic version

E. A woman with an uncomplicated postmature pregnancy

Most babies in the OP position will rotate during labour although the labour is often prolonged (which will result in the use of oxytocin out of the pool).

The woman with a high BMI should not plan to deliver in the pool because if there is a problem such as maternal collapse or shoulder dystocia the midwife may not be able to get her out of the pool quickly enough.

The main issue for the rhesus disease mother is going to be the baby's haemoglobin and bilirubin levels, and as long as the midwife can obtain blood samples from the cord after delivery, labouring in the birthing pool should be safe.

If an ECV is successful the pregnant woman can be treated the same as any other mother with a cephalic presentation.

4.7 **An obese woman has just received a spinal anaesthetic for a forceps delivery in theatre and her legs have been raised in the obstetric stirrups. She complains of feeling short of breath and a heavy feeling in both her arms.**

What is the most likely cause of her symptoms?

A. Amniotic fluid embolism

B. Hypotension

C. Hyperventilation

D. Myocardial infarction

E. ***Rising spinal block**

This combination of symptoms raises the possibility that the local anaesthetic is rising up the cerebrospinal fluid in the subdural space and paralysing the intercostal muscles. The anaesthetist will check the level of the block and get ready to intubate her should the spinal rise any higher.

4.8 Which of these obstetric complications is a recognised indication for assisted vaginal delivery (shortening the second stage of labour with forceps or ventouse)?

A. Macrosomia

B. *Maternal cardiac disease

C. Maternal hypotension

D. Prematurity

E. Previous third-degree tear

Mothers who are pushing actively are performing the Valsalva manoeuvre frequently, which is probably not a good idea if she has cardiac problems. Instrumental delivery is associated with an increased risk of third-degree tear so should only be used if there is failure to progress or fetal compromise in women with a previous third-degree tear.

4.9 A previously fit woman is in labour at 36 weeks' gestation and her temperature is noted to be 39°C. The CTG indicates that the baby is becoming distressed and the registrar on call wishes to perform a caesarean section, suspecting chorioamnionitis.

The woman refuses to give consent for the operation and the midwife looking after her thinks that she may be confused on account of her high temperature.

Select the best course of action in this situation:

A. Ask her husband to sign the consent form

B. *Assess her capacity to understand and process clinical information

C. Get a court order to force her to have the caesarean

D. Proceed without consent in the baby's best interests

E. Use the Mental Health Act to justify proceeding with caesarean delivery

If the woman is judged to have capacity to process information and make sound decisions, you cannot force her to have a caesarean even if her baby dies as a result.

The baby has no rights in law until it is born and the interests of the mother take precedence.

4.10 An obstetric anaesthetist will be unwilling to site an epidural until they have seen a recent normal platelet count and clotting screen for a woman whose pregnancy is complicated by:

A. Induction of labour

B. *Intrauterine fetal death

C. Maternal diabetes

D. Previous caesarean section

E. Twin pregnancy

IUFD puts the patient at risk of disseminated intravascular coagulation. If an epidural is inserted in the presence of this condition, there is an increased risk of a haematoma in the restricted space within the spinal canal which could lead to paralysis.

4.11 An ambulance is summoned by a community midwife who is conducting a home delivery for a multiparous woman who has had two normal deliveries before. Halfway through the first stage of labour the patient has become increasingly distressed and is complaining of severe abdominal pain.

The pain continues between contractions, which are occurring every 3 minutes and the midwife has noticed that the uterus is tender and hard on palpation.

Which of the following is the most likely complication?

A.   Chorioamnionitis
B.   *Concealed placental abruption
C.   Obstructed labour
D.   Hyperstimulated labour
E.   Uterine rupture

Fresh vaginal bleeding is suggestive of abruption or uterine rupture. Rupture is uncommon – unless oxytocin (or prostaglandins) are being used to stimulate contractions – but if the uterus ruptures the contractions usually cease.

4.12 You are in a labour room trying to cope with a severe postpartum haemorrhage whilst waiting for the registrar to arrive. The inexperienced student midwife hands you a selection of drugs to choose from to try and stop the uterine bleeding. Which of these drugs has she picked up in error?

A.   *Atosiban
B.   Carboprost
C.   Ergometrine
D.   Misoprostol
E.   Oxytocin

Atosiban is used to stop contractions in the management of preterm labour.

4.13 A woman books for antenatal care in her fourth pregnancy. Her obstetric history includes three previous deliveries by caesarean section. She is predisposed to which obstetric complication?

A.   Cord prolapse
B.   Haemorrhage
C.   *Placenta accreta
D.   Pre-eclampsia
E.   Unstable lie

The risk of placenta praevia increases with increasing number of sections and the chance of that low-lying placenta invading the myometrium and becoming accreta increases markedly with each subsequent caesarean. This is one of the main reasons for trying to keep the caesarean section rate down.

4.14 The most important reason that administration of ergometrine to control postpartum haemorrhage is contraindicated in a woman with pre-eclampsia is:

A.   It is likely to make her vomit profusely
B.   It does not work as well as oxytocin
C.   It gives a sustained effect rather than a quick onset of action
D.   *It is likely to increase her blood pressure
E.   It could decrease her intracranial pressure

Ergometrine does make patients vomit and has a sustained effect but the main reason for not giving it to pre-eclamptic patients is the potential effect on blood pressure. Several patients – whose stories are described in the triennial maternal mortality reports – died because their blood pressure was significantly raised by third-stage administration of syntometrine, and they subsequently died from massive intracranial bleeding.

4.15 As a junior doctor on the labour ward, it often feels as though you are being asked to insert an intravenous line on every woman in labour. Which of the following pregnant women does not need a cannula when she is admitted?

A.   A woman with an uncomplicated pregnancy delivering her sixth baby

B.   A primigravid woman whose haemoglobin was 95 g/l 2 weeks ago

C.   A woman who had a postpartum haemorrhage in her last delivery

D.   ***A woman who had a forceps delivery for fetal distress in her previous pregnancy**

E.   A woman who had an emergency caesarean for fetal distress in her last pregnancy

The issue here is which of these women is likely to have a PPH, need a blood transfusion, or end up in theatre for an emergency section. For any of these reasons, she could need a cannula and a 'group and save' blood test doing when she is labouring. The only woman on the preceding list who is not in this situation is the woman who needed a forceps delivery last time. She is likely to have a normal delivery with no complications this time.

4.16 Having had a massive postpartum haemorrhage following the delivery of her first baby a 34-year-old woman has received 8 units of blood, 2 units of cryoprecipitate, and fresh frozen plasma during the previous couple of hours. She has developed pulmonary oedema with an oxygen saturation of 55 per cent.

Currently her temperature is 37.5, pulse is 110 bpm, blood pressure 90/40 mmHg, and urine output is reduced to only 5 mls per hour.

The clotting screen is normal and her haemoglobin is currently 95 g/l.

What is likely to be the cause of this clinical situation?

A.   ***Adult respiratory distress syndrome**

B.   Bacterial contamination of the blood transfused

C.   Blood-borne viral infection

D.   Delayed transfusion reaction

E.   Inadequate transfusion

The pulmonary oedema with a low oxygen saturation is the key to this diagnosis, although the some of the clinical information given would also fit sepsis.

4.17 You are looking after a woman in labour who has had two fetal blood samples done already because of an abnormal CTG trace, the results of which are normal so far. The obstetric anaesthetist is keen for her to have an epidural inserted thereby avoiding a general anaesthetic if emergency delivery becomes necessary later. The most important reason for avoiding GA in labour is:

A.   General anaesthetic in an emergency takes longer than topping up an epidural

B.   Epidural can lower her blood pressure and improve placental perfusion

C. The mother does not have to be kept 'nil by mouth' in labour

D. *** The mother is at risk of Mendelssohn's syndrome (aspiration pneumonitis)**

E. Ventouse delivery is more difficult under GA because the mother cannot push

The effect of progesterone is to relax smooth muscle therefore the lower oesophageal sphincter is relaxed in pregnancy and there is reduced gastric emptying. This leads to a high chance of a pregnant woman aspirating during induction of anaesthesia and developing pneumonitis. Before the widespread use of regional anaesthesia by trained obstetric anaesthetists, this was a common cause of maternal death.

It is true that ventouse delivery is more difficult under GA but this is not as important as avoiding maternal death. Epidural may lower her blood pressure but this will reduce rather than improve placental perfusion, so it is important to make sure that the baby is not hypoxic before she has her epidural.

4.18 When performing a fetal blood sample in the first stage of labour it is preferable to place the mother in the left lateral position for which the following reason:

The midwife is more easily able to support the mother's legs

A. Necessary equipment for the procedure can be placed on the bed within reach

B. ***Placental perfusion is improved by relieving pressure on maternal vena cava**

C. The baby may be lying on the placenta thereby compressing the umbilical cord

D. The cervical os is easier to access with the amnioscope

E. The midwife is more easily able to support the mother's legs

The main reason is to improve placental perfusion by preventing the weight of the gravid uterus compressing the inferior vena cava thereby reduced venous return. It has nothing to do with the comfort of the midwife or obstetrician.

4.19 Whilst on labour ward you notice a commotion in one of the delivery rooms and hear someone shouting for help with shoulder dystocia.

Which of the following procedures may help the birth attendants deliver the baby in this life-threatening situation?

Delivering the anterior arm of the baby

A. Delivering the anterior arm of the baby

B. Fundal pressure on the uterus

C. Lovsett's manoeuvre

D. Mauriceau-Smellie-Veit manoeuvre

E. ***McRobert's manoeuvre to hyperflex the maternal hips**

Hyperflexion of the maternal hips changes the incline of her pelvis and makes more room for the impacted shoulder stuck behind the symphysis pubis to enter the pelvis.

If you want to relieve the situation by delivering an arm, it is the posterior arm that may be accessible as the anterior one is stuck in the abdomen. Mauriceau-Smellie-Veit and Lovsett's manoeuvres are for delivering a breech baby. We do not do fundal pressure because of the risk of rupturing the uterus (although this is done in some Third World countries), but suprapubic pressure would help especially if it was applied behind the baby's anterior shoulder.

4.20 A primigravid woman has been in labour for nearly 20 hours and actively pushing for 90 minutes so a decision is made to perform an assisted vaginal delivery on account of delay in the second stage.

The woman is at increased risk of which complication?

A. Cervical dystocia
B. Fetal distress
C. Inverted uterus
D. Paravaginal haematoma
E. ***Postpartum haemorrhage**

The uterus does not contract so well after delivery when labour is prolonged and she is at increased risk of PPH due to uterine atony. This risk is increased if there is an element of infection that may be the case after prolonged labour.

Extended Matching Questions

A	Amniotomy
B	Elective caesarean section
C	Electronic fetal monitoring
D	Emergency caesarean section
E	Intermittent auscultation
F	Request a clotting screen
G	Routine elective episiotomy
H	Titrated synthetic Oxytocin infusion
I	Vaginal examination in theatre with the operating team standing by
J	Ventouse delivery

The following clinical scenarios apply to women delivering in a hospital obstetric unit. In each case, select the most appropriate management plan.

Each option may be used once, more than once, or not at all.

4.21 A primigravid 32-year-old woman presents early in the first stage of spontaneous labour at 38 weeks of gestation, contracting once every 10 minutes. Her membranes have just ruptured spontaneously and fresh meconium is seen in the liquor.

C Electronic fetal monitoring

Meconium in the liquor becomes more likely as gestation advances, especially in postmature babies. It is, however, sometimes a sign of hypoxia especially if the pregnancy has not reached term, so in any labour where meconium is noted it is imperative to commence electronic fetal monitoring to look for other signs of hypoxia.

4.22 During vaginal examination in a woman's third labour, the midwife finds the cervix to be 8 cm dilated and feels a pulsatile cord alongside the fetal head. The head is below the ischial spines and in the OA position.

D Emergency caesarean section

This is a cord prolapse, so delivery of the baby must be expedited. As the cervix is not fully dilated the delivery must be by emergency caesarean section, with a birth attendant lifting the presenting part off the cord until the operator can get the baby out.

4.23 A primigravid woman had an uncomplicated pregnancy so far under mid-wifery care and presents with a heavy vaginal bleed at 39 weeks of gesta-tion. The uterus is nontender and the baby is well grown with a cephalic presentation, four-fifths palpable. The condition of both mother and baby is stable, but she is contracting strongly every 3 minutes and the blood continues to trickle from the vagina.

I Vaginal examination in theatre with the operating team standing by

The baby's head should be engaged after 37 weeks in a primiparous woman, so that the fact that it is four-fifths palpable makes you wonder why and in this situation in which there is vaginal bleeding a low-lying placenta is likely. An alternative would be to arrange an USS but it is not on the option list, and because it sounds as if she is in labour, vaginal examination is more appropriate as an initial plan.

4.24 Having been admitted to labour ward 4 hours previously experiencing three contractions every 10 minutes, a low-risk primigravid patient is examined and her cervix is found to be 6 cm dilated with intact membranes. She mobilises in her labour room using nitrous oxide for analgesia and 4 hours later the cervix is 7c m dilated.

A Amniotomy

This is primary dysfunctional labour and is common in primigravid women. Although you might choose the oxytocin infusion from the list, this works better if the membranes have been ruptured, so amniotomy is the first thing to do here. There is also a theoretical risk of amniotic fluid embolism if oxytocin is used to augment labour with intact membranes.

4.25 A midwife calls you in to a delivery room because of a small vaginal bleed in a low-risk primigravid woman whose labour has been progressing nor-mally. The midwife is auscultating the baby's heartbeat, which has been 70 bpm for 5 minutes. The mother's pulse is 90, her blood pressure is stable, and the cervix is 8 cm dilated.

D Emergency caesarean section

This is likely to be a placental abruption, so cross-matching blood and getting a clotting screen done are both reasonable options. However, the baby is bradycardic so the overwhelming urgency is to deliver the baby quickly to avoid brain damage, and therefore emergency caesarean section is the most appropriate option.

A	Arrange emergency caesarean section
B	Check airway and administer oxygen by facial mask
C	Check plasma glucose level
D	Commence electronic fetal monitoring
E	Contact the consultant haematologist on call
F	Cross-match blood
G	Counsel about postpartum sterilisation
H	Perform a vaginal examination
I	Rapid IV administration of 1 litre crystalloid
J	Request urgent USS
K	Site IV cannula and check haemoglobin

These clinical scenarios relate to an emergency situation involving a woman on the labour ward in the third trimester of pregnancy. In each case, choose the most appropriate initial management plan.

Each option may be used once, more than once, or not at all.

4.26 A 28-year-old woman with type 1 diabetes attends triage on labour ward early one morning at 30 weeks of gestation because of an antepartum haemorrhage. She collapses in the waiting room and when you attend to sort out the situation she appears confused and is asking where she is.

C Check plasma glucose level

When someone collapses our immediate response is Airway, Breathing, Circulation *(ABC); however this patient is talking therefore ABC is unnecessary. In a diabetic the most likely problem is hypoglycaemia, so her blood sugar would be the first thing to do.*

4.27 A 34-year-old woman is admitted to delivery suite at term in her eighth pregnancy. She has delivered six live children previously. On examination the cervix is 7 cm dilated and she is involuntarily pushing.

K Site IV cannula and check haemoglobin

The main risk for this 'grand multip' is postpartum haemorrhage so you need to be prepared for that. It is unlikely that you will need to cross-match blood unless she has become anaemic – but the PPH risk will have been identified as a risk factor antenatally so this should not have happened. Discussion of sterilisation does not seem appropriate when delivery is imminent!

4.28 The labour ward is very busy when a young primigravid woman is admitted at 38 weeks of gestation with contractions. Earlier, in antenatal clinic she was found to have a breech presentation confirmed by scan and is awaiting a consultant outpatient appointment arranged for tomorrow. On admission she experiences spontaneous rupture of membranes and the cervix is found to be 6 cm dilated.

A Arrange emergency caesarean section

The 'Term Breech' trial showed that babies with breech presentation do better if delivered by caesarean section. Now she has ruptured her membranes and is in labour, we must proceed with delivery.

4.29 A woman who has just delivered twins collapses in the delivery room at the end of the second stage. The placenta is still in situ and the midwife tells you that she has just noticed a large amount of blood in the bed. The patient is unresponsive and has a tachycardia of 120 bpm.

B Check airway and administer oxygen by facial mask

Although you are clearly dealing with a massive postpartum haemorrhage and there are several relevant things on the list that must be done urgently, an obstructed airway will kill her before you have had chance to do any of them. The airway always takes priority. There are other disastrous conditions that could result in the same clinical picture such as an amniotic fluid embolism.

4.30 Having been admitted with a fresh antepartum haemorrhage, a primiparous patient is diagnosed with a placental abruption at 34 weeks of gestation. Both mother and baby are stable at the moment, but the haematology technician has just contacted you to say that the clotting screen you sent to the lab an hour ago is not normal.

E Contact the consultant haematologist on call

Placental abruption can cause disseminated intravascular coagulation and if she is developing this severe complication, you will need the urgent help of the consultant haematologist to decide on the appropriate clotting factors to deal with the clotting abnormality.

A	Cryoprecipitate
B	Iron infusion
C	Iron injections weekly
D	Oral iron
E	Platelet transfusion
F	Recombinant Factor VIIa
G	Transfuse 'O negative' blood
H	Transfuse type-specific blood
I	Transfuse cross-matched blood
J	Transfuse blood from cell saver

Each of these clinical scenarios describes a pregnant woman whose clinical condition is or could be compromised by haemorrhage; for each patient pick the best management option given the information that you are presented with.

Each option may be used once, more than once, or not at all.

4.31 During a routine caesarean section under spinal anaesthetic the consultant you are assisting unexpectedly comes across a low-lying placenta and the woman loses 2,500 ml blood before the baby is delivered and the placenta is removed from the uterus. Her haemoglobin done the previous day is 105 g/l. Her blood pressure has dropped to 70/40 and she has become unresponsive to questions.

G Transfuse 'O negative' blood

This woman is in hypovolaemic shock and needs the 'O negative' blood stored on every labour ward. Unless you were expecting placenta praevia, there will only be a 'group and save' in the lab for this woman. The maternal mortality reports often criticise management of severe haemorrhage as 'too little, too late'.

4.32 A primigravid woman has a blood test at 36 weeks of gestation and is found to have a haemoglobin level of 69 gm/l. She has not been taking the iron tablets prescribed by her GP because of severe nausea, and has tried three different preparations.

B Iron infusion

There is still enough time for her to increase her haemoglobin to reasonable levels before labour if she can get her iron stores replenished. If she can't tolerate oral iron, it must be parenteral and oral iron will only increase her haemoglobin at about 1 gm per month anyway. There is an increased risk of skin discolouration and pain at the injection site with intramuscular iron. This needs to be balanced with the risk of anaphylaxis and a possible increased risk in venous thrombosis with intravenous iron dextran. Intramuscular iron requires a test dose and a Z track technique of injection so for the majority of women IV iron is preferred according to the British Committee for Standards in Haematology.

www.transfusionguidelines.org

4.33 A 31-year-old primigravid woman is known to have β thalassaemia and has a haemoglobin level of 80 g/l by the time she reaches 38 weeks of gestation. She is symptomatic, feeling very tired, and slightly breathless.

I Transfuse cross-matched blood

It will not be long before this woman is in labour so transfusion should be considered even if she is not symptomatic. Anaemia related to haemoglobinopathy should be managed by blood transfusion with advice from a haematologist. Women with haemoglobinopathy may have a problem with iron overload.

Source: RCOG Green-top Guideline number 47, 'Blood Transfusions in Obstetrics' (2015).

4.34 You are the junior doctor on labour ward assisting the registrar dealing with a manual removal of placenta under general anaesthetic. During the last 15 minutes the woman started bleeding heavily and so far has lost 3 litres of blood. The consultant obstetrician has been called and the 2 units of blood stored on the labour ward have already been transfused. Her heart rate is 120 bpm and her blood pressure is 90/50 mmHg.

H Transfuse type-specific blood

The haematology laboratory will be able to supply type-specific blood in about 20 minutes but a full cross-match takes longer. She is becoming haemodynamically unstable and therefore type-specific blood should be transfused pending the fully cross-matched units.

4.35 A 35-year-old woman pregnant with twins attends antenatal clinic at 28 weeks of gestation for a growth scan. She has a routine blood test done and her haemoglobin is 90 g/L.

D Oral iron

There is plenty of time for this woman to increase her haemoglobin with oral iron and you don't need to worry about parenteral iron (even though twins often arrive early and there is a chance she might go into labour anytime).

A	Attempt to turn the baby (version) for vaginal delivery
B	Arrange an emergency caesarean section
C	Arrange an elective caesarean section
D	Ask the anaesthetist to site an epidural
E	Conduct an assisted vaginal delivery with ventouse or forceps
F	Conduct a breech extraction
G	Obtain a fetal blood sample from the scalp
H	Obtain a fetal blood sample from the cord
I	Obtain maternal serum for cross-matching blood
J	Obtain maternal serum for a clotting screen
K	Perform a vaginal examination to exclude cord prolapse
L	Put up a syntocinon drip to increase the contractions
M	Rupture the membranes with an amnihook

As the junior doctor on the labour ward you have been called to assist the midwives with the management of labouring women experiencing a complication.

In each scenario, choose the most appropriate immediate action that you think the obstetric team (not necessarily you personally) should take.

Each option may be used once, more than once, or not at all.

4.36 One hour after administration of a prostaglandin pessary to induce labour for postmaturity, a primigravid woman is found to be having more than six contractions in 10 minutes. You are asked to site an intravenous cannula whilst the midwife removes the pessary. Although the contractions lessen in frequency to 3 in 10 the baby becomes bradycardic and you can hear that the fetal heart rate has been running at 90 bpm for 4 minutes so far.

B Arrange an emergency caesarean section

The prostaglandin pessary has caused hyperstimulation of the uterus. If it does not resolve on removing the pessary, you could give her a drug such as Terbutaline to relax the uterus, however this option isn't in the list.

As there is a persistent bradycardia, this baby must be delivered with all haste to avoid possible cerebral palsy. The confounding option is to check for cord prolapse as a possible cause of the bradycardia, but because the membranes are intact this would be termed a cord presentation, and therefore the most likely cause of the bradycardia is uterine hyperstimulation. The practicalities are that you only have a few minutes to save the baby hence the correct option is caesarean section.

4.37 A 21-year-old primigravid woman was admitted in spontaneous labour 6 hours previously when the cervix was 7 cm dilated and has been relaxing in the birthing pool, coping without formal analgesia. The liquor is clear and intermittent auscultation of the fetal heart is reassuring. The cervix is now 8 cm dilated and the baby appears to be lying in the OP position.

L Put up a syntocinon drip to increase the contractions

This woman has primary dysfunctional labour with delay in the first stage due to malposition of the fetal head, with ruptured membranes. There are no concerns about the condition of the baby and the problem should respond to oxytocin.

4.38 A multiparous woman has delivered her first twin vaginally 15 minutes ago, and there is no sign of the second twin appearing although the contractions are continuing every 2 minutes. On examination it is apparent that the second twin is lying transversely in the uterus.

A Attempt to turn the baby (version) for vaginal delivery

We often use a syntocinon drip in between the delivery of the first and second twin to ensure that contractions continue. However the second twin is lying transversely and the options are caesarean section or that a version must be performed to convert to a longitudinal lie. As she is multiparous, the second option is quicker and safer than a second-stage caesarean section and, therefore external version is the correct answer even though some obstetric trainees do not have the practical skill or experience to perform version.

4.39 A rather frightened 17-year-old primigravid woman is in spontaneous labour and the cervix is 6 cm dilated. The midwife has noted meconium in the liquor and there are late decelerations on the CTG. The woman has asked for more analgesia and the midwife says that she is becoming more and more uncooperative.

G Obtain a fetal blood sample from the scalp

You might be thinking that this woman needs an epidural but before that is offered, there is a need to address the suspected fetal distress by performing a fetal blood sample. An epidural may drop her blood pressure resulting in reduced placental perfusion and worsening the situation for the fetus. Likewise, if the baby is already acidotic an emergency caesarean may be indicated so the prime imperative is to establish fetal well-being with a fetal blood sample.

4.40 A multiparous woman who has had three previous uncomplicated vaginal births is admitted in advanced labour at term and to everyone's surprise the presentation of the baby is found to be breech, station at the ischial spines, and the cervix 9 cm dilated. The membranes rupture just after the vaginal examination and the liquor is clear. The midwife commences a CTG trace that shows occasional early decelerations.

K Perform a vaginal examination to exclude cord prolapse

The first stage of labour is progressing well and she is nearly ready for second stage, so a vaginal breech delivery is likely. However, the cause of the early decelerations should be considered – it cannot be head compression because the presentation is breech. Cord prolapse is more common with breech presentation so this obstetric emergency must be excluded before anything else is done. If there is a clinical suspicion of fetal distress, then caesarean section may well be the next course of action as fetal blood samples cannot be taken from the breech.

A	Abruption of the placenta
B	Cervical laceration
C	Disseminated intravascular coagulation
D	Placenta accreta
E	Placenta praevia
F	Retained succenturiate lobe of placenta
G	Rupture of the uterus
H	Uterine atony
I	Vasa praevia
J	Velamentous insertion of the cord

Given the clinical information provided, select the most likely diagnosis for each of these obstetric patients experiencing vaginal bleeding.

Each option may be used once, more than once, or not at all.

4.41 A woman has just delivered her first baby and whilst the midwife is inspecting the placenta she has a brisk vaginal bleed of about 600 ml. Maternal observations are stable and the uterus feels well contracted. The midwife points out to you that there are blood vessels running through the membranes.

F Retained succenturiate lobe of placenta

This situation sounds like a velamentous insertion of the cord where the vessels are attached to the membranes instead of being inserted directly into the placenta. However, if the vessels are running off the edge of the membranes, they must be carrying blood to something, which suggests an extra lobe of placenta. If it is left in the uterus, it will cause haemorrhage and/or infection and must be retrieved.

Uterine atony is the confounding option but those blood vessels are the key to this answer.

4.42 A primigravid woman aged 21 presents to labour ward at 39 weeks of gestation because of a brisk painless vaginal bleed of about 100 ml following intercourse. The uterus is nontender with a transverse fetal lie. The fetal heart is steady at 140 bpm.

E Placenta praevia

The fact that the baby is lying transversely at 39 weeks in a primigravid woman is a clue to the possibility that the placenta is in the way. Also the bleeding is painless, which suggests praevia, as placental abruption is usually associated with pain.

4.43 You are called to see a primigravid woman who has started bleeding halfway through the first stage of labour, losing 200 ml in a couple of minutes. Despite her epidural she seems to be in a great deal of pain and there are unmistakeable signs of severe fetal distress on the CTG.

A Abruption of the placenta

It is very rare for a primigravid patient to have a ruptured uterus and the only other cause of pain on this list is abruption. Both would cause an abnormal CTG. Ruptured uterus is usually associated with a uterine scar such as previous caesarean section or myomectomy. The unscarred uterus can rupture in multiparous women with obstructed labour particularly with syntocinon use, but again this is very rare in the United Kingdom.

4.44 During her second labour a 35-year-old woman starts to lose fresh blood per vaginam. Her first baby was delivered by caesarean section because of fetal distress related to chorioamnionitis at 6 cm dilatation in the first stage. This time the cervix has reached 7 cm dilatation but the contractions have stopped.

G Rupture of the uterus

Cessation of contractions is an ominous sign that suggests rupture of the uterus especially in a woman who is labouring with a previous section scar. Other features of scar rupture are bleeding, as in this case, pain continuing between contractions, CTG abnormalities, a sudden change in the presentation as the baby is expelled from the uterus into the abdominal cavity, or even fetal death.

4.45 The midwife looking after a primigravid woman in labour at term ruptured the membranes 5 minutes ago with an amnihook to speed up the progress of the first stage of labour, as cervical dilatation has been stuck at 5 cm for the last 4 hours. You are called because the midwife is concerned that the liquor is very heavily bloodstained. The uterus is nontender, contracting 4 in 10 minutes and the fetal heart rate has risen from a baseline of 120 before amniotomy to 180 bpm with late decelerations.

I Vasa praevia

Your first thought might be that the midwife has lacerated the cervix with the amnihook and that is where the bleeding is coming from. However there are ominous signs of the CTG that suggest that the baby is in trouble and the tachycardia may be occurring because of acute fetal blood loss. This is a very rare situation but there are only minutes to save the baby's life before it exsanguinates and suspected vasa praevia should be mentioned to the resuscitating paediatrician as they should give blood to the baby early on or resuscitation may be unsuccessful.

A	Administer oral benzylpenicillin
B	High vaginal swab on admission
C	Induction of labour and intrapartum IV benzylpenicillin
D	Prescribe intrapartum IV benzylpenicillin
E	Prescribe intrapartum IV erythromycin
F	Prescribe intrapartum IV clindamycin
G	Prescribe intrapartum IV metronidazole
H	Reassure the patient that no action is necessary
I	Vaginal cleansing with chlorhexidine on admission in labour

Each of these pregnant women has been found to be carrying group B streptococcus on vaginal swabs at some stage in this or a previous pregnancy. For each patient select the most appropriate management plan to prevent early-onset neonatal group B streptococcal disease.

Each option may be used once, more than once, or not at all.

4.46 A primigravid woman has been admitted to labour ward for elective caesarean delivery for persistent breech presentation. She had a swab taken last week by her GP that has grown group B streptococcus.

H Reassure the patient that no action is necessary

This is an elective caesarean and you should assume that there are intact membranes therefore the guidance given in the Green-top Guideline is that antibiotic treatment is unnecessary for the prevention of early onset neonatal group B streptococcal (GBS) disease.

4.47 A woman is admitted in established labour at term. An MSU done 2 weeks ago when she had abdominal pain grew group B streptococcus.

D Prescribe intrapartum IV benzylpenicillin

The background risk of neonatal early onset GBS disease is 0.5/1000 births. The risk rises to 2.3/1000 births if GBS is detected in the current pregnancy and its presence in the urine means that there is heavy colonisation leading to a significantly increased risk. This justifies antibiotic treatment in labour and benzylpenicillin is the first line drug of choice. The intravenous route is preferred due to variable absorption of oral antibiotics during labour.

4.48 At 37 weeks of gestation a multiparous woman is admitted with prelabour rupture of the membranes. She was found to have group B streptococcus on a high vaginal swab done a few weeks previously when she was seen in another maternity unit in Skegness on holiday.

C Induction of labour and intrapartum IV benzylpenicillin

Routine care would be to offer induction of labour 24 hours after prolonged rupture of the membranes (PROM); however, the risk of ascending GBS infection in colonised women with PROM justifies immediate induction with IV antibiotic cover. The aim is to ensure that the first dose of IV antibiotics is given at least 2 hours prior to delivery. IV antibiotics should be continued every 4 hours through-out labour until delivery. If the delivery takes place within 2 hours of the first dose of antibiotics, then the baby needs IV treatment instead.

4.49 A woman presents in spontaneous labour at term with her second baby. In her previous pregnancy she had a swab done in the first trimester that grew group B streptococcus; then she delivered at term and the baby was fine. She has not had any swabs done in this pregnancy.

H Reassure the patient that no action is necessary

If GBS was detected in a previous pregnancy the chance of the woman being colonised in this pregnancy rises from the background incidence of 21 per cent to around 38 per cent. However, the risk of early onset neonatal GBS only rises from 0.5/1000 to 0.9/1000 births and therefore the guidance is to only offer antibiotics to women with a previously affected child.

4.50 A woman is admitted in established labour at 38 weeks with ruptured membranes. Her previous baby developed meningitis after delivery that was subsequently found to be due to group B streptococcus. Following that delivery, she developed a rash when she was given penicillin in the puerperium to prevent her developing endometritis.

F Prescribe intrapartum IV clindamycin

We frequently meet patients claiming to have a penicillin allergy when in fact they had a gastrointestinal upset or a Candida infection following treatment, however a clear description of a rash should be taken seriously and the guideline recommends clindamycin as an alternative to benzylpenicillin for women colonised by GBS.

Source: RCOG Green-top Guideline, No. 36, 'The Prevention of Early Onset Neonatal Group B Streptococcal Disease'. Published 2012.

This guideline was introduced following a Cochrane review and discussion by the UK National Screening Committee, as it is routine practice to screen for group B streptococcal colonisation in the United States. The review concluded that it was not necessary to copy the United States in this regard, but that women who are at higher risk of colonisation should be offered IV penicillin in labour (clindamycin if they are allergic to penicillin).

Curriculum Module 5

Answers

Single Best Answer Questions

5.1 A woman who delivered her first baby 2 days ago is having problems breast-feeding on account of sore nipples. She is considering bottle feeding instead and the midwife asks you see her on a home visit.

Which of the following statements is correct advice regarding breast-feeding in her situation?

A. She could give the baby a bottle as well as breast-feeding
B. *She should continue to breast-feed to avoid milk stasis
C. She should stop breast-feeding until the soreness has resolved
D. She will need antibiotics to continue breast-feeding
E. Sore nipples mean that she is already developing mastitis

The organisms that cause mastitis can enter through cracks or fissures in the nipples, but it is important to continue to empty the breast as mastitis is due to milk stasis with superimposed infection. Cracked nipples should be treated with lanolin ointment and breast-feeding continued to prevent mastitis.

5.2 A baby born to a mother who has used cocaine in pregnancy is at increased risk of which problem?

A. Hypoglycaemia
B. Jaundice
C. *Low birth weight
D. Nasal septum defect
E. Neonatal abstinence (withdrawal) syndrome

Cocaine use in pregnancy is a serious issue for the fetus, causing placental insufficiency and abruption. Recreational drug use is common amongst women of childbearing age and it is possible that they may consult their GP for advice when they find out they are pregnant.

Neonatal abstinence syndrome does not occur in babies exposed to cocaine alone in utero, although they may suffer withdrawal if the cocaine is taken in the context of other drugs of dependence, for example, heroin.

5.3 A woman who delivered her first baby 8 hours ago asks for an urgent home visit from her GP because she is in severe pain and cannot pass urine. She had a normal birth with no stitches and was sent home 6 hours postpartum, when it seemed that all was well. On examination the vulva looks swollen.

Which is the most likely diagnosis?

A. Acute attack of herpes
B. Anaphylactic reaction
C. ***Paravaginal haematoma**
D. Perineal abscess
E. Thrombosed vulval varicosities

Paravaginal haematomas usually develop slowly during the first couple of hours after delivery and are extremely painful. There may be a large amount of blood in the haematoma by the time it presents with vulval swelling as most of the haematoma is in the paravaginal space and may not be noticed unless you digitally examine the vagina.

Although acute herpes infection can cause retention of urine it would be unusual for it to present in the immediate postpartum period and signs of it would have been noticed in labour.

It is too early for an abscess to form.

A thrombosed varicosity is unlikely to cause retention of urine, although retention can sometimes happen just due to pain or after delivery. In the immediate postpartum period, midwives will catheterise a woman who has not passed urine by 6 hours after delivery.

5.4 **For babies born to obese women without diabetes mellitus, which of the following risks is increased?**

A. Hypoglycaemia
B. Jaundice
C. ***Macrosomia**
D. Polyhydramnios
E. Transient tachypnoea of the newborn

Macrosomia leads to issues like shoulder dystocia and birth trauma. Polyhydramnios occurs as a consequence of diabetes.

Source: CMACE/RCOG joint guideline, 'Management of Women with Obesity in Pregnancy' (2010).

5.5 **A woman who is HIV positive has just been delivered of her first baby by caesarean section.**

Which of these statements is correct advice regarding the care of the neonate?

A. Cord blood should be sent for viral load
B. ***She should be advised against breast-feeding the baby**
C. The baby should not have any invasive tests such as blood tests
D. The baby does not need antiretroviral therapy
E. The baby should be isolated from the mother until she has stopped bleeding

All neonates should receive antiretroviral therapy within 4 hours of birth, and HIV tests on the baby are performed at 1 day, 6 weeks, and 12 weeks of age.

A confirmatory HIV antibody test is performed at 18 months of age. If these tests are negative (and the baby is not being breast-fed) the parents can be informed that the baby is HIV negative. Breast-feeding doubles the risk of mother-to-child transmission.

Source: British HIV Association Guideline for the management of HIV infection in pregnant women. Published 2012, reviewed 2014. www.bhiva.org

5.6 You are asked to review a woman on the postnatal ward because the midwives suspect that she has had a pulmonary embolus 48 hours after an emergency caesarean section for slow progress in labour.

She complains of shortness of breath but no pleuritic chest pain. On examination her legs are of normal size and she is wearing antiembolism stockings.

Which of these statements is correct regarding her management?

A. Anticoagulation should be delayed as it may cause her section wound to bleed

B. Await the results of a lower-limb Doppler study

C. Breathlessness is the only symptom so pulmonary embolus is unlikely

D. She cannot breast-feed if you prescribe heparin

E. *She should be fully anticoagulated whilst awaiting the results of tests

If you suspect that a woman has a pulmonary embolus from her history and examination, you should not delay anticoagulation – it can always be stopped if investigations are negative. She is not likely to bleed excessively from anywhere more than 6 hours after her surgery. The maternal mortality reports highlight how easy it is to misdiagnose thromboembolism, and we should be wary if a woman is breathless as this is sometimes the only symptom.

Neither heparin nor warfarin is contraindicated during breast-feeding.

Source: RCOG Green-top Guideline, No. 37b, 'The Acute Management of Thrombosis and Embolism during Pregnancy and the Puerperium' (2015).

5.7 When a baby is born to a diabetic mother on insulin, although there is a risk of neonatal hypoglycaemia, it is recommended that babies stay with their mothers if possible.

In which circumstance may admission to the special care baby unit be avoided?

A. The baby can be fed every 2 hours on the postnatal ward

B. The baby can be tube fed on the postnatal ward

C. *The baby can maintain blood glucose levels >2 mmol/L before feeds

D. The baby feeds well orally

E. The baby has no clinical signs of hypoglycaemia before feeds

Women with diabetes should feed their babies within 30 minutes of birth and then every 2 to 3 hours until feeding maintains prefeed capillary glucose levels >2 mmol/L because of the risk of hypoglycaemia due to the baby's endogenous hyperinsulinaemia. Tube feeding or even intravenous dextrose may be needed if the baby cannot feed effectively orally.

Source: NICE Guideline, No. NG3, 'Diabetes in Pregnancy; Management from Preconception to the Postnatal Period' (2015).

5.8 A woman is admitted 2 days after a normal delivery with severe sepsis and the on-call obstetric consultant advises you to institute the 'sepsis six' care bundle.

Which of these statements is correct regarding this clinical pathway?

A. Administer facial oxygen whatever the pO_2

B. Intravenous fluids should be used if the woman appears clinically dehydrated

C. ***Lactate levels >2 mmol/L mean severe sepsis**

D. Oral antibiotics are adequate if she is not vomiting

E. The 'bundle' must be undertaken within 6 hours of diagnosis

The 'sepsis six' bundle involves

1. Measuring the arterial blood gas and administering oxygen if required
2. Take blood cultures
3. Commence intravenous antibiotics
4. Start intravenous fluid resuscitation
5. Take blood for haemoglobin and lactate levels
6. Measure the urine output hourly

The suggestion is that the bundle is undertaken within an hour of diagnosis.
Source: UK Sepsis Trust (2013); MBRRACE report (2014).

5.9 The day after her forceps delivery under epidural anaesthesia, you are asked to see a woman who has a severe continuous headache that has come on gradually and has been worsening over the previous few hours. The midwifery staff on the postnatal ward telephone to expedite your attendance as they are becoming concerned about her condition. She seems to be developing an acute confusional state.

Her pulse, BP, and temperature are all normal, and there are no focal neurological signs.

Select the most likely diagnosis for her headache:

A. ***Cerebral vein thrombosis**

B. Dural tap

C. Meningitis

D. Migraine

E. Subarachnoid haemorrhage

Migraines are described as a pulsating headache whereas this one is continuous. Non-focal neurological symptoms such as behavioural changes are a 'red-flag' symptom that suggests a serious intracranial cause for the headache such as cerebral venous thrombosis. Dehydration that often occurs during labour is a predisposing factor to cerebral vein thrombosis, as is pregnancy.

Subarachnoid haemorrhage classically comes on very suddenly – described as a 'thunderclap' headache, and this was a subacute onset, but this is still on the differential list.

Meningitis is less likely as she is not pyrexial.

Postpartum headaches are often blamed on leakage of spinal cerebrospinal fluid due to inadvertent dural tap during epidural insertion, but the anaesthetist will know if this has happened and these patients do not usually develop an acute confusional state. In the latest MBRRACE report a couple of women died because their headaches were misdiagnosed as spinal headaches and no further investigation was carried out.

Source: MBRRACE report (2015).

5.10 You review a postpartum woman at home who has been discharged following a caesarean section 3 days ago. She was given antibiotics in labour and tells you that the baby was admitted to the neonatal intensive care unit shortly after delivery. He is very unwell with meningitis.

What is the most likely infective organism?

A. Candida Albicans

B. E. Coli

C. Group A Streptococcus

D. ***Group B Streptococcus**

E. Staphylococcus Aureus

Source: RCOG Green-top Guideline, No. 36, 'Prevention of Early Onset Neonatal Group B Strep Disease' (2012) describes Group B Strep as 'the most common cause of early neonatal sepsis and meningitis'.

5.11 A woman has just delivered her second baby yesterday and requests sterilisation before she goes home. Her partner is not keen for her to have this done as he is having trouble coping with their toddler and wants her to go home immediately. Whilst you are counselling her about puerperal sterilisation, which of the following statements is correct about this situation?

A. ***Clip sterilisation is more likely to fail if it is done now as the fallopian tubes are thicker**

B. If she is sterilised now it will take longer for the uterus to involute

C. Laparoscopic sterilisation is feasible immediately postpartum

D. Puerperal sterilisation requires the written consent of both partners

E. She should defer the decision 24 hours for further discussion to avoid regret

Puerperal sterilisation is feasible but not using the laparoscope as the fundus of the uterus is still high – a 'mini-laparotomy' will be needed with the incision just below the umbilicus to reach the tubes. The failure rate is higher as it is more difficult to get the whole fallopian tube securely included in the clip. The chance of her changing her mind is also higher, and it is worth pointing out that if the decision is delayed until after the baby's first birthday, the chance of cot death declines and regret is less likely.

5.12 A woman is recovering on the postnatal ward following an emergency caesarean section. On the third day she complains of discomfort and swelling in her right leg, which is clearly larger than the left leg, with a tender calf. The most appropriate medication whilst awaiting the results of further investigation is:

A. Enoxaparin 20 mg daily

B. Enoxaparin 40 mg daily

C. ***Enoxaparin 1mg per kg twice daily**

D. Graduated compression stockings

E. Loading dose of Warfarin

You need to protect her against thromboembolism whilst you are awaiting the results of investigations. Twenty and forty milligrams are prophylactic doses rather than treatment so this is not enough heparin. In pregnancy the advice is still to give twice-daily treatment doses despite the change in management for nonpregnant patients on medical wards to use once-daily treatment doses. It is better to use heparin rather than warfarin as it is easier to manage and TED stockings alone are not enough.

5.13 A diabetic woman who has been on insulin since the age of 11 years has just delivered her first baby. Which of these statements contains correct advice regarding the management of her diabetes in the puerperium?

A. Breast-feeding is contraindicated because of the risk of hypoglycaemia

B. Glucose tolerance test should be arranged for 6 weeks postpartum

C. Insulin should be stopped for 24 hours in case she becomes hypoglycaemic

D. She needs a sliding scale for 24 hours

E. ***She should immediately revert to her prepregnant dose of insulin**

Most diabetic mothers need extra insulin during pregnancy but the requirement reduces after delivery so she should return to her original dosage as soon as she has delivered and you can stop the sliding scale at that point. The 6-week GTT is for gestational diabetics.

5.14 A community midwife asks you to attend a home delivery because she cannot determine the sex of the baby. On examination the newborn infant is well but the genitalia are ambiguous with a small phallus and some scrotal-like development of the skin. Which is the most appropriate course of action?

A. Advise the parents to choose a name that could be either male or female

B. Reassure the parents that the child is male with undescended testes

C. Send a referral letter to paediatric clinic so karyotyping can be arranged

D. ***Send the baby into hospital for urgent paediatric review**

E. Take the baby's blood for 17-hydroxyprogesterone levels

This baby is likely to be a girl with congenital adrenal hyperplasia due to 21-hydroxylase deficiency. The ambiguous genitalia are due to exposure to high levels of androgen in utero.

Although there will be high levels of 17-hydroxyprogesterone in the baby's blood, it is important to check that the baby does not have the salt-losing form of this condition, which can lead to severe dehydration and death so hospital admission is advisable.

5.15 A woman consults you in surgery about feeling very low in mood for the last 4 weeks. She is experiencing bouts of crying, is off her food, and having trouble sleeping. She delivered her first baby 6 weeks ago and is very upset that she has had to give up breast-feeding as she felt unable to cope.

What is the most appropriate course of action to deal with her symptoms?

A. Admit her urgently to a 'mother and baby unit'

B. Inform her that her symptoms are very common and will resolve shortly

C. Inform her that she has a mental illness and should see a psychiatrist

D. Refer to a breast-feeding counsellor

E. ***Suggest that she takes an antidepressant and monitor her progress**

This woman clearly has a mild depressive illness and it is not just about the breast-feeding. However, she does not need formal psychiatric input at this stage.

5.16 You have just finished assisting at a difficult caesarean section during which the woman sustained a massive haemorrhage. She is at present on the High Dependency Unit having a blood transfusion but her condition seems to have stabilised and her husband is at her bedside looking after the newborn baby.

His mother came into hospital with them but only one person was allowed into the operating theatre with her.

In the hospital cafe you meet the mother-in-law who is anxiously waiting for news and asks you why the delivery is taking so long.

You must deal with her enquiry but what should you tell her?

A.   That the mother and baby are both fine

B.   That she is not on labour ward but you are not allowed to tell her why

C.   ***That you will send the husband to give her information**

D.   The delivery has been complicated but everything is alright now

E.   To go to the High Dependency Unit to see the new mother and baby

This is an ethical challenge. It is a breach of confidentiality even to acknowledge that the patient is in the hospital but the mother-in-law came in with her, so it is slightly ridiculous to pretend otherwise. However, you are absolutely not allowed to give her any information – family dynamics can sometimes be surprisingly awkward – and the safest thing to do is to send the husband to tell his mother what is going on.

5.17 The highest risk factor for puerperal psychosis is:

A.   A history of postnatal depression in a previous pregnancy

B.   ***A previous history of bipolar disorder**

C.   Eating disorder as a teenager

D.   Family history of puerperal psychosis

E.   Personality disorder

A family history of puerperal psychosis is a risk factor but the highest risk is for those patients with a personal history of severe mental illness (which gives about a 50 per cent chance of developing puerperal psychosis).

Further reading: NICE Clinical Guideline CG192 'Antenatal and postnatal mental health: clinical management and service guidance' Published 2014, updated 2015.

5.18 On the evening shift you go to the postnatal ward and find that the midwives have been waiting for you to complete a list of prescribing tasks they have been saving up.

Which task takes priority?

A.   A woman who delivered a stillborn baby this morning is waiting for a prescription for cabergoline to suppress lactation.

B.   A woman who had a caesarean section 3 days ago is ready to be discharged and is awaiting a prescription for analgesic drugs to take home.

C.   ***A woman who has just been readmitted with puerperal sepsis is waiting for antibiotics. Her temperature is 35.8°C, BP 90/60 mmHg, and pulse 120 bpm.**

D. A woman who suffered a major postpartum haemorrhage yesterday is waiting for you to prescribe a blood transfusion. Her haemoglobin is 60g/l.

E. A woman who had an emergency caesarean section 2 hours ago is waiting for a prescription of low molecular weight heparin prophylaxis.

The woman with sepsis is urgent because her clinical condition is serious, as evidenced by her low temperature and blood pressure. She shouldn't even be on the postnatal ward and transferring her to a high dependency ward would be a priority too. She should get her antibiotics immediately as she may deteriorate rapidly.

Source: RCOG Green-top Guideline, No. 64b, 'Bacterial Sepsis Following Pregnancy' (2012).

5.19 A 34-year-old primigravid Jehovah's Witness signed an advance directive refusing blood transfusion when she first booked for antenatal care. She has just been readmitted a week postpartum with a massive haemorrhage and is on the operating table where the consultant is having difficulty stopping the bleeding. Her haemoglobin is currently 30 g/L and her life hangs in the balance.

Which of the following statements is correct regarding the management of this situation?

A. Her husband can give consent for her to have a blood transfusion

B. Transfuse her without consent because it is in her best interests

C. Get an emergency court order to transfuse

D. *Respect advance directive and withhold transfusion*

E. Transfuse her own blood from the cell saver

Unfortunately, there is nothing you can do if she has signed an advanced directive unless you can prove that she was not of sound mind when she did that. This must be one of the most distressing situations medical staff can find themselves in, but she cannot be rescued by a blood transfusion.

5.20 A woman was delivered of her first baby using forceps because of fetal distress in the second stage of labour. The baby is doing fine but the mother sustained a third-degree tear that has been repaired by your consultant. When debriefing her about the third-degree tear, which of the following statements is true?

A. If she has another baby she will need a caesarean section

B. *She will be given antibiotics and laxatives postpartum*

C. She is very likely to be incontinent of flatus in the future

D. The tear will have involved the anal mucosa as well as the sphincter muscle

E. Third-degree tears do not occur with normal deliveries

Third-degree tears usually heal very well and it is uncommon for women to have problems with anal incontinence afterwards. Studies show that 60 to 80 per cent of women are asymptomatic at 12 months postpartum. These tears can happen during a normal birth but are more common with assisted delivery (forceps more so than ventouse). We are uncertain how to advise women to deliver in the next pregnancy and some obstetricians only advise caesarean of she has residual symptoms after the previous repair such as incontinence of flatus or faeces. There is a paucity of research evidence in this area.

Source: RCOG Green-top Guidelines, No. 26, 'Operative Vaginal Delivery' (2011) and No. 29 'The Management of Third- and Fourth-Degree Perineal Tears' (2015).

Extended Matching Questions

A	COC
B	Condoms
C	Copper intrauterine device
D	Depot medroxyprogesterone acetate
E	Diaphragm
F	Female sterilisation
G	Levonorgestrel intrauterine system
H	POP
I	Spermicide gel
J	Vasectomy

These clinical scenarios describe mothers requesting contraceptive advice in the postpartum period. Select the most appropriate method of contraception for each woman.

Each option may be used once, more than once, or not at all.

5.21 Having just delivered her first baby a 15-year-old schoolgirl is very keen to avoid getting pregnant again.

D Depot medroxyprogesterone acetate

LARCs (long-acting reversible contraception) are recommended for teenagers as they need secure contraception. The best option from the list is to give her Depo-Provera®, which you would review after 2 years. In the long term she would do well to consider an implant.

5.22 A 40-year-old woman who was delivered by caesarean section yesterday has now had two children. She wishes to start secure contraception immediately before she leaves hospital but does not want to rule out having another child in the future.

H POP

As she is over 35 years, the POP is a safer option than the combined pill although she may opt for that if the side effects of the POP become a problem. COC would also add to the risk of DVT which is high because of her age and recent pregnancy as well as the caesarean section.

5.23 A 35-year-old woman with a BMI of 45 attends for her postnatal checkup with her first baby. She conceived after IVF treatment because of infertility due to polycystic ovarian syndrome.

She still has some frozen embryos in storage but does not want to conceive again just yet as she has been advised to lose a great deal of weight first.

G Levonorgestrel intrauterine system

This patient is at risk of endometrial hyperplasia due to her PCO and if she wishes to use contraception a Levonorgestrel IUS is a good idea because it will protect her against that problem until she is ready to conceive again.

5.24 Having used the pill with no problems in the past, a 25-year-old wishes to restart contraception after delivering her first baby a week ago. She had a normal delivery, her lochia is normal, and she is successfully breast-feeding.

H POP

She is likely to be keen to use the pill again but will need the POP instead of the combined pill whilst she is breast-feeding. Exogenous estrogen interferes with milk production.

5.25 A woman who used to suffer from premenstrual syndrome wishes to have a secure form of contraception after delivering her first baby. She has decided that she is very sensitive to hormones and requests a method that does not involve using hormones.

C Copper intra-uterine device

The only secure method of contraception without hormones on the list is the copper coil. Barrier methods have too high a Pearl index to be described as secure.

A	Arrange a district nurse to supervise dressings
B	Arrange a visit from a breast-feeding peer support group
C	Arrange readmission to the obstetric unit for review
D	Arrange urgent admission to the emergency medical ward
E	Ask the community midwife to visit at home
F	Prescribe broad spectrum antibiotics
G	Send her in to A&E
H	Take the sutures out and allow the wound to drain

These clinical scenarios describe recently delivered women who have developed complications. In each case, select the most appropriate management plan. Each option may be used once, more than once, or not at all.

5.26 A woman who had a caesarean section 2 days ago was discharged home yesterday. She has asked for a home visit this morning because there is copious sero-sanguinous fluid discharging from the wound.

C Arrange readmission to the obstetric unit for review

The nature of the discharge suggests the possibility of wound dehiscence although it could be a wound infection or haematoma about to discharge: this patient needs reviewing at the hospital.

5.27 Two days after a normal delivery, a primiparous women telephones the surgery to report heavy vaginal bleeding with clots.

C Arrange readmission to the obstetric unit for review

This patient either has retained products of conception or endometritis or both. She needs readmission and possibly an evacuation of uterus.

5.28 You are asked to do a home visit to look at the caesarean wound of a patient who has been out of hospital for 4 days. She has an absorbable subcuticular suture in situ in the skin and there is a spreading cellulitis around the scar.

F Prescribe broad spectrum antibiotics

This is a superficial spreading wound infection rather than an abscess. Antibiotics should resolve the problem providing they will cover Staph aureus. The distracter is H 'take the suture out'.

5.29 A primiparous patient who delivered 4 days ago is having problems with breast-feeding due to pain. On examination her nipples are cracked and sore but there is no unusual swelling of the breasts.

E Ask the community midwife to visit at home

Cracked nipples are very painful and this woman is going to need extra help to continue breast-feeding. Peer support can be very helpful but she is likely to need clinical help until the situation improves. It is not an abscess so she does not need admission. It is not mastitis so she does not need antibiotics.

5.30 The community midwife is doing a home visit for a woman who has been discharged from hospital 2 days after a forceps delivery. She is struggling with breast-feeding and has asked for help. The midwife telephones you because she has noticed that the woman's left leg is swollen.

C Arrange readmission to the obstetric unit for review

She probably has a DVT so she needs to go back into hospital for investigation and anticoagulation. As she is trying to establish breast-feeding, she will want to take the baby in with her and the obstetric unit is more likely to admit her baby too.

A	Blood transfusion
B	Evacuation of retained products of conception
C	Examination under anaesthetic
D	Full blood count
E	Intravenous antibiotics
F	Norethisterone 5 mg tds
G	Oral antibiotics
H	Pelvic USS
I	Reassure the patient
J	Resuture the perineum

These clinical scenarios relate to women in the puerperium with problems following a vaginal delivery. For each scenario select the most appropriate course of action from the preceding list.

Each option may be used once, more than once, or not at all.

5.31 You are seeing a 24-year-old woman in your GP surgery for her postnatal check. She had a normal vaginal delivery 6 weeks ago with a small second-degree perineal tear. She is breast-feeding and is feeling well. She tells you that she still has a pink loss vaginally but there have been no clots and the loss is not offensive.

I Reassure the patient

Lochia is a red loss initially, then becomes red/brown followed by pink, and finally becomes a white discharge. The mean duration of lochia is 24 days but 13 per cent of women will still have pink or red lochia at 8 weeks postpartum. Unless the lochia is increasing in amount, associated with clots, or offensive then this is unlikely to indicate infection or retained products of conception so the patient can be reassured that it will settle spontaneously.

5.32 You are the junior obstetric doctor on call overnight and at midnight are asked to see a woman who has been readmitted 3 days after the delivery of her third child. Over the last few hours her lochia has become heavier and she is passing clots vaginally. Her observations are pulse 90 bpm, blood pressure 125/85, temperature 37.5°C, and respiratory rate 14. The midwife has already taken a high vaginal swab.

E Intravenous antibiotics

The change in her lochia associated with a pyrexia and tachycardia suggests that she has either sepsis or retained placental tissue. The initial management is to treat aggressively with intravenous antibiotics. She does also need an USS but this should be done by an experienced practitioner. It is unlikely that this would be available out of hours so this isn't the correct answer. A full blood count could be helpful but the scenario in the preceding text is one of sepsis rather than postpartum haemorrhage, which is why IV antibiotics is the correct answer here.

5.33 The midwives ask you to review a woman on the postnatal ward 1 day after delivery. She had a right medio-lateral episiotomy, which was repaired by the registrar, and now she is complaining of severe perineal pain so she can't sit comfortably. On examination her temperature is 36.5°C, pulse 75 bpm, and blood pressure 110/65 mmHg. The episiotomy sutures are intact and the perineum is bruised with a 3 cm swelling underlying the sutures. The vaginal sutures are also intact and there is no swelling in the vagina.

G Oral antibiotics

Perineal haematomas usually present within 24 hours of delivery. This is a small haematoma as it is less than 5 cm and therefore, unless it is rapidly enlarging, it is likely to resolve spontaneously. The blood is an obvious focus for infection, hence the need to treat with oral antibiotics. The indications for taking the woman to theatre are if the haematoma is large, if she is haemodynamically unstable, or if the haematoma is infected.

5.34 Eight hours after delivery a woman who has just arrived on the postnatal ward suddenly starts to bleed heavily per vaginam, losing another 200 ml on top of the 300 ml estimated blood loss at delivery. Her predelivery haemoglobin done on admission in labour was 115 g/L. The notes indicate that the placenta was removed in pieces after the cord came off during controlled cord traction.

B Evacuation of retained products of conception

It is likely that there is still some placental tissue in this woman's uterus and if nothing is done to remove it, she is likely to bleed again. Having experienced a blood loss of 500 ml in total, she is unlikely to need blood transfusion unless she continues to bleed and the point of evacuating the uterus is to stop her bleeding. USS will not help here.

5.35 A woman is readmitted by her community midwife because she is worried about the appearance of the perineal wound a week after delivery. On examination you find that the wound has broken down and the tissues are covered in a sloughy yellow-green exudate that smells offensive.

G Oral antibiotics

If the wound is resutured while it is infected like this, it will not heal and will break down again. It is best to let it heal by secondary intention, and the oral antibiotics will speed this process.

A	Bimanual pressure to compress the uterus
B	Controlled cord traction (Brandt Andrews method)
C	Ergometrine 500 micrograms IM
D	Evacuation of uterus
E	Inject carboprost (Hemabate®) into the uterus
F	IV infusion of 40 units of oxytocin over 4 hours
G	IV dose of 40 units of oxytocin stat
H	Manual removal of placenta
I	Place a Bakri balloon into the uterine cavity

Each of these obstetric patients has either bled heavily after delivery or is at risk of doing so, and this question refers to the prevention or treatment of postpartum haemorrhage. Choose the most appropriate management plan for each woman.

Each option may be used once, more than once, or not at all.

5.36 A 35-year-old woman has just had an emergency caesarean section for failure to progress in labour and the baby weighed 4.8 kg. During the delivery the blood loss was estimated at nearly a litre but she is no longer bleeding actively. As they are suturing the skin at the end of the operation, the registrar asks you to prescribe something to keep the uterus contracted.

F IV infusion of 40 units of Oxytocin over 4 hours

Ergometrine does have a sustained effect compared with Oxytocin, but in this case we want the effect to last much longer so the 4-hour option is best.

5.37 A woman has delivered her third baby at home 2 hours ago but the community midwife has transferred her in to hospital because she has not been able to deliver the placenta despite active management of the third stage. There is quite a big blood clot in the bed that amounts to about 600 ml.

H Manual removal of placenta

The distracter answer here is controlled cord traction but the midwife will already have been doing this and failed. As it is 2 hours since delivery and she has already lost quite a bit of blood, she needs to go to theatre urgently for manual removal of placenta.

5.38 A woman is urgently brought back to labour ward 6 hours after a normal delivery because she suddenly bleeds heavily vaginally, losing 500 ml in a couple of minutes. Looking through her previous notes you see that a succenturiate lobe was mentioned on her anomaly scan at 21 weeks of gestation.

D Evacuation of uterus

Unless the succenturiate lobe was found at delivery it is probably still in the uterus so this woman needs an evacuation.

5.39 You are the only doctor on labour ward when a woman who was being induced for pre-eclampsia unexpectedly starts pushing and rapidly delivers the baby and placenta. She has a brisk postpartum haemorrhage of 500 ml. She has already had 10 units of oxytocin given as the baby was delivering and you have put up an oxytocin infusion with another 40 units so she is now nearing the maximum dose. The registrar is in the gynaecology emergency theatre dealing with a woman in extremis due to a ruptured ectopic pregnancy and you are waiting for the obstetric consultant to arrive from home. She continues to bleed heavily, so you must select the best course of action to save her life.

A Bimanual pressure to compress the uterus

This is an emergency situation in which squashing the uterus between your hands can slow the bleeding down for long enough for the consultant to arrive and take over. Compressing the uterus against the sacrum abdominally may also have the same effect. You cannot give her Ergometrine because it can cause an uncontrolled rise in her blood pressure (although if you don't stop this woman bleeding, her blood pressure is going to drop dramatically shortly).

5.40 The midwives ask you to put up an intravenous infusion on a woman who is bleeding heavily after delivery of her placenta. You are sure the bleeding is coming from the uterus but every time the senior midwife stops massaging the uterus the bleeding starts again. You are having trouble getting a cannula into a vein so you send for the anaesthetist and ask the midwife to continue rubbing the fundus. The registrar is on the way but you need to give something quickly to make the uterus contract.

C Ergometrine 500 micrograms IM

As you have not yet got IV access, intramuscular ergometrine is the obvious answer. We do also use carboprost but IM, not directly into the uterus.

A	Arterial blood gas
B	Blood cultures
C	CT pulmonary angiogram
D	CT brain
E	Chest x-ray
F	D-dimer
G	Electrophoresis
H	Haemoglobin
I	LFT daily until results are normal
J	LFT 10 days after delivery
K	Liver ultrasound
L	Lumbar puncture
M	Pelvic x-ray
N	Pulmonary V/Q scan

These clinical scenarios relate to postpartum women with complicated pregnancies experiencing problems or seeking advice after delivery. For each woman, select the most appropriate initial investigation that will help you make a diagnosis.

Each option may be used once, more than once, or not at all.

5.41 You are asked to see an unwell 27-year-old woman on the postnatal ward who delivered yesterday. She is complaining of a fronto-occipital headache that is so severe that she can hardly move and is associated with nausea. She had an epidural in labour that was initially ineffective and whilst it was being resited the dura was inadvertently punctured. Her temperature is 38°C.

L Lumbar puncture

Although the most likely cause of this woman's headache is a so-called spinal headache, she might also have meningitis. If there are no indicators of infection, she could have a 'blood patch' done to stop the CSF leak that will cure her headache. The distracter is CT brain.

5.42 A woman whose labour was induced for obstetric cholestasis has returned home from hospital and you are asked to review her by the community midwife. She asks you what tests she needs now that the baby is safely delivered.

J LFT 10 days after delivery

The diagnosis of cholestasis is made if the LFTs return to normal after delivery and other causes such as hepatitis have been ruled out. The distracter is daily

LFTs and ultrasound of liver (which will already have been done antenatally to rule out gallstones, etc.).

Source: RCOG Green-top Guideline, No. 43, 'Obstetric Cholestasis' (2011).

5.43 A woman with sickle cell disease is on the postnatal ward after a caesarean section for the delivery of her first baby. She complains of pain at the top of her right leg near the hip joint and cannot stand up comfortably. There is no swelling of either leg on examination.

M Pelvic x-ray

Women with sickle cell disease are at risk of avascular necrosis of the femoral head, although you would be initially concerned about the possibility of DVT or sickle crisis. Having had a caesarean section, she is likely to be fully anticoagulated for 6 weeks prophylactically.

Source: RCOG Green-top Guideline, No. 61, 'Management of Sickle Cell Disease in Pregnancy' (2011).

5.44 Following an unsuccessful attempt at induction of labour over 3 days, a primigravid woman has an emergency caesarean section at 42 weeks of gestation. The baby has been admitted to the SCBU with meconium aspiration and you are asked by the SCBU staff to review the mother there the following day because she has become increasingly short of breath.

A Arterial blood gas

Postoperative pulmonary embolism (PE) is still a major cause of death in pregnant women. A woman with risk factors should be commenced on treatment dosage of low molecular weight heparin if there is a suspicion of a PE whilst awaiting further investigation. The symptoms and signs can be subtle such as shortness of breath or an unexplained tachycardia, and a drop in oxygen saturation may be an important clue.

5.45 A primigravid woman has a rather prolonged second stage but achieves a normal delivery of a 4 kg baby after pushing really hard for 2 hours. Shortly after delivery she becomes progressively short of breath and complains of mild left-sided chest pain on inspiration. On examination there is decreased air entry on the left side of her chest. Her midwife brings the saturation probe from theatre and tells you that her oxygen levels are normal.

E Chest x-ray

This sounds like a pneumothorax and a chest x-ray is appropriate especially as you already know that her oxygen saturation is normal. The other distracters are the more expensive chest imaging such as CT pulmonary angiogram and V/Q scan used to diagnose pulmonary embolism.

A	Elective caesarean section at 37 weeks
B	Elective caesarean section at 39 weeks
C	External cephalic version
D	Induce labour before term
E	Vaginal birth and consider episiotomy

F	Vaginal birth with CTG monitoring
G	Vaginal birth with oxytocin drip
H	Take low-dose aspirin 75 mg in next pregnancy
I	Terminate the pregnancy

These clinical scenarios relate to women who have recently delivered and have returned to the hospital postnatal clinic for debriefing. In each case, select the most appropriate advice regarding her next pregnancy.

Each option may be used once, more than once, or not at all.

5.46 After being induced for severe pre-eclampsia at 34 weeks of gestation, a primigravid woman is delivered by emergency caesarean section for fetal distress at 8 cm dilatation. She is thinking of embarking on another pregnancy in about a year's time as her husband is keen to have another baby soon.

H Take low-dose aspirin 75 mg in next pregnancy

Although you need to have the discussion about VBAC with this woman, it would be beneficial to try and prevent her getting early onset pre-eclampsia again as she is more likely to have a vaginal birth if the pregnancy is uncomplicated and the baby well grown. The distracter is vaginal birth with monitoring.

5.47 After a very prolonged first stage of labour, the registrar unsuccessfully attempts a forceps delivery in theatre for a primigravid woman who has been pushing for 2 hours. The position of the baby's head was OA at the ischial spines with moulding++. A caesarean section was performed after three strong pulls during which there was no descent of the fetal head. The baby weighed 3.8 kg and was 2 weeks overdue.

B Elective caesarean section at 39 weeks

The clinical details here are suggestive of cephalo-pelvic disproportion, which may well recur in a subsequent pregnancy unless she spontaneously labours early for some reason. The distracter is induction of labour before term but we prefer not to induce women with section scars as the drugs used increase the risk of scar rupture.

If she did present in spontaneous labour before term in her next pregnancy, she could attempt a vaginal birth with continuous monitoring.

5.48 Halfway through her labour, when the membranes ruptured at 5 cm dilatation, a primigravid woman was found to have a breech presentation and therefore had her first baby delivered by caesarean section. You note from the operation notes that there was a bicornuate uterus that might lead to another breech presentation next pregnancy. Choose the best course of action if the next baby is breech too.

B Elective caesarean section at 39 weeks

The distracter is external cephalic version that is contraindicated when there is a major uterine malformation and relatively contraindicated if there is a scar on the uterus.

Source: RCOG Green-top Guideline, No. 20a, 'External Cephalic Version (ECV) and Reducing the Incidence of Breech Presentation', (2006; reviewed 2010).

5.49 During a forceps delivery performed for fetal distress, a primigravid woman sustains a third-degree tear. At her follow-up appointment the perineum has healed well and she has made a full recovery with no symptoms related to the anal sphincter. She wishes to discuss plans for her next birth.

E Vaginal birth and consider episiotomy

We are unsure as to how to advise women who have sustained a third-degree tear previously. If she has residual symptoms such a faecal incontinence, most obstetricians would suggest elective section but there is no hard evidence to back up that opinion – it is merely a worry that next time a repeat third-degree tear might make things worse. A compromise (also not evidence-based) is to offer an elective episiotomy next time.

Source: RCOG Green-top Guideline, No. 29, 'The Management of Third- and Fourth-Degree Perineal Tears' (2015).

5.50 Having reached 8 cm cervical dilation in her first labour, a primigravid woman was delivered by emergency caesarean section because of a fetal bradycardia associated with fresh vaginal bleeding. The labour was progressing well up to that point but unfortunately the bradycardia turned out to be due to placental abruption and the baby did not survive. She does not feel strong enough to contemplate another pregnancy just yet, but is wondering about the mode of delivery next time.

F Vaginal birth with CTG monitoring

This is slightly difficult because we might be considering induction before term (as soon as the baby's head is safely engaged in the pelvis, reducing the risk of cord prolapse) in a woman who had suffered a placental abruption before. However, induction will increase the risk of scar rupture, so the correct answer here is vaginal birth with monitoring, which is safer if labour is spontaneous rather than induced.

Curriculum Module 6

Answers

Single Best Answer Questions

6.1 A nulliparous 22-year-old woman presents with a 4-month history of inter-menstrual and postcoital bleeding. She is healthy with no other medical problems and is using the withdrawal method for contraception.

Select the most appropriate investigation:

A. Cervical cytology
B. *Endocervical chlamydia swab*
C. Hysteroscopy
D. Pregnancy test
E. Transvaginal ultrasound scan

Chlamydia causes cervicitis that can make the cervix bleed. In this age group, this is the most likely diagnosis.

Speculum examination of the cervix is appropriate as cervical cancer is possible but unlikely at this age and she is too young for a smear anyway.

Endometrial or ovarian pathology are rare causes of abnormal bleeding at the end of the differential diagnosis list.

6.2 An asymptomatic nulliparous 49-year-old woman attends for a routine cervical smear. The practice nurse finds it very difficult to access the cervix because it is pushed backwards and sideways into the left fornix by a 10 cm diameter pelvic mass.

Which is the mass most likely to be?

A. Bowel cancer
B. Diverticular abscess
C. Full bladder
D. Ovarian cyst
E. *Uterine fibroid*

The only pathologies that would produce a pelvic mass without symptoms are ovarian cyst and fibroid. It is more likely to be fibroid because of the way the anatomy is distorted, as an ovarian cyst this large would rise out of the pelvis and become an abdominal mass.

If the mass was related to the bowel, she would have some symptoms such as alteration in bowel habit or pain. Retention of urine is uncommon in women, but they usually have symptoms such as frequency or dribbling incontinence to draw attention to the bladder. A full bladder would not alter the anatomy of the pelvis so that the cervix is pushed laterally either.

6.3 A 16-year-old woman presents to the surgery with primary amenorrhoea. She has some development of secondary sexual characteristics and is 146 cm tall with a BMI of 28.

Which of these investigations is the most relevant to make a diagnosis for her amenorrhoea?

A. FSH and LH levels

B. *Karyotype

C. Pregnancy test

D. Serum testosterone

E. USS of pelvis

The most likely diagnosis is Turner syndrome because of her short stature.

6.4 Some women present to their GP seeking HRT around the time of the menopause to get rid of their vasomotor symptoms. Many of these women are still menstruating.

Which of these statements is correct if HRT is prescribed in these circumstances?

A. HRT is first-line management in a patient at risk of osteoporosis

B. It protects against unwanted pregnancy in perimenopausal women

C. Period-free HRT is the most suitable formulation for menstruating women

D. *Prescribe the lowest possible estrogen dose for the shortest possible time

E. The risk of breast cancer is not increased if she only uses HRT for 5 years

Although the use of HRT is disputed in the press at the moment, the International Menopause Society guidelines currently state that we should use the lowest effective dose, tailor the treatment to the individual, use treatment for as long as there is symptomatic benefit and awareness of risks, and evaluate the risk/benefit balance on an annual basis to decide whether to continue therapy.

She must have sequential HRT, not period-free, otherwise she will get irregular bleeding and you will have to refer her for investigation.

6.5 Which of the following is a feature of the HPV?

A. *Genital warts are associated with subtypes 6 and 11

B. Infection causes intermenstrual bleeding

C. The virus can produce painful ulcers on the vulva

D. There are four different subtypes: HPV 6, 11, 16, and 18

E. Vaccination against HPV prevents cervical cancer

There are many different subtypes but these four are the most significant clinically. HPV causes cervical cancer, CIN, or genital warts – depending on the subtype – but vaccination will only prevent 70 per cent of cervical cancers. Painful ulcers on the vulva will be herpes, not HPV. Both wart virus and CIN on the cervix are asymptomatic.

6.6 A first-year degree student attends the university GP practice complaining of period pains that are severe enough to prevent her from going to lectures during the first 2 days of each period. Mild analgesic tablets have not helped. She is otherwise healthy and uses condoms for contraception.

Which is most appropriate management option?

A. Co-codamol tablets
B. *COC
C. Prostaglandin synthetase inhibitors
D. Refer for diagnostic laparoscopy
E. Utero-sacral nerve ablation

Conservative measures for treating dysmenorrhoea include heating pads, mild analgesics, sedatives or antispasmodic drugs, and outdoor exercise. In patients with dysmenorrhoea there is a significantly higher than normal concentration of prostaglandins in the endometrium and menstrual fluid. Prostaglandin synthase inhibitors such as indomethacin, naproxen, ibuprofen, and mefenamic acid are very effective in these patients. However, for patients with dysmenorrhoea who are sexually active, COC are the first-line management as they will provide needed protection from unwanted pregnancy as well as effectively alleviating the dysmenorrhoea.

Very few women in this age group have pathology in the pelvis such as endometriosis, and laparoscopy should be reserved for refractory cases.

Source: NICE Guideline, 'Dysmenorrhoea' (revised 2014).

6.7 A 42-year-old woman is diagnosed with a complete hydatidiform mole that was initially treated by surgical evacuation of the uterus. The Regional Trophoblastic Centre then treated her with methotrexate due to rising beta-hCG levels.

She is currently using barrier contraception but is worried about her age and wishes to become pregnant again as soon as possible.

What advice should she be given about when it is safe to discontinue all methods of contraception?

A. She may discontinue at any time
B. She may discontinue when hCG levels normalise
C. She should wait 6 months from the date of evacuation
D. She should wait 6 months from when hCG levels normalise
E. *She should wait 12 months from completion of treatment

Green-top Guideline 38 states that women who have had chemotherapy should wait a year from the completion of their treatment. If she had not had chemotherapy, she would be advised to avoid conception until her follow-up was complete, which will be 6 months from the date of evacuation (if the hCG levels return to normal within 56 days) or 6 months from subsequent normalization of the hCG levels if this takes longer than that.

Source: RCOG Green-top guideline 38 'Gestational Trophoblastic Disease' (2010).

6.8 An 18-year-old student is referred to gynaecology clinic because she has experienced increasingly heavy irregular periods during the previous year. Her menarche occurred aged 14 and her periods were initially normal.

Her BMI is 38 and abdominal examination is unremarkable. She declines pelvic examination because she is a virgin.

Select the most likely diagnosis in her case:

A. Anovulatory cycles
B. Pelvic inflammatory disease
C. ***Polycystic ovarian syndrome**
D. Thrombocytopaenia
E. Von Willebrand disease

Anovulatory cycles do cause irregular heavy bleeding but this would have started at puberty and should have resolved by this age; so although this is a distracter, polycystic ovarian syndrome is a more likely diagnosis.

She will not have PID if she has never been sexually active. Clotting disorders are rare and will normally present with menorrhagia at puberty.

6.9 A woman having a hysterectomy for fibroids after the age of 45 years may be advised by her gynaecologist to have her ovaries removed at the same time.

Identify the main reason for suggesting that she consider oophorectomy:

A. So that she can have postoperative estrogen-only replacement therapy
B. To avoid ovarian cysts in the future
C. To eliminate premenstrual syndrome
D. To prevent metabolic effects of polycystic ovarian syndrome, for example, diabetes
E. ***To prevent ovarian cancer**

She could have postoperative estrogen-only HRT if she needed it – as she has had her uterus removed she no longer needs progesterone to protect her endometrium, so that answer is a red herring. She would not get PMS if she had her ovaries removed but this a red herring too. It would avoid ovarian cysts in the future but the main issue is to avoid ovarian cancer, which often presents at an advanced stage. It doesn't completely protect them 100 per cent as some patients get primary peritoneal cancer, which behaves in the same way. There is no evidence that the metabolic effects of PCO can be prevented but the stem does not describe a patient with PCO anyway.

6.10 A woman telephones your surgery for advice about vomiting in pregnancy. She thinks that she is 6 weeks pregnant and is just starting to feel nauseous. She is very worried because she had her last pregnancy terminated at 10 weeks because of severe hyperemesis.

Regarding her situation, which is the best advice to give her?

A. Antiemetics are not available without a prescription in the United Kingdom
B. It is better to try and manage symptoms by dietary manipulation
C. ***Preemptive prescription of antiemetics has been shown to reduce the incidence of hyperemesis**
D. Risk of recurrence of hyperemesis is less than 1 per cent
E. She needs a higher dose of folic acid than normal

Cyclizine and promethazine are available without prescription and there is a great deal of evidence that they are safe in pregnancy but because of the lawsuits surrounding thalidomide, all antiemetics carry a warning about not taking them in pregnancy without consulting a doctor. Prescribing antiemetics before the condition develops or extremely early as soon as the patient feels nauseous has been shown to prevent hyperemesis developing and we should be considering this to reduce hospital admissions.

Source: The Obstetrician and Gynaecologist, 'Severe Nausea and Vomiting of Pregnancy' 13 (2) (2011).

6.11 A 68-year-old woman with a BMI of 30 presents to her GP with a history of urinary urgency and frequency almost every hour with occasional urge incontinence. She must wear a pad all the time and rarely leaves the house as a result. Vaginal examination reveals no prolapse and urinalysis is negative.

Which one of the following management options is most likely to ameliorate her symptoms?

A. Colposuspension operation
B. Electrical stimulation of pelvic floor muscle
C. Weight loss
D. Prescription of duloxetine
E. ***Bladder drill (retraining)**

This patient probably has detrusor instability from the symptoms, although you are not told the results of a bladder pressure study (which would be the next step if you were looking after this woman because the bladder is an unreliable witness).

Colposuspension and duloxetine are treatments for genuine stress incontinence. Pelvic floor physiotherapy (including electrical stimulation) and weight loss may help but the best treatment here for instability is bladder drill.

6.12 A 38-year-old woman attended for a routine cervical smear during which an asymptomatic polyp is noted on the surface of the cervix. The result of the smear was normal.

In counselling her about the polyp, which one of the following statements is true?

A. It could be caused by chlamydia
B. ***It is unlikely to be associated with endometrial pathology**
C. It is most likely to be a nabothian follicle
D. It is associated with HPV infection
E. It should be removed because it is likely to be malignant

If the polyp is obviously an endometrial polyp – bright red and coming through the cervix instead of being on the surface – then there might be further polyps within the uterus. Cervical polyps are usually benign and not associated with endometrial problems. Nabothian follicles sit within the substance of the cervix; they are mucus-retention cysts.

6.13 When you are on call for gynaecological emergencies in your hospital, you are frequently asked to organise management for women attending the Early Pregnancy Clinic. Which one of these statements is correct regarding the management of miscarriage?

A. Expectant management is the treatment of choice if the uterus is septic
B. Histological proof that the uterus contained trophoblastic tissue will always exclude ectopic pregnancy
C. Medical management is associated with an increased incidence of pelvic infection

D.   Perforation of the uterus during surgical evacuation is more likely in incomplete rather than missed miscarriage

E.   ***Women having a surgical evacuation should be screened for chlamydia**

There is a reduction in clinical pelvic infection after medical evacuation compared with surgical (7.1 per cent vs. 13.2 per cent p < 0.001). The chance of a patient developing an infection after surgical evacuation with subsequent fertility problems can be reduced if screening for chlamydia is undertaken routinely. If the uterus is already septic, she is at risk of systemic sepsis and the uterus should be evacuated with antibiotic cover. Ectopic cannot be completely excluded by finding trophoblastic tissue in the uterus although the chance of a coexistent ectopic and intrauterine pregnancy – heterotopic pregnancy – is rare (somewhere between 1 in 10,000 to 1 in 30,000 pregnancies).

In missed miscarriage the cervix is often tightly closed and difficult to dilate making perforation of the uterus much more likely during surgical evacuation. Having said that, surgical evacuation is more effective than medical management in this group of patients.

Further reading: NICE Guideline CG154 'Ectopic pregnancy and miscarriage: diagnosis and initial management' (2012).

6.14   A woman has been fully investigated after her third first-trimester miscarriage and all the results are normal. In this situation in which there is unexplained recurrent miscarriage, which of the following interventions have been shown to be effective in reducing the risk of further miscarriage?

A.   Cervical cerclage

B.   hCG injections

C.   Metformin treatment

D.   Progesterone supplements

E.   ***Psychological support and regular scans**

The only intervention that has been shown to reduce the risk of further miscarriage in couples with unexplained recurrent miscarriage is support and counselling even though there is no clear understanding of the mechanism of action of this.

Source: NICE Clinical Guideline, No. CG 154, 'Ectopic Pregnancy and Miscarriage: diagnosis and initial management' (2012).

6.15   A routine 'dating' scan arranged by the midwife at 11 weeks of gestation shows that a primigravid woman has suffered a missed miscarriage. The sac contains a fetus about 9 weeks' size but there is no fetal heart pulsation seen. She was not expecting this as she has not had any bleeding at all during the pregnancy, so is extremely upset and would like to deal with the problem as quickly as possible.

Select the best management plan in her case:

A.   Admit to hospital for medical management with methotrexate

B.   ***Evacuate the uterus with cervical preparation**

C.   Expectant management with another scan in 2 weeks to see if she has miscarried

D.   Give 800 micrograms of misoprostol

E.   Prescribe mifepristone orally and follow up after 2 weeks

The quickest way to complete this episode for her is surgical management. Missed miscarriages are different from other miscarriages because there has been no

bleeding and often the cervix is tightly closed, being difficult to dilate at evacuation. Expectant management is not as successful compared with incomplete miscarriage and if medical management is chosen the dose of misoprostol prescribed is usually higher (800 micrograms instead of 600). NICE guidance recommends that Mifepristone should not be offered as treatment. Methotrexate is used for ectopic pregnancy.

Source: NICE Guideline, No. CG154, 'Ectopic Pregnancy and Miscarriage: diagnosis and initial management' (2012).

6.16 A 24-year-old woman whose scan reveals PCO consults you about management of her facial hirsutism. Her serum testosterone is within normal limits and she does not wish to conceive.

Which of these treatments for PCO is the most appropriate management option?

A. Clomifene citrate

B. ***Co-cyprindiol COC**

C. Cyproterone acetate

D. Metformin

E. Ovarian drilling

Clomifene, metformin, and ovarian drilling are all treatments designed to produce ovulation so are used to treat fertility problems. Cyproterone is an anti-androgen that can be used in large doses (when it might cause menstrual irregularity and liver tumours although it is effective against hirsutism) or small doses in the form of the co-cyprindiol pill – the latter will be more suitable because she needs contraception.

6.17 In your GP surgery you see a diabetic woman aged 49 years who seeks treatment for irregular heavy menstrual bleeding. Her pelvis feels normal on examination and speculum reveals a healthy cervix.

Which of the following statements about her management is correct?

A. LH/FSH levels are a useful investigation

B. Serum ferritin should be measured as well as haemoglobin at the first visit

C. ***She should be referred to gynaecology clinic**

D. Testing for coagulation disorders should be done prior to commencing treatment

E. Tranexamic acid can be prescribed as first line therapy

This woman should be referred because the bleeding is irregular, which makes the chances of serious endometrial pathology higher. Diabetes is a risk factor for endometrial cancer.

It is unlikely that a coagulation disorder will present in this age group – the problem will have been noticed at menarche. LH and FSH levels do not reliably go up until she has finished menstruating; therefore they are a good test to diagnose premature menopause in a woman with secondary amenorrhoea but do not predict the menopause.

6.18 You are seeing a 48-year-old woman for a preoperative checkup. She is due to have a hysterectomy for fibroids next week and is thinking of having her normal ovaries removed at the same time as the uterus. She wishes to discuss the possible benefits and problems associated with a surgical menopause. Which one of her ideas about the bilateral oophorectomy operation is actually correct?

A. Oophorectomy will not affect her libido

B. She will need sequential HRT to get rid of her menopausal symptoms

C. It will completely prevent her from getting any gynaecological cancer in later life

D. ***She should consider oophorectomy if her mother had ovarian cancer**

E. Oophorectomy will increase the operating time substantially

The loss of the testosterone-producing ovaries could decrease her libido and some women ask for testosterone replacement therapy because of this. She will be able to take estrogen-only HRT instead of sequential HRT (with all its progestogen side effects) as she has no uterus. It will not completely protect her against ovarian cancer as there are patients who develop a condition called primary peritoneal cancer, which looks and behaves like ovarian cancer even though their ovaries have been removed. Removing the ovaries does not add anything to the operating time and family history is a strong predisposing factor for ovarian cancer.

6.19 A 23-year-old woman with a BMI of 50 attends your GP surgery to discuss her fertility problems because she and her husband have been trying to conceive for 18 months. She has irregular periods with a cycle varying from 35 to 42 days and the ovulation predictor kits she has purchased from the chemist indicate that she is not ovulating. Her husband has two children from his previous marriage.

Which of the following is the most appropriate piece of advice?

A. Continue trying for 6 more months then you will refer her to infertility clinic

B. Commence taking folic acid 10 mcg daily

C. Make an appointment for her husband to arrange a semen analysis

D. Prescribe clomifene citrate to be taken on days 2 to 6 of the cycle

E. ***To avoid pregnancy until she has lost weight**

She is likely to be anovulatory because of her weight and fertility treatments do not work well in women with such a high BMI. In addition, pregnancy poses a great risk to her health when she is at risk of developing problems such as diabetes, hypertension, pre-eclampsia, and so forth. In the recent CMACE maternal mortality report more than half the patients who died were morbidly obese.

6.20 A young woman attends her GP's surgery with a positive pregnancy test after 7 weeks of amenorrhoea. She is anxious because has suffered two previous early pregnancy losses; a miscarriage at 10 weeks followed by an ectopic pregnancy that was managed surgically. Which course of action is most appropriate?

A. Admit to gynaecology ward

B. Arrange midwifery booking

C. ***Refer for early scan**

D. Refer to antenatal clinic

E. Take blood for serum hCG in the surgery

The main worry here is the ectopic pregnancy history, which carries a recurrence risk of 10 per cent, so she needs an early scan to confirm intrauterine pregnancy.

Extended Matching Questions

A	Ascorbic acid
B	Clomifene citrate
C	Danazol
D	Depo-Provera®
E	Dianette®
F	LHRH analogues
G	Medroxyprogesterone acetate
H	Mefenamic acid
I	Tamoxifen
J	Tibolone
K	Tranexamic acid

Each of these clinical scenarios describes a woman presenting to her GP requesting help with menstrual problems; for each patient pick the most appropriate treatment option given the information that you are presented with.

Each option may be used once, more than once, or not at all.

6.21 A 22-year-old nulliparous lady who is not currently sexually active seeking treatment for menorrhagia and primary dysmenorrhoea

H. Mefenamic acid

This woman does not need contraception therefore your choices are between mefenamic and tranexamic acid. Mefenamic acid is better for this patient as it would also treat her dysmenorrhoea.

6.22 An obese teenager with acne and frequent heavy periods seeking secure contraception

E. Dianette®

This girl may have PCO but in any case she has androgenic problems in terms of her acne. She needs secure contraception and a cyproterone containing combined pill will give her that as well as helping with her skin.

6.23 A 34-year-old overweight woman with irregular heavy bleeding whose endometrial biopsy reveals cystic hyperplasia with no atypia

G. Medroxyprogesterone acetate

Endometrial hyperplasia should be treated with progestogen. The usual management plan is for her to take it for 6 months and then have a repeat endometrial biopsy to check that it has been adequately treated. A Mirena® would also be suitable although it is not licensed for this.

If there had been atypia on the histology report, she should have a hysterectomy as this is a premalignant condition and some of these women already have endometrial cancer.

6.24 A 30-year-old woman with three children has just undergone a third termination of pregnancy without complications. She has attended the surgery twice in the past for help with her menorrhagia and dysmenorrhoea.

D. Depo-Provera®

This woman clearly needs a secure method of contraception as well as help with her periods. Depo-Provera® would be an appropriate option to deliver both, although the effect on her periods may be unpredictable.

6.25 A sterilised 32-year-old woman whose menorrhagia has not responded to treatment with nonsteroidal antiinflammatory drugs

K. Tranexamic acid

This woman does not need contraception and if her period problems do not respond to mefenamic acid, tranexamic acid is the next option.

A	Anterior colporrhaphy operation
B	Antibiotics
C	Biofeedback
D	Bladder drill (retraining)
E	Helmstein bladder distension
F	Injection of phenol into the bladder trigone
G	Sacrocolpopexy operation
H	Supervised pelvic floor physiotherapy
I	TVT operation

Each of these scenarios describes a woman presenting to gynaecology clinic with urinary incontinence; for each patient pick the most appropriate treatment option given the clinical information.

Each option may be used once, more than once, or not at all.

6.26 Eighteen months after a colposuspension operation for stress incontinence, a 60-year-old woman presents with a recurrence of her incontinence. She brings with her the results of a private urodynamic study that she had done after surfing the Internet. This shows that she has a compliant bladder on filling in a sitting position, but when she stands up there is demonstrable leakage of urine associated with spikes of high detrusor pressure measurements >30 cm water.

D Bladder drill

This woman has an unstable bladder – likely to be a de-novo problem following her stress incontinence surgery. The first-line management would be bladder drill; anticholinergics could also help but we haven't given you this option.

6.27 Less than a week after her bladder pressure study where she was diagnosed as having detrusor instability, a 51-year-old postmenopausal woman comes to the surgery seeking treatment on account of a marked deterioration in her symptoms of dysuria, urinary frequency, and urgency with urge incontinence.

B Antibiotics

Urinary tract infection is a complication of a bladder pressure study because of the catheterisation involved.

6.28 Six months after the normal vaginal birth of her first child, a 37-year-old teacher complains of urinary incontinence when doing her aerobic classes. On examination she does have a moderate cystocoele and minor rectocoele but no uterine descent.

H Supervised pelvic floor physiotherapy

A young woman with a minor prolapse like this is likely to respond to intensive physiotherapy.

6.29 A bladder pressure study excludes detrusor instability in a 55-year-old woman with a mixed picture of stress and urge urinary incontinence. Her symptoms are getting worse with frequent leakage despite intensive supervised pelvic floor physiotherapy.

I TVT operation

If her symptoms have not responded to physiotherapy, she should consider surgery and the TVT is the only operation on the list that fits the bill.

6.30 A fit 62-year-old woman has had a vaginal hysterectomy done years ago for menorrhagia. She presents with 'something coming down' and on examination of the external genitalia you can see the vaginal vault protruding.

G Sacrocolpopexy operation

The only treatment option on this list that would deal adequately with vault prolapse is this operation where the vaginal vault is fixed to the sacral promontory.

A	Appendicitis
B	Ectopic pregnancy
C	Haemorrhage into an ovarian cyst
D	Incomplete miscarriage
E	Missed miscarriage
F	Normal intrauterine pregnancy
G	Partial hydatidiform mole
H	Threatened miscarriage
I	Urinary tract infection

These clinical scenarios describe women presenting with pain in early pregnancy. For each case select the most likely diagnosis.

Each option may be used once, more than once, or not at all.

6.31 A 23-year-old woman comes in to the Gynaecological Admission Unit complaining of left iliac fossa pain. She is very tender on the left side of her abdomen and on pelvic examination you find cervical excitation. She has had 7 weeks of amenorrhea and her serum βhCG is 5,000 IU/ml. The transvaginal ultrasound scan shows a small, empty, rounded structure (thought to be a gestational sac) in the uterus.

B Ectopic pregnancy

The history and examination findings would make you suspect ectopic pregnancy. The rounded structure in the uterus on the scan could just as easily be a decidual ring as there are no contents in the 'gestational sac' and does not rule out ectopic.

6.32 A week after her 12-week dating scan, a 24-year-old woman presents to A&E with an acute onset of central abdominal pain and nausea. On examination you find severe lower abdominal tenderness with generalised guarding and rebound. Her white cell count is 14×10^6/l, and urinalysis is negative.

A Appendicitis

Just because someone is pregnant does not mean that their symptoms must be related to the pregnancy. Appendicitis can be difficult to diagnose in more advanced pregnancy because the position of the appendix can alter.

6.33 An obese 35-year-old who had her Mirena® IUS removed 5 months ago on account of breast tenderness attends her GP to complain of lower abdominal discomfort and that her breast tenderness persists. She remains amenorrhoeic. On examination you can feel a mass in her lower abdomen above the symphysis pubis.

F Normal intrauterine pregnancy

The mass could be an ovarian cyst but in the absence of contraception it is more likely to be a pregnant uterus.

6.34 A 21-year-old woman is admitted to A&E by ambulance having collapsed while out shopping. On arrival at hospital she is complaining of shoulder tip pain, and examination shows a tender abdomen with guarding. She had a copper coil fitted just after the delivery of her 2-year-old son, and thinks her last menstrual period was 2 weeks ago although it was lighter than usual.

B Ectopic pregnancy

The fact that she has collapsed and has shoulder tip pain suggests ectopic.

6.35 A primigravid woman presents to the Early Pregnancy Unit with a history of 11 weeks' amenorrhea, minor lower abdominal discomfort, and a small amount of vaginal bleeding. A urine pregnancy test is positive. Pelvic examination reveals no tenderness and the uterus is the correct size with a closed cervical os.

H Threatened miscarriage

You won't know whether it is a viable pregnancy or not until you get the scan result. The absence of pelvic tenderness makes ectopic less likely and the fact that the uterus is the right size for dates means that the diagnosis is not likely to be missed miscarriage either.

A	Adenomyosis
B	Appendicitis
C	Chronic pelvic inflammatory disease
D	Endometriosis
E	Interstitial cystitis
F	Irritable bowel syndrome
G	Ovarian cyst
H	Polycystic ovarian syndrome
I	Urinary tract infection
J	Uterine fibroids

These clinical scenarios describe nonpregnant women presenting in the gynaecology clinic with lower abdominal or pelvic pain. For each case select the most likely diagnosis.

Each option may be used once, more than once, or not at all.

6.36 A 22-year-old student with an 18-month history of noncyclical intermittent lower abdominal pain and deep dyspareunia. She is tender in both adnexae and the uterus is retroverted.

C Chronic pelvic inflammatory disease

As her pain is noncyclical, this suggests PID rather than endometriosis.

6.37 As well as experiencing deep dyspareunia for 6 months, a 48-year-old woman has pain when her bladder is full, which is associated with urinary frequency and nocturia.

E Interstitial cystitis

Interstitial cystitis produces pain that is always worse when the bladder is full and is often mistaken for endometriosis and chronic PID. The bladder will be very tender on bimanual examination, and it is sometimes refractory to treatment. It is diagnosed at cystoscopy.

6.38 After years of being on the pill, a 35-year-old woman has developed gradually increasing severe dysmenorrhoea, intermittent pelvic pain, and dyspareunia in her first pill-free year. On examination her uterus is normal size but both adnexae are tender.

D Endometriosis

The pill often protects women from the manifestations of endometriosis until they stop taking it in later life.

6.39 A woman who has had five normal deliveries complains of increasingly severe secondary dysmenorrhoea. Her periods are regular but becoming heavier. The uterus is bulky and very tender on pelvic examination.

A Adenomyosis

If the uterus is very tender on examination this suggests adenomyosis, which is more common in multiparous women. It produces severe secondary dysmenorrhoea. If the uterus is irregularly enlarged, this suggests fibroids instead.

6.40 A 24-year-old woman has been using the pill since her teenage years to control her heavy periods as well as for contraception. She seeks help on account of intermittent pain in both iliac fossae associated with abdominal bloating and deep dyspareunia.

F Irritable bowel syndrome

The bloating is the clue to this diagnosis. There is a useful description of the management of women with pelvic pain in the RCOG Green-top Guideline, No. 41, 'The Initial Management of Chronic Pelvic Pain' (2012).

A	Reassurance only
B	Repeat pelvic ultrasound at beginning of next cycle
C	Repeat pelvic ultrasound in 3 months
D	Repeat serum CA125
E	Routine referral to a gynaecological oncologist
F	Routine referral to a gynaecologist
G	Serum CA125 and repeat pelvic USS
H	Serum CA125 and urgent (2-week wait) referral to gynaecologist
I	Urgent (2-week wait) referral to gynaecological oncologist
J	Urgent (2-week wait) referral to gynaecologist

Each of these clinical scenarios relates to a woman presenting in a GP surgery with an ovarian cyst. In each case select the most appropriate management plan for that patient.

Each option may be used once, more than once, or not at all

6.41 A 54-year-old postmenopausal woman presents to your surgery with irregular vaginal bleeding over the last 6 months. An USS shows an endometrial thickness of 8 mm and large bilateral multiloculated ovarian cysts. There are no other abnormal features on the scan.

H. Serum CA125 and urgent (2-week wait) referral to gynaecologist

The cysts and the thickened endometrium might be related (granulosa cell tumours secreting estrogen and causing endometrial stimulation) but in any case she requires a 2-week wait referral because she may have endometrial cancer. The CA125 will help work out the RMI, which guides the treatment plan for the ovarian cysts. It might not be malignant, so referral to a gynaecologist initially rather than oncology is indicated.

6.42 A 27-year-old woman gives a history of long-standing dysmenorrhoea and deep dyspareunia. A pelvic ultrasound shows a unilocular 4 cm diameter cyst on the left ovary consistent with a 'chocolate cyst'.

F. Routine referral to a gynaecologist

This woman probably has endometriosis and should be referred for further investigation and management of her symptoms. CA125 doesn't usually help that much with the diagnosis as it is often mildly raised in cases of endometriosis.

6.43 A 19-year-old woman attends surgery with right iliac fossa pain, nausea, and vomiting. Her last menstrual period was 3 weeks before and an USS shows a 3 cm diameter right ovarian cyst with internal echoes consistent with haemorrhage. Her pain settles with simple analgesia.

C. Repeat pelvic ultrasound in 3 months

This cyst is likely to disappear over the next few months as the most likely diagnosis is an ovulatory cyst. The beginning of the next cycle is a little too early to rescan to check it has disappeared. Persistence of the cyst would require referral.

6.44 A 39-year-old woman complains of left iliac fossa pain radiating down her left leg. The ultrasound shows a 9 cm diameter complex cyst on her left ovary and her CA125 level is 470.

I. Urgent (2-week wait) referral to gynaecological oncologist

The high CA125 level increases the chance of this cyst being malignant therefore she requires urgent referral to a gynaecology oncology service.

6.45 A 65-year-old woman presents to the surgery with loss of appetite and abdominal distension, 12 years after her menopause. It started with a bout of 'gastroenteritis' that has just settled. You organise a CA125 level, which is slightly raised at 55, and an USS of the pelvis, which is normal.

D. Repeat serum CA125

This scenario has become increasingly common since the recommendation that GPs 'think ovarian cancer' and request CA125 levels on women presenting with nebulous distension symptoms. The problem is that other conditions such as bowel problems (diverticulitis, gastroenteritis, inflammatory bowel disease) can also raise the levels. In this case a repeat CA125 level is indicated as it will have decreased if the bowel problem has resolved. If the level is increasing a repeat ultrasound is indicated to see if anything is developing on the ovaries.

A	Ergometrine infusion over 4 hours
B	Evacuation of uterus on routine consultant list tomorrow
C	Evacuation of uterus immediately on emergency list
D	Evacuation of uterus after cervical priming
E	Gemeprost pessaries

F	Intravenous antibiotics
G	Methotrexate injection
H	Mifepristone and misoprostol
I	Oxytocin infusion over 4 hours
J	Repeat βHCG level in 48 hours

These clinical scenarios describe women experiencing complications in the first trimester of pregnancy. For each case, select the most appropriate management plan for that patient.

Each option may be used once, more than once, or not at all.

6.46 Having developed hyperemesis, a 39-year-old primigravid patient has an USS during her hospital admission that shows a 'snowstorm appearance'. You are asked to review the scan and plan management when you take over the night shift at 8 pm.

B Evacuation of uterus on routine consultant list tomorrow

The scan shows the typical appearance of a hydatidiform molar pregnancy. She requires a careful evacuation of the uterus to remove all the abnormal tissue and histological classification of the type of molar pregnancy. These are difficult evacuation operations to perform and a senior surgeon is required.

Follow-up with βHCG measurements is arranged in conjunction with the appropriate National Gestational Trophoblast Disease Surveillance Centre.

The distracters are immediate evacuation or cervical preparation, but not medical evacuation.

6.47 A 20-year-old shop assistant presents to early pregnancy unit at 7 weeks gestation in her second pregnancy complaining of left-sided abdominal pain. She had an ectopic pregnancy a year ago that was treated by laparoscopic right salpingectomy. Her BP and pulse are normal and scan shows an empty uterus with a mixed echo mass in the left adnexa that is 2 cm in diameter. The βhCG level is 2,150 iu/ml and haemoglobin is 117 g/l.

G Methotrexate injection

This woman only has one fallopian tube left and the clinical information suggests that she has another ectopic pregnancy in that remaining tube. Her only chance of achieving a pregnancy in the future without assisted conception is to retain that tube so medical management of ectopic is more appropriate than surgical here. Awaiting a repeat βHCG level before organising treatment is not sensible because the diagnosis is clear.

6.48 A routine 'dating' USS shows that a 21-year-old woman who had a ventouse delivery for her previous child 9 months ago, has suffered a missed miscarriage.

D Evacuation of uterus after cervical priming

The history indicates that there was no warning symptom that might have prompted earlier investigation. With missed miscarriage, the cervix is more resistant to dilatation so cervical priming is needed and surgical evacuation is preferred to medical management.

6.49 On admission to the gynaecology ward, you note that a young woman admitted with bleeding at 10 weeks of gestation has a temperature of 38.5°C and a tender uterus. There is a small amount of bleeding on speculum examination but the cervical os is open and you can see what looks like a gestation sac protruding through.

F Intravenous antibiotics

The pyrexia and tenderness suggest a diagnosis of sepsis and although the uterus needs to be evacuated at some point, administering antibiotics is the first priority.

6.50 At 2 am you are summoned to A&E urgently to see a 23-year-old woman who is having a miscarriage. There is a great deal of blood all over the bed and someone has initiated an intravenous infusion as she is hypotensive. On speculum examination you must remove clots from the vagina to visualise the cervix and find that the cervical os is wide open.

C Evacuation of uterus immediately on emergency list

You must do something to stop her bleeding and the best way to do this is to evacuate the uterus, which needs doing as an emergency because of the severity of her bleeding.

Curriculum Module 7

Answers

Single Best Answer Questions

7.1 If a 15-year-old schoolgirl consults you in the surgery for contraception provision, select the most appropriate statement:

A. She should be advised to have a cervical smear as she has become sexually active

B. She cannot attend a family planning clinic until she reaches the age of 16 years

C. There are unlikely to be child protection issues if she is deemed competent to give consent for treatment

D. You must inform her parents or legal guardians before prescribing

E. *You should enquire about her sexual history regarding partners

If you think she is mentally competent to understand the implications of the course of action she is embarking on and the complications and side effects of the proposed contraceptive method, then she can give consent. Obviously it is better if her parents are aware of the situation but you cannot insist on that. You should enquire about the age of her partner(s) because you may need to consider child protection issues and you also have a duty of care to consider the possibility of sexually transmitted diseases. Even though she has become sexually active at a very young age, she does not have a smear until the age of 25 years under the current screening programme rules.

7.2 Which of these statements is correct regarding the health of women who are using the combined pill for contraception?

A. *An alternative method should be used if they are planning a long high-altitude trek

B. A family history of breast cancer is a contraindication

C. The risk of mortality from large bowel cancer is increased

D. The failure rate in typical use rather than in ideal use is <1 per cent

E. The risk of venous thromboembolism is about the same as in pregnancy

High-altitude trekking (above 4,500 metres) is associated with an increased risk of VTE and if planning to do this for more than a week, women should plan to change their contraceptive method.

Women with a family history of breast cancer already have an increased risk compared to the background risk but there is no evidence that taking the COC increases this risk.

A large cohort study found a significantly lower mortality from bowel cancer in COC users. Typical use represents actual use involving inconsistent or incorrect

pill taking as opposed to perfect or ideal use. The failure rate with ideal use is 0.3 per cent but in real life it is more like 9 per cent.

The risk of VTE in COC users is about 10 times less than pregnancy (29 per 10,000 women years against 300–400 per 10,000 women years).

Source:

Clinical Guidance, Faculty of Sexual and Reproductive Healthcare website www .fsrh.org

7.3 A woman comes to the GP surgery requesting referral for female sterilisation as she has had trouble with various other forms of contraception. She is not in a stable relationship currently but has had six pregnancies: five children and one ectopic pregnancy.

Which of these statements is correct regarding sterilisation?

A. A history of previous ectopic pregnancy is a contraindication to laparoscopic sterilisation

B. If she regrets her decision, reversal involves laparoscopic clip removal

C. Mirena® IUS has a much lower Pearl index than sterilisation

D. Sterilisation carries a lifetime failure rate of 1 in 2,000

E. *There is a future risk of ectopic pregnancy

If she regrets having it done, a laparotomy will be needed to reconstruct the fallopian tubes and restore patency as the portion of the tube under the clip is irretrievably crushed. Reversal operations are rarely available on the NHS.

In terms of contraceptive reliability (Pearl index) sterilisation is about the same as Mirena.

The chance of a sterilisation operation failing in a woman's lifetime is reckoned to be about 1 in 200 and, if it does fail, there is a substantial chance of the pregnancy being tubal.

7.4 Which three compounds can be found as the estrogen component in combined oral contraception formulations?

A. Conjugated equine estrogen, estriol, estradiol valerate

B. Estriol, estradiol valerate, ethinylestradiol

C. Mestranol, estriol, estradiol valerate

D. *Mestranol, estradiol valerate, ethinylestradiol

E. Mestranol, estriol, ethinylestradiol

Conjugated equine estrogen is used in HRT preparations. Estriol is the estrogen produced by the placenta in pregnancy and used to be measured as a placental function test many years ago. The others are all used in COCs.

7.5 A 15-year-old girl attends the GP surgery requesting contraception as she is sexually active using condoms but is very worried about pregnancy and wishes to use something much more secure. She has no relevant past medical history and you deem her to be Fraser competent to make decisions on her own behalf.

Select the best first line contraception for her:

A. Combined pill

B. Depot medroxyprogesterone acetate

C. *Etonogestrel implant

D. Levonorgestrel IUS

E. Progestogen-only pill

The COC, POP, and implant are all UKMEC 1 and are recommended as first-line treatment for young women. There is evidence that the failure rate of the POP and COC are higher in teenagers and the discontinuation rate at 1 year is higher than in older women. Therefore, the best answer is etonogestrel implant. Both Depot Provera and the levonorgestrel IUS are UKMEC 2 for use in teenagers, and are not first-line choices.

Source: UK Medical Eligibility Criteria for Contraceptive Use (UKMEC), Faculty of Sexual and Reproductive Healthcare website www.fsrh.org

7.6 A 52-year-old woman had a Mirena IUS® inserted 5 years ago for treatment of menorrhagia as well as contraception. She has been amenorrhoeic since it was inserted and is requesting HRT for menopausal symptoms.

What is the most appropriate advice to give her regarding her Mirena IUS® and contraception?

A. If her Mirena IUS® is removed she should use barrier contraception for another 2 years

B. *In terms of her contraceptive needs the Mirena IUS® is effective for another 2 years*

C. Remove the Mirena IUS® as it will have run out of levonorgestrel

D. The Mirena IUS® can be removed as HRT is adequate contraception

E. The Mirena IUS® should be left in place so she can use estrogen-only HRT

The problem is that you do not know when this woman became menopausal as she is amenorrhoeic due to the Mirena, so the difficulty is with her ongoing contraceptive needs.

The Faculty of Sexual and Reproductive Health (FSRH) advises that although the license for the Mirena IUS® specifies replacement every 5 years, after the age of 45 women can retain the Mirena IUS® for up to 7 years and only need replacement of the IUS if they haven't become menopausal. If you are not sure whether they are menopausal or not, measure FSH on two occasions six weeks apart. If the result is more than 30iu/l, they are likely to be menopausal. If the IUS is used for more than 5 years to provide contraception in this scenario, then you need to record the discussion and agreement in the medical notes.

Over the age of 40 but under the age of 50 using a nonhormonal method of contraception a period of 2 years of amenorrhoea is required before cessation of the contraception can be recommended. Over the age of 50 in a similar situation 1 year of amenorrhoea is required.

HRT is not contraceptive. If the IUS is used to oppose estrogen-only HRT the licence is 4 years, not 5 years so this IUS should be replaced.

Source: Contraception for Women Aged Over 40 years. Faculty of Sexual and Reproductive Health Clinical Effectiveness Unit. (2010) www.fsrh.org

7.7 You are asked to review a woman on the Day Case Unit who had a laparoscopic sterilisation yesterday. She has had four children between the ages of 6 months and 4 years, all delivered by caesarean section.

The nurses are concerned because she maintains that she is still not well enough to go home, although your consultant saw her last night after the operating list had finished and discharged her. When you examine her, you notice that the dressing on her suprapubic incision is wet.

Select the most appropriate course of action:

A. Arrange an ultrasound
B. Enquire sensitively about home circumstances
C. Increase her analgesia
D. Prescribe antibiotics
E. *Request a cystogram

The main issue is to realise that something has gone wrong during the operation as she should be well enough to go home by now. The lower incision may have perforated the bladder because it is stuck there due to her previous sections and the best way to diagnose that is with a cystogram.

7.8 A woman who has had two children has a Mirena IUS® fitted at the hospital. She attends the surgery for a checkup 6 weeks later but on speculum examination you cannot find the coil strings.

Which of the following statements is correct regarding counselling her about the situation?

A. An x-ray is better than an USS to locate the coil
B. She cannot be pregnant if the coil is in the uterus
C. *She is not currently covered for contraception
D. The coil could not have been extruded per vaginam without her noticing
E. The next step is to try and retrieve the coil strings with a thread retriever

Until you know where the coil is, she cannot assume that she has a secure method of contraception. The coil could be in the uterus and the strings could have disappeared because the uterus is enlarging (she is pregnant) or because the strings are alongside the coil in the cavity. Alternatively, it could have fallen out of the uterus or have perforated the uterus at insertion. You need to ascertain her LMP and exclude pregnancy before proceeding further. A scan will show whether the coil is in the uterus, and if it is not an x-ray is then indicated to see if the coil has perforated the uterus and is somewhere in her abdomen.

7.9 In the surgery you are counselling a woman who is considering using a POP for contraception. Which is correct information about these preparations?

A. *Additional measures are not required if the method is initiated on days 1 to 5 of the menstrual cycle
B. She can expect a couple of kilos weight gain associated with POP use
C. She should stop taking POP prior to major surgery to avoid thromboembolism
D. There is a link between POP use and breast cancer
E. The window for missed pill taking is only 3 hours for all formulations

If the POP is initiated after day 5 of the menstrual cycle or if the woman is amenorrhoeic, additional measures are recommended for 48 hours.

All progesterone methods including injectables are suitable for women having major surgery or immobilised, for example, due to lower limb trauma. The missed pill window is 3 hours except for Cerazette® where it is 12 hours. There is no published evidence linking the POP with breast cancer or weight gain.

7.10 When advising women about methods of postcoital emergency contraception?

A. The copper device should be fitted within 10 days of unprotected intercourse

B. The levonorgestrel pill (Levonelle®) can only be used once in a cycle

C. Ulipristal (EllaOne®) works primarily by altering the endometrium to prevent implantation

D. Use of the coil may predispose to ectopic, but not the oral methods

E. *Women with poorly controlled asthma should avoid ulipristal (EllaOne®)

Ten days is too late for coil insertion – implantation could have occurred by then.

Repeated doses of levonorgestrel can be used during the same cycle on a named patient basis but are likely to interfere with her bleeding pattern. Ulipristal works by inhibiting ovulation mainly but there is some effect on the endometrium too.

There is a risk of ectopic pregnancy with progesterone methods, so if she experiences pain subsequently, she might have an ectopic and it needs investigating further.

Ulipristal can provoke an asthma attack.

7.11 Which is the single best course of action if a woman presents to your surgery at 12 weeks of gestation having conceived with an IUCD in situ?

A. Do serial βHCG estimations to exclude ectopic pregnancy

B. Repeat the pregnancy test to check for miscarriage

C. *Remove the coil if the strings can be visualised

D. Request an x-ray to localise the coil

E. Take triple swabs as infection is likely in this situation

An USS is better than a repeat pregnancy test to check for viability of the pregnancy.

The reason for removing the coil is that the risk of miscarriage is higher if it stays in the uterus and there is an increased risk of sepsis, risking the health and possibly even the life of the mother.

X-ray is contraindicated especially in the first trimester of pregnancy.

Although screening for infection is reasonable, the best answer is to remove the coil.

If this pregnancy were ectopic it is likely to have caused symptoms by the time the pregnancy has reached 12 weeks and in any case at this gestation USS is a better investigation than serial βhCG in excluding ectopic pregnancy. We tend to use serial βhCG much earlier in pregnancy (<6 weeks) if the gestation is too early to see an intrauterine sac on scan.

7.12 A woman whose pelvic USS indicates that she has polycystic ovarian syndrome consults you because she does not wish to conceive for a couple of years. She has sought help previously for management of her facial hirsutism and her serum testosterone is within normal limits.

Select the most appropriate management option in her case from this list:

A. Clomifene citrate

B. *Co-cyprindiol (cyproterone acetate and 35 mcg ethinylestradiol)

C. Cyproterone acetate

D. Levonorgestrel releasing intrauterine system

E. Metformin

As this woman is requesting contraception, your options are co-cyprindiol or the IUS, because the other preparations are not contraceptive. The IUS will not treat her hirsutism.

7.13 Which one of the following statements about laparoscopic female sterilisation is correct?

A. Applying two clips to each tube is advisable to improve efficacy

B. Diathermy sterilisation increases the chances of successful reversal

C. The clips are made of nickel so can't be used if a woman is allergic to base metal

D. The operation is usually done under local anaesthetic

E. ***The patient should regard it as an irreversible method of contraception**

Some women seem to think that you can just remove the clips from the tubes and they will be fertile again. The reversal operation involves a painstaking re-anastomosis of each tube with a variable success rate, depending on many factors including the length of tube remaining after reversal. Diathermy destroys the structure of the tube along most of its length thereby reducing the chance of successful reversal. Applying two clips to the tube can cause a hydrosalpinx to form between the clips, which could be painful – better to ensure correct application of one clip (to the tube, the whole tube and nothing but the tube).

The operation can be done under local but takes much longer and requires a stoical patient!

7.14 A 28-year-old woman who is virgo intacta wishes to start contraception in advance of her marriage, which is arranged for a few months' time. She has polycystic ovarian syndrome that was diagnosed when she saw a gynaecologist with oligomenorrhea, and she is worried that she will develop hirsutism, which would spoil her wedding photographs.

From this list, select the most appropriate form of contraception for her in these unusual circumstances:

A. Cerazette®

B. Dianette®

C. ***Marvelon®**

D. Nexplanon®

E. NuvaRing®

Hirsutism is a secondary issue to contraception for this woman, but combined hormonal contraception increases the level of sex hormone binding globulin, which over time can reduce the level of free testosterone and improve hirsutism. Dianette should only be used if she has significant hirsutism and other options are not tolerated or effective because of the potential effects of cyproterone on the liver.

Progesterone – only contraception would have no effect on the potential hirsutism.

As she is virgo intacta NuvaRing® would not be suitable in her case.

7.15 A woman has unprotected intercourse with a stranger at a party 2 days before she consults you for emergency contraception. She has since heard that he is HIV positive and she has made herself an appointment with the local GUM Clinic this afternoon.

Choose the best option for emergency contraception in her case:

A. EllaOne®

B. Levonelle 1500®

C. Marvelon®

D. Mirena®

E. ***Multiload Cu 375®**

The woman is at risk of both unplanned pregnancy and contracting HIV. She will require postexposure HIV prophylaxis, and these drugs are inhibitors of liver enzyme inhibitors so oral hormonal emergency contraception methods are not recommended. The Multiload Cu375® can be inserted up to 120 hours after unprotected intercourse.

Neither Mirena® and Marvelon® are licensed for emergency contraception.

Without the HIV problem, Levonelle® could be used up to 72 hours and EllaOne® up to 120 hours after unprotected intercourse.

Source: UK Guideline for the use of postexposure prophylaxis for HIV following sexual exposure,

www.bashh.org.documents/4076.pdf

www.fsrh.org/pdfs/CEUguidanceEmergencyContraception11.pdf.

7.16 A woman who is using a copper IUD for contraception has had a cervical smear that shows the presence of actinomyces-like organisms. She has no pelvic pain or vaginal discharge and on examination her pelvis is normal. Her LMP was 2 weeks ago and she had sexual intercourse yesterday.

Which is the most appropriate management option for this woman?

A. Leave the IUD in place and arrange an USS to exclude pelvic abscess

B. ***Leave the IUD in place and reassure**

C. Remove the IUD and prescribe emergency contraception

D. Remove the IUD and prescribe penicillin

E. Remove the IUD and repeat the smear

Actinomycosis is an uncommon infection that cannot be diagnosed on routine swab culture. The infection is diagnosed on cytology or histology because of the presence of hyphae with sulphur granules. It can colonise the oral, gastrointestinal, and genitourinary tracts and is associated with the presence of a foreign body in the female genital tract.

It can cause abscesses that sometimes resemble tumours, and pathology books describe the organism as 'the great mimicker' as the lesion can be mistaken for cancer until the histology is revealed.

If the woman is asymptomatic you do not need to do anything and the IUD can be left in place. If she has pelvic pain, tenderness, or a mass the device must be removed and referral for urgent gynaecological opinion is indicated.

Source: For further reading: www.patient.co.uk/doctor/Actinomycosis.htm.

7.17 A neurology consultant colleague has written to you about an epileptic patient on your surgery list whose compliance with her phenytoin medication is poor so that she is having frequent fits. She attends surgery asking for contraceptive advice, having found a new partner.

What is the best method of contraception for her?

A. Cerazette®
B. Evra®
C. Marvelon®
D. ***Mirena®**
E. NuvaRing®

Phenytoin is an enzyme inducer and all forms of contraception on the list are metabolised in the liver except for Mirena®. She is a poor tablet taker as well and you want to avoid pregnancy in someone on Phenytoin.

7.18 Which of the following statements is true of abortions performed in the United Kingdom?

A. ***More than 90 per cent of terminations are performed in the first trimester below 13 weeks of gestation**
B. Patients are not usually screened for STIs if undergoing medical rather than surgical termination
C. Patients are routinely scanned to check the gestational age of the pregnancy
D. Simultaneous sterilisation should be carried out on request if the patient is having a general anaesthetic
E. Subsequent subfertility can be reliably prevented by administering routine antibiotic prophylaxis effective against chlamydia

Scanning is available in most termination clinics but not routinely recommended unless there is a discrepancy between the gestational age and clinical findings. The risk of infection is the same for medical and surgical termination.

Government statistics collected for 2012 showed that 91 per cent of terminations are carried out below 13 weeks in the United Kingdom, presumably due to the increasing use of early medical termination. Antibiotic prophylaxis does not always prevent subsequent pelvic inflammatory disease especially if no contact tracing is undertaken or if the patient is noncompliant with treatment.

Some patients who are sterilised at the same time regret having it done especially if they experience regret about the termination, and it may not be advisable to make such an important decision when under pressure. Many women who have a termination replace the unwanted pregnancy with another one within months. The failure rate of sterilisation is higher when it is undertaken during pregnancy as the tubes are hypertrophied and there is a risk that a clip will not completely occlude the tubes.

7.19 A 40-year-old woman with mild learning difficulties needs contraception because she is having a sexual relationship with another patient in the same residential accommodation. An USS is requested because her periods are known to be heavy and this reveals multiple small submucosal fibroids distorting her uterine cavity.

Select the most appropriate form of contraception in her case:

A. Copper IUD
B. Hysterectomy

C.   Mercilon®

D.   Mirena®

E.   *Nexplanon®

Long-acting reversible contraception offers the best option because her learning difficulties might result in noncompliance. An assessment of mental capacity would be needed when taking consent. As her uterine cavity is distorted Nexplanon® would be more suitable than Mirena®.

7.20 Which of the following statements is not true about the use of the combined oral contraceptive pill?

A.   It will reduce primary dysmenorrhoea

B.   It ameliorates the symptoms of premenstrual syndrome

C.   ***It is associated with an increased risk of pelvic inflammatory disease**

D.   It reduces the incidence of benign breast disease

E.   It reduces the risk of ovarian cancer in later life

There is known to be a positive effect on the incidence of benign breast disease and pelvic inflammatory disease and the COC is recognised as an effective treatment for women with PMS or dysmenorrhoea. Ovarian cancer is linked to 'incessant ovulation', for example, early menarche and late menopause.

Extended Matching Questions

A	COC
B	Depot medroxyprogesterone acetate
C	Etonogestrel subdermal implant
D	Female sterilisation
E	Intrauterine contraceptive device
F	Levonelle®
G	Levonorgestrel intrauterine system
H	Male condom
I	POP
J	Vasectomy

These clinical scenarios relate to women attending your surgery for contraceptive provision. In each case select the most appropriate method for her.

Each option may be used once, more than once, or not at all.

7.21 An 18-year-old student is about to go abroad on a 'gap year' and wishes to organise effective contraception whilst she is away. She has regular periods and no relevant medical or family history

C. Etonogestrel subdermal implant

It may be difficult for this student to access supplies of contraception whilst she is away so a long-acting method with a low Pearl index seems appropriate.

7.22 The development of a latex-allergy rash on the vulva results in a 38-year-old woman requesting a change in her contraceptive plans. She has four children and has consulted you recently for heavy periods.

G. Levonorgestrel intrauterine system

The IUS is ideal as she would get treatment for her menorrhagia as well as contraceptive cover.

7.23 A 17-year-old hairdresser has just had her second termination of pregnancy. Both pregnancies occurred as a result of running out of supplies of the pill.

C. Etonogestrel subdermal implant

Feckless and erratic use of contraception is common amongst teenagers and this is a situation in which long-acting progestogens are more suitable.

7.24 At her postnatal appointment, a 38-year-old mother of three children seeks advice about a reliable method of contraception. She had severe breast tenderness on the POP and is therefore not keen on taking any hormones.

E. Intrauterine contraceptive device

She would have the choice of an IUCD or permanent methods such sterilisation if she doesn't wish to take hormones in any form. The question says reliable rather than permanent and many doctors recommend delaying permanent methods of contraception until the baby is aged one and the risk of cot death is minimal.

7.25 A 32-year-old woman attends gynaecology clinic, having been referred by her GP for sterilisation. She reveals that her husband and father of her two children has just found out about her extramarital affair and left the family home. Her lifestyle is rather chaotic and she needs a very secure method of contraception.

G. Levonorgestrel intrauterine system

Choosing an irreversible permanent method does not seem appropriate for a woman whose husband has just left her, as she is likely to find herself in a new relationship at some stage in the future when she may regret having been sterilised. The IUS has a similar Pearl index to sterilisation but is obviously reversible.

A	3 months
B	6 months
C	12 months
D	24 months
E	5 years
F	7 years
G	10 years
H	15 years
I	20 years

These statements refer to a 47-year-old woman seeking contraceptive advice. Choose the most appropriate time option given the clinical information in each scenario.

Each option may be used once, more than once, or not at all.

7.26 If the 47-year-old woman chooses the Mirena® how long will it be effective as a contraceptive in her particular case?

F   7 years

The licence is only for 5 years but a woman of 47 will be much less fertile when she reaches 52 and could continue to rely on it for another 2 years. As this time limit is 'off licence' you would have to discuss this fully with the patient and record that discussion in the notes.

7.27 If the 47-year-old woman chooses a nonhormonal method, how long should she continue to use the method if she has her menopause (last ever period) next year?

D   24 months

The time recommended depends on the age at which she has her last ever period. If a woman reaches her menopause under the age of 50 years, a time span of two years of amenorrhoea is required before cessation of contraception because there could still be some residual ovarian activity. Over the age of 50 years a time span of 1 year will be sufficient.

7.28 The 47-year-old woman makes an informed decision to choose the combined pill as she has no cardiovascular risk factors. When she eventually stops taking the pill, for how long after cessation could she expect a protective effect against ovarian cancer?

H   15 years

No method is contraindicated on age alone. The combined pill may increase the risk of breast cancer, but it has a protective effect against both endometrial and ovarian cancer that lasts for up to 15 years from cessation of use.

7.29 If the 47-year-old woman makes an informed decision to choose the combined pill, how soon should you check her blood pressure after initiating the prescription?

B   6 months

7.30 If the 47-year-old woman makes an informed decision to choose the combined pill, how often should she attend for blood pressure checks?

C   12 months

Source: Contraception for Women Aged Over 40 years. Faculty of Sexual and Reproductive Health Clinical Effectiveness Unit. (2010) www.fsrh.org

A	Administer a gonadotrophin releasing hormone (GnRH) analogue
B	Commence antibiotics
C	Commence the COC

D	Commence oral progestogens for 25 days
E	Continue with the next pack of the COC without a pill-free period
F	Insert an IUD
G	No intervention is required
H	Remove the IUD
I	Use condoms as an additional form of contraception

These clinical scenarios relate to women seeking advice in the Family Planning Clinic in your surgery. For each case, select the most appropriate management plan.

Each option may be used once, more than once, or not at all.

7.31 A 26-year-old woman using Depot medroxyprogesterone acetate who has a BMI of 27 kg/m^2 is suffering from breakthrough bleeding. This is now causing relationship difficulties as she does not want to have intercourse when she is bleeding and she is annoyed that she needs to carry pads around with her all the time. She wishes to control the bleeding if possible.

C Commence the COC

When there is breakthrough bleeding with Depot medroxyprogesterone acetate one suggestion is to commence the COC for 2 to 3 months after excluding causes of bleeding such as sexually transmitted infection.

Source: http://www.fsrh.org/pdfs/CEUGuidanceProgestogenOnlyInjectables09.pdf.

7.32 A 32-year-old woman attends surgery because she is feeling unwell and on examination she has a large boil in her left armpit after shaving. You prescribe flucloxacillin 500mg qds for 7 days. She is using Microgynon® for contraception and has five pills left in her pack.

G No intervention is required

The latest advice states that neither continuation of the combined pill pack nor additional contraception is required when antibiotics are commenced even within a week of the pill-free week. The only situation in which an additional method needs to be considered is when the use of antibiotics results in diarrhoea, except if the antibiotic is an enzyme inducer, for example, rifampicin.

7.33 A 29-year-old woman attends surgery. She has a BMI of 34 kg/m^2. She has bought the anti-obesity drug orlistat over the counter at a chemist and is worried as she has developed severe diarrhoea since taking it. You discover that she is using Mercilon® for contraception but she has not had sexual intercourse since the commencement of orlistat.

I Use condoms as an additional form of contraception

In the presence of diarrhoea then additional contraception is recommended.

Source: fsrh.org/pdfs/CEUGuidanceCombinedHormonalContraception.pdf.

7.34 A 27-year-old woman attends surgery because she has discovered that she is 8 weeks pregnant having had a scan in the local hospital where she went complaining of severe nausea. This confirmed an intrauterine pregnancy and she has a Multiload Cu 375® in place. She is shocked to find herself pregnant but wishes to continue with the pregnancy.

H Remove the IUD

If an intrauterine pregnancy occurs with an IUD in situ, then the advice is that the IUCD is removed if the pregnancy is less than 12 weeks' gestation unless the strings cannot be seen.

7.35 A 34-year-old woman attends your surgery. She has a Nova T 380® copper intrauterine device in situ for contraceptive purposes. She had a casual sexual encounter with a stranger 4 days ago and now she is suffering from abdominal pain. On examination she is apyrexial, a yellow discharge is noted, and the uterus is tender to palpate.

B Commence antibiotics

If PID is suspected but not confirmed the advice from the Faculty of Family Planning and Sexual Health is to commence appropriate antibiotics and leave the IUD in place.

Source: http://www.fsrh.org/pdfs/CEUGuidanceIntrauterineContraceptionN.

A	At any time in the menstrual cycle
B	After 3 weeks
C	After 6 weeks
D	After 8 weeks
E	After 12 weeks
F	After 3 months
G	After 3 years
H	After 5 years
I	After 7 years
J	Day 1–5 of cycle
K	Day 19 of cycle
L	Day 21 of cycle

Each of these clinical scenarios relate to women requesting contraceptive advice. For each patient select the single most appropriate advice to give from the list above.

Each option may be used once, more than once, or not at all.

7.36 An 18-year-old woman attends for repeat emergency contraception having had a second episode of unprotected intercourse in this menstrual cycle. You offer her levonorgestrel 1.5mg orally and counsel her about the need for contraception. She is keen to have the etonogestrel implant (Nexplanon®) inserted and asks you when is the most appropriate time that this can be done.

J Day 1–5 of cycle

The advice from the FSRH is that the progestogen implant can be started imme-diately after EC for women who are likely to continue to have unprotected inter-course but the disadvantage is the difficulty in removing the implant if EC fails and she is pregnant. They therefore recommend bridging contraception with oral contraceptives until pregnancy has been excluded and then proceeding with the Nexplanon® in days 1–5 of her next period.

7.37 A 23-year-old woman has opted to use medroxyprogesterone acetate injection (Depo-Provera®) for contraception. She enquires when she will need her second injection.

E After 12 weeks

The license for Depo-Provera® clearly states an injection interval of 12 weeks and if longer than 12 weeks and 5 days, that pregnancy must be ruled out. The answer is not 3 months because 3 calendar months can be longer than 12 weeks.

7.38 A 45-year-old woman attends for replacement of her levonorgestrel intrau-terine system (Mirena IUS®), which she uses both for contraception and control of her heavy menstrual bleeding. She is currently amenorrhoeic with the IUS in place. She asks you when she will need the next IUS if she hasn't gone through the menopause.

I After 7 years

The FSRH advises that although the license for the Mirena IUS® specifies replacement every 5 years, after the age of 45 women can retain the Mirena IUS® for up to 7 years and only need replacement if they haven't become menopausal or have an FSH greater than 30iu/l on 2 occasions.

7.39 A 25-year-old woman is requesting the COC for contraception postnatally. She had a normal vaginal delivery and is bottle feeding her baby. When should she commence the COC?

B After 3 weeks

The COC is licensed for postnatal use from day 21 after delivery in women who are not breast-feeding. Delaying longer than that increases the risk of unplanned pregnancy as ovulation may occur as soon as 21 days after delivery, how-ever if the COC is commenced before this there is an increased risk of venous thromboembolism.

7.40 A 25-year-old woman attends your surgery requesting to commence the COC for the first time. She has been amenorrhoeic for some time but her pregnancy test is negative. When can she commence her pill?

A At anytime in the menstrual cycle

FRSH recommend that the COC may be commenced any time within the cycle but with 7 days of additional contraception or 9 days for estradiol valerate/dienogest pill (Qlaira®)

A	Copper IUCD delayed until chlamydia swab results available
B	Copper IUCD with chlamydia antibiotic prophylaxis
C	Depot medroxyprogesterone acetate injection
D	Levonorgestrel (Levonelle®) 1.5 mg oral dose
E	Levonorgestrel intrauterine system (Mirena®)
F	Nexplanon® etonogestrel implant
G	No prescription needed; reassure
H	Ulipristal acetate (EllaOne®) 30 mg oral dose
I	Repeat ulipristal acetate (EllaOne®) 30 mg oral dose

These clinical scenarios relate to women seeking emergency contraception. For each case, select the most appropriate method.

Each option may be used once, more than once, or not at all.

7.41 A 35-year-old woman presents to her local police station the morning after an alleged rape and is seen at the SARC. She has had a full infection screen done and thinks that her last period was about 12 days ago. She does not usually use contraception as she has never been sexually active and is very distressed at the thought of possible pregnancy as a result of the attack.

H Ulipristal acetate (EllaOne®) 30 mg oral dose

This woman does not need ongoing contraception; otherwise the IUCD would have the lowest failure rate. Ulipristal seems to have a lower failure rate than levonorgestrel, although both could be used within this time frame.

7.42 The same 35-year-old woman returns to the SARC 3 hours later having just vomited in the car on the way home.

I Repeat ulipristal acetate (EllaOne®) 30 mg oral dose

Women should be advised to seek medical advice if they vomit within 3 hours of taking ulipristal (2 hours if they have taken levonorgestrel).

7.43 Three months after her first delivery, a woman is still fully breast-feeding her baby. She has not had a period yet and thought that she didn't need to use contraception at all so had unprotected intercourse 2 days ago. It took her a long time to get pregnant and you suspect that her subfertility might have been due to previous episodes of pelvic inflammatory disease related to proven chlamydia infection.

D Levonorgestrel (Levonelle®) 1.5 mg oral dose

She cannot take ulipristal because of feeding her baby (breast-feeding is not recommended up to 36 hours after taking it) and her gynaecological history precludes the use of a copper IUCD as first choice. She does need ongoing contraceptive advice too.

7.44 A 24-year-old woman normally uses Depot medroxyprogesterone acetate for contraception but has forgotten to return for her usual injection, which is now over a month overdue. She has been amenorrhoeic since she started on Depot medroxyprogesterone acetate 3 years ago and she is keen to continue using it because her periods had been heavy previously. She had unprotected intercourse 3 days ago.

H Ulipristal acetate (EllaOne®) 30 mg oral dose

It is too late for her to use levonorgestrel as this is only licensed for use within 72 hours. She should have a pregnancy test done now anyway as you would have no idea whether she was already pregnant or not.

7.45 On return from her holidays, a teenage woman seeks help 4 days after a condom failure abroad. She is now on day 18 of an irregular cycle and uses a Ventolin inhaler several times a day for her asthma (which has been severe enough to necessitate hospital admission in the past).

B Copper IUCD with chlamydia antibiotic prophylaxis

It is too late for her to use levonorgestrel as this is only licensed for use within 72 hours and she cannot use ulipristal because of her asthma. You should not wait for the results of the chlamydia swab – and you might also counsel her about being screened for other STIs if she has had sex with a stranger on holiday – so it is best to prescribe prophylaxis alongside inserting a copper IUCD straight away.

Source: Faculty of Sexual and Reproductive Healthcare 'Clinical Guidance on Emergency Contraception' (updated January 2012) www.fsrh.org

A	24 hours
B	72 hours
C	120 hours
D	Anytime in the cycle
E	Day 1–5 of the menstrual cycle
F	Day 1–7 of the menstrual cycle
G	Five days after expected ovulation
H	Immediately
I	Next expected menses
J	2 weeks
K	3–4 weeks

The following clinical scenarios relate to timing of commencement of contraceptive methods. For each scenario select the most appropriate option.

Each option may be used once, more than once, or not at all.

7.46 A 19-year-old drug user had a vaginal delivery yesterday and the baby has been taken into care. She has a chaotic lifestyle and this was her third unplanned pregnancy. She is happy to have an etonogestrel implant but is keen to leave hospital and asks you when is the soonest that the device can be inserted.

H Immediately

The UKMEC guidance recommends inserting the etonogestrel implant between 21 and 28 days postpartum in non-breast-feeding women but also advises that the implant can be inserted immediately if the woman is unlikely to attend for medical care and is at risk of pregnancy. Given her lifestyle and drug habit it is far better to take the opportunity to insert the implant now and accept that she may have irregular bleeding initially.

7.47 A 19-year-old woman has just completed the second part of a medical abortion. Following counselling she has requested the etonogestrel sub-dermal implant (Nexplanon®) for ongoing contraception. When should she have this inserted?

H Immediately

FRSH recommend that the progesterone-only implant can be inserted on the day of surgical abortion or the second part of a medical abortion or immediately following miscarriage. No additional contraception is required unless the method is started more than 7 days after the abortion or miscarriage, at which time additional contraception is required for 7 days.

7.48 A woman using medroxyprogesterone acetate (Depot medroxyprogesterone acetate) for contraception has forgotten to attend her appointment for her next injection. She telephones the surgery to make another appointment and asks how much time she has before she cannot rely on the injection for effective contraception.

C 120 hours

If the woman is more than 5 days late when she attends for her injection (more than 89 days after the previous dose) she should use another method of contraception for 14 days as she is not protected against pregnancy.

7.49 A 32-year-old woman has been using a POP for a year following the birth of her second child. She has stopped breast-feeding now and is unhappy with the intermenstrual bleeding that she has with the POP. She is keen to switch to the COC and asks how long after finishing her POP packet she should start the COC.

H Immediately

The advice in the British National Formulary is to start the COC without a break after the last POP and to use additional contraception, for example, condoms for 7 days.

7.50 A 16-year-old woman requests emergency contraception for her first episode of unprotected intercourse due to condom failure. She is in a steady relationship and is keen to start the COC. When would you advise her to start taking the COC?

H Immediately

The FSRH advises that although starting the COC immediately after EC is unlicensed, it is preferable to start the pill immediately but to recommend avoiding intercourse or to use condoms as well for 7 days. The advantages of 'quick starting' COC is to reduce the time in which she is at risk of pregnancy, to ensure she remembers the advice given on starting the COC, and to avoid 'waning enthusiasm' for contraception.

Exam Paper 1

Extended Matching Questions

A	Anomaly scan at 20 weeks of gestation
B	Laparoscopy
C	Midstream urine specimen for culture
D	Repeat USS in 1 week
E	Repeat USS in 1 month
F	Routine booking scan
G	Serum βhCG assay
H	Serum lactate
I	Serum progesterone levels
J	Thyroid function test
K	Viability scan

These pregnant women have been admitted to hospital with excessive vomiting. Select the most appropriate investigation for each patient.

Each option may be used once, more than once, or not at all.

1   A 39-year-old primigravid woman is admitted to hospital with vomiting at 8 weeks of gestation. Her USS shows a 'snowstorm' appearance.

Answer   [   ]

2   A primigravid woman is admitted to hospital with intractable vomiting for the first time at 16 weeks of gestation. She has seen her midwife a few times during the pregnancy already and everything seemed to be fine.

Answer   [   ]

3   Having been treated for hyperemesis twice before, a primigravid woman is readmitted with further vomiting at 13 weeks of gestation. She is very dehydrated and her urine contains a great deal of ketones but nothing

else. On her first admission at 8 weeks she had a scan that showed a twin pregnancy.

Answer [ ]

A	Chorioamnionitis
B	Pelvic girdle pain
C	Placental abruption
D	Preterm labour
E	Pyelonephritis
F	Red degeneration of fibroid
G	Torsion of ovarian cyst
H	Urinary tract infection
I	Uterine rupture

The following clinical scenarios relate to women experiencing pain in pregnancy. For each case suggest the single most likely diagnosis.
Each option may be used once, more than once, or not at all.

4   A 35-year-old African woman presents at 34 weeks of gestation with severe continuous abdominal pain. There is no vaginal bleeding or history suggestive of ruptured membranes and fetal movements are normal. On examination the uterus is irregular, large for dates, and tender over the fundus. The cardiotocograph is reassuring.

Answer [ ]

5   A woman presents at 28 weeks of gestation feeling unwell with generalised abdominal pain for the last 12 hours. She gives a history of losing fluid per vaginam intermittently over the preceding 3 days. Fetal movements are present but reduced. On examination she is apyrexial and normotensive but has a tachycardia of 120 bpm. On examination the uterus is tender and the symphysis-fundal height is 24 cm.

Answer [ ]

6   A 20-year-old woman in her first pregnancy presents to the labour ward complaining of a sudden onset of severe abdominal pain 6 hours ago. She hasn't felt any fetal movements since the pain started. There is no history of vaginal loss or bleeding. On examination her blood pressure is 170/110 mmHg, pulse 100 bpm, and she is apyrexial. Urinalysis shows protein++++. On abdominal palpation the uterus is hard and tender and the fetal heart cannot be detected.

Answer [ ]

A	Await result of fetal anomaly scan at 20 weeks of gestation
B	Inform the woman that Down syndrome is confirmed
C	Inform the woman that Down syndrome is excluded
D	Inform the woman that the risk for this pregnancy is low
E	Nuchal translucency scan at 11–13 weeks of gestation
F	Offer amniocentesis
G	Offer chorionic villus sampling
H	Offer cordocentesis
I	Serum screening at 15–17 weeks of gestation

These clinical scenarios relate to women seeking prenatal testing for Down syndrome. For each woman select the most appropriate option.

Each option may be used once, more than once, or not at all.

7   A 38-year-old woman has a nuchal translucency test at 11 weeks of gestation and the risk of Down syndrome is calculated at 1 in 80. She requests a diagnostic test to be done as soon as possible.

Answer   [ ]

8   A primigravid 40-year-old woman is 10 weeks pregnant after many years of fertility investigations and she consults an obstetrician in private practice for antenatal care. She is concerned about the risk of having a baby affected by Down syndrome and wishes to have a diagnostic test with lowest possible risk of miscarriage.

Answer   [ ]

9   A 36-year-old woman presents late for antenatal care at 15 weeks' gestation in her first pregnancy because she was unaware that she was pregnant on account of irregular cycles. She has serum screening only done for Down syndrome and the result shows a 1 in 5,000 risk of the pregnancy being affected.

Answer   [ ]

A	Delivery by caesarean section at 37 weeks of gestation is recommended
B	Elective caesarean section carries less fetal risks than vaginal birth
C	Emergency caesarean section in labour is as safe as elective section
D	Induction of labour is contraindicated

E	Induction of labour is recommended at 40 weeks of gestation
F	Pregnancy could continue to await spontaneous labour
G	The risk of scar rupture/dehiscence in labour is 10 per cent
H	Vaginal delivery is contraindicated for maternal reasons
I	Vaginal delivery is only possible if expected fetal weight is <4000 g

Each of these pregnant women is seeking advice about the management of her delivery. Select the most appropriate advice in each case.

Each option may be used once, more than once, or not at all.

10 A 22-year-old woman attends antenatal clinic at 36 weeks of gestation in her second pregnancy worried about her mode of delivery. Her current pregnancy is uncomplicated and she previously had an elective caesarean section for placenta praevia.

Answer [ ]

11 A 25-year-old woman attends your clinic at 37 weeks of gestation in her first pregnancy to discuss mode of delivery. She is anxious because scan confirms a breech presentation and she refuses to consider external cephalic version.

Answer [ ]

12 A 34-year-old primigravid woman with a singleton uncomplicated pregnancy attends your clinic wishing to discuss mode of delivery. She is 38 weeks pregnant, having conceived following her third cycle of IVF. She has no complications and the baby is well grown.

Answer [ ]

A	Anorexia nervosa
B	Anovulatory cycles
C	Asherman's syndrome
D	Haematocolpos
E	Juvenile type Granulosa cell tumour of the ovary
F	Kallman's syndrome
G	Munchausen's syndrome by proxy
H	Polycystic ovarian syndrome
I	Pregnancy
J	Sheehan's syndrome

These teenagers are referred by their GPs to gynaecology outpatients with amenorrhoea. Select the most likely diagnosis based on the clinical information given. Each option may be used once, more than once, or not at all.

13 Six months of secondary amenorrhoea in a 19-year-old professional model whose periods started at 12 years of age. She has a BMI of 16. Examination of the abdomen and pelvis is normal.

Answer [ ]

14 Secondary amenorrhoea of 4 months' duration followed by a week of intermittent light vaginal bleeding in a shy 18-year-old shop worker who weighs 68 kg. She has a mass palpable in the suprapubic region arising from the pelvis.

Answer [ ]

15 A 15-year-old girl who has not yet started menstruating complains of lower abdominal pain for 3 days. You note that she has been admitted to hospital twice already during the previous 3 months with pain and suspect that she is avoiding school as exams are imminent. Her younger sister also has frequent episodes of pain but attained menarche recently at the age of 14 years.

Answer [ ]

A	Admission to isolation ward
B	Admission to maternity ward
C	Advise termination of pregnancy
D	Prescribe antibiotics
E	Prescribe acyclovir
F	Reassurance that no action necessary
G	Send blood for varicella zoster IgG levels
H	Varicella zoster immune globulin (VZIG)
I	Varicella zoster vaccination

These clinical scenarios relate to chickenpox in pregnancy.
Select the most appropriate management option for each pregnant woman. Each option may be used once, more than once, or not at all.

16 A woman whose first pregnancy is 28 weeks advanced is in the surgery for a routine check with the midwife. She sees a poster about chickenpox in pregnancy on the surgery wall and realises that she was exposed to a toddler with chickenpox 6 weeks ago at a birthday party. She had chickenpox herself as a child and is currently well.

Answer [ ]

17 A newly qualified teacher is exposed to chickenpox at 20 weeks of gestation when a child in her class is sent home from school unwell with a fever and a rash. She did have some routine screening tests when she started her job 6 months ago but was not given any results. She visits her GP that afternoon, who contacts occupational health and discovers that the teacher is not immune to varicella zoster.

Answer [ ]

18 A woman whose current pregnancy is 15 weeks advanced takes her 3-year-old daughter to the GP because the child is unwell with a maculopapular rash. The GP diagnoses chickenpox.

Answer [ ]

A	CT scan of the pelvis
B	Barium enema
C	Diagnostic laparoscopy
D	Erythrocyte sedimentation rate
E	Faecal occult blood test
F	Laparoscopy and dye test
G	MRI scan of the pelvis
H	Serum estradiol levels
I	Transvaginal ultrasound scan
J	Triple swabs

Each of these clinical scenarios describes a woman presenting in primary care with pain that is likely to be gynaecological in origin. For each patient pick the most appropriate investigation given the clinical information provided.

Each option may be used once, more than once, or not at all.

19 An 18-year-old woman presents to her GP with cyclical pain for the previous 9 months. She is not yet sexually active and her mother had similar problems before starting a family.

Answer [ ]

20 An 18-year-old biology student presents to the University Student Health Centre for contraceptive advice. She mentions that she has experienced severe deep dyspareunia for several weeks and wishes to stop using Depo-Provera® as she has read that it can cause low estrogen levels, which she thinks is responsible for her problem.

Answer [ ]

21   When she attends the surgery for a routine smear a 51-year-old woman mentions to the practice nurse that she has had lower abdominal pain for several months associated with bloating and episodes of diarrhoea. Her symptoms have not responded to mebeverine which one of your colleagues has prescribed recently. The nurse arranges for her to have a CA125 blood test and the result is 66 U/l.

Answer [ ]

A	Cervical biopsy
B	Cervical smear at 3 months' postpartum
C	Colposcopy within 4 weeks
D	Counselling regarding increased risk of preterm labour
E	High vaginal swab
F	LLETZ
G	Repeat cervical smear in 12 months
H	Routine colposcopy
I	Routine smear for liquid-based cytology
J	Urgent smear for liquid-based cytology
K	Urine or endocervical swab for chlamydia trachomatis screen

These scenarios relate to women who have presented for cervical screening.
   Select the most appropriate management plan for each woman based on the clinical information given.
   Each option may be used once, more than once, or not at all.

22   A 26-year-old nulliparous woman recently had her first cervical smear, which is reported as showing severe dyskaryosis. She tells you she is delighted to have discovered that she is about 8 weeks pregnant.

Answer [ ]

23   A 26-year-old nulliparous woman complains of postcoital bleeding for the last 3 weeks. She has been recently assessed at the colposcopy clinic because of her second smear showed mild dyskaryosis.

Answer [ ]

24   A 26-year-old nulliparous woman attends for contraceptive advice. She has never had a cervical smear but as the whole family attend your GP practice you are aware that her sister had a hysterectomy for cervical cancer at the age of 28 years.

Answer [ ]

A	Abdominal x-ray (KUB) to look for calculus
B	Creatinine clearance
C	Flexible cystoscopy
D	FSH and LH levels
E	Intravenous urogram (IVU)
F	Micturating cystogram
G	Renal perfusion study
H	Serum urea and electrolytes
I	Three early-morning urine specimens for culture
J	Urodynamics (bladder pressure study)

Each of these clinical scenarios describes a woman presenting in primary care with urinary symptoms.

Select the most appropriate investigation based on the clinical information given.

Each option may be used once, more than once, or not at all.

25 A perimenopausal woman who is seeing you for hormone replacement therapy complains of urge and stress incontinence that is beginning to affect her social life as she cannot leave home without a pad.

Answer [ ]

26 Since arriving in the country 3 months ago, a 47-year-old immigrant agricultural worker has experienced urinary frequency and urgency. She is at risk of losing her job as she cannot continue to work in the fields on account of her symptoms. She is still menstruating regularly but wonders if she is menopausal because she has night sweats. Pelvic examination reveals a minor cystocoele and a tender bladder.

Answer [ ]

27 The nurse running your smoking cessation programme sends a 61-year-old woman to see you on account of long-standing urinary incontinence that is made worse by her chronic cough. On testing her urine, you find microscopic haematuria.

Answer [ ]

A	Arrange to see the woman on her own to ask her about domestic abuse
B	Arrange an independent translator and ask about domestic abuse
C	Ask the relatives if she is experiencing domestic abuse

D	Ask the community midwife to visit her at home
E	Contact the adult safeguarding team
F	Contact the police
G	Discuss child protection issues with the on-call social work team
H	Encourage the woman to confide in a close relative if she is being abused
I	Give the woman a card with contact numbers of agencies and refuges
J	Offer immediate admission to hospital

You are concerned about the possibility of domestic violence in each of these women who are attending the hospital for antenatal care.

Select the best course of action in each case.

Each option may be used once, more than once, or not at all.

28 Whilst performing an anomaly scan at 20 weeks of gestation, the ultrasonographer notices several bruises of different colours on the abdomen of a timid 17-year-old primigravid woman. Her 25-year-old boyfriend is also present to watch the scan and when she is asked questions (such as her address and date of birth) he supplies the answers.

Answer [ ]

29 At 02.30 hours in the morning a 19-year-old primigravid woman presents to labour ward with postcoital bleeding. Her pregnancy is 32 weeks of gestation and she is unaccompanied.

On examination you notice that she has a 'black eye' and some circular bruises on her arms. Speculum examination reveals a tear in the posterior vaginal fornix that is not actively bleeding and the cervix is healthy. The baby is moving well, the uterus is not tender, and the cardiotocograph is normal.

Answer [ ]

30 A 26-year-old immigrant woman attends antenatal clinic at 34 weeks with her sister-in-law who translates for her, as she speaks no English at all. This is her first pregnancy and she is having growth scans on account of recurrent ante-partum haemorrhage. The growth of the baby is fine, but when you are auscultating the fetal heart you notice some circular lesions on the maternal abdomen that look like cigarette burns.

Answer [ ]

A	Advise against flying
B	Advise against travel after 32 weeks of gestation
C	Advise against travel after 36 weeks of gestation

D	Aspirin 75 mg for duration of flight and several days afterwards
E	Avoid flying in first trimester
F	Graduated compression stockings
G	Hydration and mobilization during flight
H	Low molecular weight heparin for duration of flight
I	Low molecular weight heparin for flight and several days afterwards
J	Reassurance/no special measures needed
K	Take out travel insurance that covers pregnancy complications

Select the most appropriate advice for a woman wishing to go on a commercial flight during pregnancy, given the clinical information provided.
Each option may be used once, more than once, or not at all.

31 A primigravid woman with an uncomplicated 22-week pregnancy and a BMI of 25 wishes to fly to New Zealand to attend a wedding. She fractured her tibia and fibula 2 days ago and is wearing a plaster on her leg but the airline has assured her that a wheelchair will be available for her use at the airport. She is concerned about the risks of air travel in pregnancy and seeks your advice.

Answer [ ]

32 A 25-year-old primigravid woman with a singleton pregnancy wishes to fly from London to Paris for a fashion show and shopping trip at 34 weeks of gestation. She seeks your advice because she is concerned about the risk of thromboembolism and is wondering about catching a train instead.

Answer [ ]

33 A primigravid woman who is pregnant with twins wishes to visit her mother in South Africa and seeks advice about when she should plan to fly.

Answer [ ]

34 A primigravid woman who has been referred to antenatal clinic at 31 weeks of gestation for management of severe anaemia with a haemoglobin of 70 gm/L, asks if she can take a short-haul flight to Italy to go on holiday the day after tomorrow.

Answer [ ]

A	Audit
B	Case-based discussion
C	Case presentation in a practice meeting

D	Lecture with PowerPoint presentation
E	Mini clinical evaluation exercise
F	Observation of the technique
G	Practical session using a patient
H	Practical simulation session using a manikin (dummy)
I	Reflective practice
J	Show a video of the technique
K	'Skills drills' session
L	Small group tutorial

Each of these scenarios describe a teaching situation in which you may encounter during your training. Select the most appropriate method for delivering the required learning objective.

Each option can be used once, more than once, or not at all.

35 A new medical student is starting in your GP practice who has never done gynaecology before. You are asked to ensure that they have been taught to do speculum examination by the end of their first week.

Answer [ ]

36 Last week you taught a new trainee how to counsel a patient who wants to be sterilised. Now you want to check whether they have learnt the principles you taught them.

Answer [ ]

A	Anaphylactic rash
B	Eczema
C	Erythema multiforme
D	Pemphigoid gestationis
E	Polymorphic eruption of pregnancy
F	Prurigo (atopic eruption) of pregnancy
G	Psoriasis
H	Striae gravidarum
I	Urticaria

These clinical scenarios relate to women seeking help with skin conditions they have developed in pregnancy. From the preceding list choose the most likely diagnosis given the examination findings.

Each option may be used once, more than once, or not at all.

37 A primigravid woman presents to her GP at 30 weeks of gestation with itching all over her abdomen. On examination she has pink linear wrinkles, and she has clearly been scratching them.

Answer [ ]

38 A primigravid woman has slightly raised papules and plaques across her gravid abdomen, thighs, and buttocks. There are no lesions around the umbilicus.

Answer [ ]

A	Amlodipine
B	Bendroflumethazide
C	Hydralazine
D	Labetalol
E	Magnesium Sulphate
F	Methyldopa
G	Nifedipine
H	Ramipril

These clinical scenarios relate to pregnant women presenting with hypertensive problems. In each case choose the most appropriate drug to treat the patient.

Each option may be used once, more than once, or not at all.

39 A 25-year-old primigravida is referred to the obstetric unit because her blood pressure is 150/100 mmHg on a routine check at 38 weeks of gestation. On admission her blood pressure is repeated twice and found to be 165/100 mgHg and 158/110 mmHg. Urinalysis reveals 2+ proteinuria.

Answer [ ]

40 A 32-year-old woman with gestational hypertension at 37 weeks of gestation has a blood pressure of 150/105 mmHg despite taking labetalol 200 mg t.d.s. for several days. She is asymptomatic and has no proteinuria.

Answer [ ]

Exam Paper 2

Single Best Answer Questions

1   A woman who has three children has unfortunately conceived whilst using a copper coil for contraception. She attends surgery after a positive pregnancy test and thinks that she is probably 7 weeks pregnant. Having talked to her husband, she is not too upset and is intending to keep the pregnancy. She feels well and has no vaginal discharge, pain, or bleeding.

Select the most appropriate course of action:

A.   Perform a full STI screen as infection is likely to cause miscarriage
B.   Prescribe a course of antibiotics prophylactically
C.   Remind the midwife that the coil needs removing at her postnatal appointment
D.   Send her for a routine booking scan mentioning the coil on the scan request form
E.   Take the coil out as there is a risk of septic miscarriage

Answer [ ]

2   As she is completing the hospital discharge paperwork for a recently delivered mother on the maternity ward one of the midwives accidentally puts her copy of the list containing details of women currently on the ward into the handheld notes, so that the patient takes the list home with her.

Which of these options is the most appropriate course of action for the midwife in charge of the ward to take?

A.   Ask the woman's community midwife to visit and retrieve the list
B.   Complete an incident form and inform the Information Governance Lead
C.   Send the police to retrieve the list from the patient's house
D.   Telephone the woman and ask her to shred the list
E.   Write to the woman and ask her to return the list

Answer [ ]

3   A 26-year-old primigravid woman has a routine appointment with her community midwife at 32 weeks of gestation. Her ankles and feet are so swollen that she has had to wear sandals instead of shoes and can no longer wear her rings. Her BP at booking was 120/70 mmHg and it is now 130/80 mmHg. Urinalysis is negative.

On examination she does have bilateral varicose veins and both ankles are mildly oedematous, but there is no redness or tenderness in either leg.

Which is the most appropriate management option?

A. Advise the use of compression stockings
B. Arrange lower-limb venous Doppler studies
C. Commence low-dose aspirin
D. Refer to an obstetrician
E. Request serum U&E and urate testing

Answer [ ]

4 A 20-year-old woman is admitted to the gynaecology ward over a bank holiday weekend with lower abdominal pain, deep dyspareunia, vaginal discharge, and a fever of 38°C. She has no gastrointestinal symptoms, is using the pill for contraception, and is halfway through a packet. On examination there is suprapubic tenderness and bimanual pelvic examination elicits cervical motion tenderness. Urinalysis is negative as is her pregnancy test.

Which of the following is the most appropriate management plan?

A. Take triple swabs and prescribe appropriate antibiotics according to sensitivities
B. Prescribe doxycycline 100 mg twice daily for 14 days
C. Prescribe metronidazole 400 mg and cephalexin 500 mg t.d.s. for 14 days
D. Prescribe metronidazole and ofloxacin 400 mg b.d. for 14 days
E. Administer azithromycin 1g intramuscular injection and refer to the GUM clinic

Answer [ ]

5 Obstetric units utilise a 'maternity dashboard' that describes items such as the caesarean section rate, the percentage of forceps deliveries, the number of home births, the number of inductions of labour, and the number of third-degree tears per month, and so forth.

The purpose of this 'dashboard' is to:

A. Check on the performance of individual obstetricians for revalidation
B. Compare the outcomes of their maternity services with other units
C. Keep track of the costs incurred on labour ward
D. Present the data to the Clinical Negligence Scheme for Trusts (CNST) inspectors
E. Reduce the risk of litigation in relation to labour

Answer [ ]

6 Following the realisation that suicide was the leading cause of maternal death in the 2000–2002 triennium, GPs are expected to be aware of issues concerning the mental health of pregnant women.

Which one of the following statements is true with regard to psychiatric problems in pregnant women?

A. A previous history of puerperal psychosis carries a recurrence risk of 5 per cent

B. A woman with a history of depression should be always be referred for a formal psychiatric opinion during pregnancy

C. The risk of suicide increases during pregnancy

D. New mothers who commit suicide are more likely to die by violent means rather than overdose

E. The Edinburgh depression scale may be used to screen for the risk of a psychotic depressive illness occurring

Answer [ ]

7   Following a ward round with the registrar on labour ward you are left with a list of tasks to do. Which job takes priority over the rest?

A. Clerking a new patient admitted with raised blood pressure at 39 weeks of gestation

B. Discharging a patient recovering after a severe postpartum haemorrhage to the postnatal ward

C. Inserting an IV line for a patient in labour with a previous caesarean scar

D. Obtaining consent for postmortem from a mother who is waiting to be discharged having delivered her stillborn baby 6 hours ago

E. Performing a fetal blood sample on account of late decelerations on the CTG at 5 cm dilatation

Answer [ ]

8   Six days after a difficult hysterectomy and bilateral salpingo-oophorectomy operation for endometriosis, a woman presents to the surgery with right loin pain. She reports that she did have some pain and 'felt shivery' when she was discharged from hospital 3 days before. She now looks very unwell with a temperature of 38°C. There is no vaginal bleeding or discharge. On examination she is tender in the right renal angle and right hypochondrium. You take a midstream urine specimen and can see that she needs readmission for antibiotic treatment.

Which of the following investigations would be the most appropriate to check for an underlying cause when she gets to hospital?

A. Computed tomography (CT) urogram

B. Laparoscopy

C. Serum amylase

D. Three swab test with methylene blue in the bladder

E. Ultrasound scan (USS) of the gallbladder and liver

Answer [ ]

9   You are clerking a new patient in gynaecology clinic with pelvic pain and trying to sort out a differential diagnosis. As well as the pelvic pain, which one of the following is a recognised symptom of endometriosis?

A. Abdominal bloating

B. Dyschezia

C. Postcoital bleeding

D.   Primary dysmenorrhoea

E.   Superficial dyspareunia

Answer [   ]

10   Two years after her last menstrual period a woman aged 51 presents with
     severe dyspareunia that is so bad that she can no longer tolerate inter-
     course. She was glad to see the end of her periods because they were
     becoming increasingly troublesome and has not experienced any vasomo-
     tor symptoms. On speculum examination the vulva and vagina look very
     atrophic and opening the speculum causes a small amount of bleeding by
     splitting the skin at the introitus.

     What is the most appropriate treatment in her case?

A.   Fenton's operation to enlarge the vaginal introitus

B.   Dilators

C.   Psychosexual counselling

D.   Transdermal estradiol and progestogen patches

E.   Vaginal estradiol pessaries

Answer [   ]

11   A postmenopausal woman presents to gynaecology clinic with an
     advanced utero-vaginal prolapse. Which of the following clinical problems
     is not likely to be attributable to the prolapse:

A.   Constipation

B.   Digitation

C.   Recurrent cystitis

D.   Ulceration of the vaginal walls

E.   Vaginal bleeding

Answer [   ]

12   Following a normal delivery a baby is unexpectedly in poor condition and
     you are the first person on the scene. His heart rate is 80 bpm and his
     extremities are blue. His body has some muscle tone and he grimaces
     when pinched but is not yet making any respiratory effort.

     What Apgar score would you give him at one minute?

A.   2

B.   4

C.   6

D.   8

E.   10

Answer [   ]

13   The main purpose of organising a bladder pressure (urodynamic) study for
     a woman whose presenting symptoms are a mixed picture of stress and
     urge incontinence with nocturia is:

A.   Check for urinary fistula

B.   Diagnose problems with bladder emptying

C. Differentiate detrusor instability from genuine stress incontinence

D. Find out whether her symptoms are due to utero-vaginal prolapse

E. Prevent subsequent medico-legal problems if she does not respond to treatment

Answer [ ]

14 You are counselling a woman about having an evacuation of uterus to deal with her first trimester miscarriage. With regard to the surgical management of miscarriage, which of these statements is correct?

A. Avoiding surgery is advisable if the uterus is septic

B. Histological proof that the uterus contained trophoblastic tissue will always exclude ectopic pregnancy

C. Medical management is associated with an increased incidence of pelvic infection

D. Perforation of the uterus during surgical evacuation is more likely in incomplete rather than missed miscarriage.

E. *Women having a surgical evacuation should be screened for Chlamydia trachomatis.

Answer [ ]

15 A woman with preexisting type 2 diabetes which was previously treated with metformin and glibenclamide switched to insulin during pregnancy to improve her blood glucose control. The insulin was stopped after delivery and she is breast-feeding her baby.

Select the most appropriate management advice during the time she is breast-feeding:

A. Avoid any oral blood glucose lowering medication whilst breast-feeding

B. Both metformin and glibenclamide can be taken whilst breast-feeding

C. Metformin should be avoided until she ceases breast-feeding

D. She should have a snack before breast-feeding

E. There is an increased risk of hypoglycaemia during breast-feeding

Answer [ ]

16 A 25-year-old woman presents to the Early Pregnancy Unit with brown vaginal discharge. She is unsure of her last menstrual period but thinks the gestational age might be about 7 weeks. The USS has shown a small sac in the uterus with no contents. On vaginal examination you find no pelvic tenderness.

What is the most suitable management plan?

A. Booking scan at 12 weeks of gestation

B. Evacuate the uterus and send the contents for histological examination

C. Laparoscopy

D. Repeat USS in 1 week

E. Serial urine βhCG assays with the next test 48 hours later

Answer [ ]

17 A 47-year-old woman presents with a 6-month history of regular heavy menstrual bleeding. She has had normal smears in the past and pelvic examination is unremarkable. Histology on a 'pipelle' sample of the endometrium and USS are reported as normal. She had a DVT following a long-haul flight in the past but is otherwise healthy.

Which of the following is the most appropriate treatment option for her menorrhagia?

A. Combined oral contraceptive pill
B. Hysterectomy
C. Levonorgestrel releasing IUS (Mirena®)
D. Norethisterone 15 mg daily from day 5–26 of menstrual cycle
E. Tranexamic acid

Answer [ ]

18 A 14-year-old schoolgirl attends the Teenage Family Planning Clinic requesting emergency contraception after a mid-cycle condom breakage.

Her parents are unaware of her sexual activity and do not approve of the relationship with her 22-year-old partner because he has another girlfriend who is currently pregnant.

She is clearly Fraser-competent.

Select the most appropriate action in this situation:

A. Referral to police because of underage sexual activity
B. Referral to social services to investigate her sexual relationship with an adult
C. Referral to GUM clinic for full sexually transmitted disease screening
D. Refuse to supply contraception until parents give consent
E. Supply contraception and arrange follow-up appointment

Answer [ ]

19 A 16-year-old woman presents to the surgery with primary amenorrhoea and a pelvic USS requested by one of your GP colleagues suggests that the uterus is absent. She has normal breast and pubic hair development and is 166 cm tall with a BMI of 23.

Which of these conditions is likely to be responsible for her amenorrhoea?

A. XYY syndrome
B. Gonadal dysgenesis
C. Mullerian agenesis
D. Kleinfelter syndrome
E. Turner syndrome

Answer [ ]

20 Having presented at 34 weeks of gestation with an antepartum haemorrhage, a multigravid woman is found to have a major degree of placenta praevia. The bleeding settles and her haemoglobin the following day is

105 gm/L with normal parameters and ferritin levels. She has experienced trouble tolerating oral iron preparations in her previous pregnancies because of constipation.

Select the most appropriate management option:

A. A blood sample should be obtained once a week for 'group and save'
B. Autologous blood deposit should be arranged
C. Prescribe parenteral iron
D. She should alter her diet to increase iron intake
E. She should have a blood transfusion to increase her haemoglobin level above 12 gm/L

Answer [ ]

21 One of the pregnant women in your practice has just been found to be HIV positive. She has just had a swab taken at the hospital as part of a routine screen and the result showing bacterial vaginosis has been faxed to the surgery. She is asymptomatic.

Select the most appropriate course of action:

A. Prescribe oral metronidazole 400 mg b.d. for 5 days
B. Repeat the swab
C. Reassure her that it will not affect the pregnancy
D. Treat her only if she develops a discharge
E. Treat with high-dose 2 g oral metronidazole

Answer [ ]

22 Vaginal birth after caesarean (VBAC) used to be known as 'trial of scar'. Which of the following signs or symptoms would prompt concern that a previous caesarean scar is dehiscing during labour in a woman having a VBAC?

A. Contractions become more painful
B. Leakage of liquor per vaginam
C. Maternal bradycardia
D. Slow progress of labour
E. Uterine contractions cease

Answer [ ]

23 A primigravid woman who is 16 weeks pregnant asks for advice because she has been exposed to a case of chickenpox 5 days ago. She cannot remember having chickenpox as a child and there is nothing about that in her records at the surgery, so a serum test was taken just after exposure that was negative for IgG antibodies. Select the most appropriate management option:

A. Administer oral acyclovir for 7 days
B. Give VZIG as soon as possible
C. Intravenous acyclovir
D. Order sputum culture and chest x-ray
E. Prescribe a course of zanamivir or oseltamivir

Answer [ ]

24 A woman has chosen to deliver her third baby at home and has gone into labour at 38 weeks of gestation. The community midwife has only just left the labour ward on her way to the house, having collected a cylinder of Entonox. The woman's husband telephones the surgery to say that her waters have just gone and he can see the cord hanging out of the vagina.

Select the most appropriate instruction to give him on the telephone:

A. Encourage his wife to start pushing
B. Push the cord back in to her vagina
C. Put her into the knee-chest position
D. Take her straight to hospital in the car
E. Wrap the cord in a warm towel

Answer [ ]

25 A nulliparous woman whose partner is HIV positive wishes to get pregnant whilst minimising her risk of HIV infection through unprotected intercourse with her partner. He is compliant with his highly active antiretroviral therapy (HAART) and is clinically well.

What advice should be given?

A. Avoid sexual intercourse until he has a plasma viral load of less than 5000 copies/ml
B. HIV transmission can be eliminated by sperm washing and intrauterine insemination
C. Prescribe broad spectrum antibiotics to cover intercourse
D. She should be prescribed HAART as well
E. Unprotected intercourse should be limited to the time of ovulation

Answer [ ]

26 An USS was performed to locate a 45-year-old woman's intrauterine copper device because the strings were not visible when she attended the surgery to have it changed. The abdominal USS report confirmed that the IUD was in the uterine cavity but also found a 5 cm complex ovarian cyst with no free fluid in the pelvis. She has no symptoms at all, so this is an incidental finding

Select the best management option:

A. Another scan in a few weeks to see if the cyst has gone
B. Change the IUD and ignore the cyst as it is <7 cm
C. Refer for diagnostic laparoscopy
D. Send blood for all the tumour markers including alpha-fetoprotein (AFP) and human chorionic gonadotrophin (hCG)
E. Serum carcinoma antigen 125 (CA125) level

Answer [ ]

27 You see a woman in clinic with urinary frequency and urgency who you suspect might have overactive bladder (detrusor instability) and counsel her about it.

Which of these statements is correct with regard to detrusor instability?

A. Bladder drill (retraining) is ineffective
B. It can be confidently diagnosed from the history without further investigation
C. It may be a symptom of multiple sclerosis
D. It will respond to oral duloxetine
E. Pelvic floor physiotherapy is not indicated

Answer [　]

28 Women with a BMI > 30 at booking are at increased risk of vitamin D deficiency and are advised to supplement their diet with 10 micrograms of vitamin D daily during pregnancy and breast-feeding.

The main reason for taking vitamin D is:

A. To prevent haemorrhagic disease of the newborn
B. To prevent intrauterine growth restriction
C. To prevent neural tube defects
D. To prevent pre-eclampsia
E. To prevent rickets in the neonate

Answer [　]

29 In the 2014 MBRRACE report on maternal deaths there was a decrease in the maternal mortality rate to 10.12 maternal deaths. What is the denominator for the maternal mortality rate?

A. The number of maternal deaths per hundred deliveries
B. The number of maternal deaths per hundred thousand maternities
C. The number of maternal deaths per million maternities
D. The number of maternal deaths per thousand maternities
E. The number of maternal deaths per thousand pregnancies

Answer [　]

30 A 45-year-old woman presenting with urinary incontinence is diagnosed with overactive bladder and starts treatment with immediate-release oxybutynin tablets. She reads on the leaflet that constipation can be a side effect.

Which of these statements is appropriate advice to give her regarding this side effect of oxybutynin?

A. Adverse effects such as constipation indicate that the treatment is starting to work
B. Constipation side effects should prompt cessation of treatment
C. Laxatives will not work if she continues to take the oxybutynin
D. Every patient should routinely take laxatives whilst they are taking oxybutynin
E. The chance of the tablets causing constipation is less than 1 per cent

Answer [　]

31 A 23-year-old woman presents to the surgery complaining of intermenstrual and postcoital bleeding. She is not using any contraception as she is trying to get pregnant.

Select the most likely diagnosis:

A.   Cervical polyp
B.   Chlamydia infection
C.   Endometrial polyp
D.   Nabothian follicle on the cervix
E.   Squamous cancer of the cervix

Answer   [   ]

32   Obstetric units often audit the decision-to-delivery interval for caesarean section as a marker of their performance. According to the 2011 NICE guideline, what should the interval be for a category 2 caesarean section where there is maternal or fetal compromise that is not immediately life threatening?

A.   30 minutes
B.   45 minutes
C.   60 minutes
D.   75 minutes
E.   No time limit for this category

Answer   [   ]

33   An immigrant woman presents late for antenatal care at 39 weeks of gestation having just arrived in the country from Latvia. The baby is presenting by the breech and external cephalic version is indicated but she cannot sign the consent form as she has no English at all.

Select the best course of action with regard to consent for the procedure:

A.   Ask her husband to sign the consent form
B.   Find a translator
C.   Get permission using a court order
D.   Give her a leaflet in Latvian to read and then ask her to sign
E.   Ignore as consent is not needed because it is not an operation

Answer   [   ]

34   A woman whose BMI is 42 books for antenatal care in her fourth pregnancy. She is 27 years old and her general health is good although she does smoke ten cigarettes daily. Her previous pregnancies and deliveries have been straightforward.

Select the most appropriate recommendation regarding low molecular weight heparin (LMWH) for thromboprophylaxis in her case?

A.   LMWH antenatally only if she develops two more risk factors
B.   LMWH for 1 week postnatally if she has a normal delivery
C.   LMWH for 6 weeks postnatally regardless of the mode of delivery
D.   LMWH is not effective enough for morbidly obese women
E.   LMWH throughout pregnancy and for 6 weeks postpartum

Answer   [   ]

35 A primigravid woman at 33 weeks of gestation is referred to the antenatal clinic because the uterine fundus is large for dates. USS reveals a very high amniotic fluid index, confirming the diagnosis of polyhydramnios.

Which is the most appropriate next investigation?

A. Cardiotocograph
B. Glucose tolerance test
C. Pass a nasogastric tube when the infant is delivered
D. Serial growth scans
E. Toxoplasmosis IgM titre

Answer [ ]

36 You are asked to review a woman who had a forceps delivery of her first baby 12 hours ago after a long labour because she is keen to go home. The midwives are unhappy to let her leave the hospital yet because she has not passed urine since delivery.

Which statement is correct with regard to the management of her bladder and urine output:

A. Dehydration is the most likely cause
B. Intermittent self-catheterisation is inadvisable straight after delivery
C. Referral to urology is indicated
D. She is at risk of long-term detrusor failure
E. Voiding problems are likely to be related to damage to her bladder from the forceps

Answer [ ]

37 The following women leave the pre-op clinic without having their full blood count (FBC) taken and the nurse asks you if they need to be called back to the clinic.

In which case does it not matter, that is, which of them does not really need to have it done before the operation?

A. 27-year-old woman having an ovarian cystectomy
B. 30-year-old woman being sterilised laparoscopically
C. 40-year-old woman having an endometrial ablation
D. 42-year-old woman having a hysteroscopy for menorrhagia
E. 50-year-old woman undergoing cystoscopy for recurrent infections

Answer [ ]

38 A woman books with a community midwife in her first pregnancy and gives a history of having being treated for manic episodes whilst at university. She has been well since and is not currently under the care of a psychiatrist or taking any medication.

Which information is correct in terms of the effect of her mental health history on the pregnancy?

A. Bipolar disorder is a strong predictor for postpartum psychosis
B. Her risk of developing puerperal psychosis is 2 per 1,000

C.   She is more likely to become mentally ill during pregnancy than postpartum

D.   She is unlikely to commit suicide once the baby is born

E.   The history of bipolar disorder will not affect the pregnancy at all

Answer [ ]

39   A 24-year-old primigravid primary school teacher is in the early third trimester when one of her pupils develops German measles. On review of the woman's previous blood tests during pregnancy, there are no rubella IgG antibodies detected.

Select the most appropriate course of action:

A.   Defer rubella vaccine until postnatal period

B.   Give rubella vaccine to her immediately

C.   Prescribe rubella immunoglobulin to reduce the chance of infection

D.   Reassure that no further action necessary at any stage

E.   Refer to hospital for a scan

Answer [ ]

40   A 39-year-old woman with a BMI of 39 requests referral to gynaecology clinic for laparoscopic sterilisation. She has four children all delivered by caesarean section and currently uses barrier contraception. She has recently been diagnosed with type 2 diabetes and gives a history of heavy intermenstrual bleeding for 6 months.

Which is the most appropriate initial management option?

A.   Arrange vasectomy instead

B.   Opportunistic cervical smear

C.   Pelvic USS

D.   Refer for endometrial biopsy

E.   Suggest Mirena® IUS insertion

Answer [ ]

41   A pregnant woman in the first trimester has just been in contact with a patient with swine flu (H1N1) and seeks advice having seen posters about the condition in your surgery. She has asthma but no other medical problems and is currently well with no respiratory symptoms at all

Which of the following is correct advice to give in this situation?

A.   Asthma is a contraindication to vaccination against swine flu

B.   She should have antiviral therapy instead of the vaccine

C.   The safety of H1N1 vaccines in the first trimester is well documented

D.   The vaccination should be offered immediately

E.   Vaccination is contraindicated in pregnancy

Answer [ ]

42   Following a course of supervised physiotherapy for stress incontinence, a 48-year-old woman still experiences frequent episodes of incontinence of urine. She is about to go to Australia for 2 months and is seeking

further help with her symptoms so that her holiday is not spoiled by incontinence.

Select the most appropriate advice:

A. Duloxetine tablets
B. Electrical stimulation to levator ani muscle
C. Oxybutynin tablets
D. Transvaginal tape procedure
E. Wear a pad

Answer [ ]

43 A Jehovah's Witness is being seen in the preoperative clinic. She is having a hysterectomy for menorrhagia and her haemoglobin is 90 gm/L.

Select the most appropriate management option:

A. Arrange a 'cell saver' for the operation
B. Cancel the operation as it is too dangerous
C. Postpone the operation and prescribe iron
D. Prescribe erythropoietin
E. Sign a Jehovah's Witness 'advance directive'

Answer [ ]

44 A woman attends surgery asking for fertility investigations as she stopped taking the pill 3 years ago and is not yet pregnant. She has a past history of an episode of pelvic inflammatory disease following a surgical termination of pregnancy as a teenager. Her partner's semen analysis is normal. Pelvic examination reveals a retroverted uterus that is slightly tender.

Which is the most suitable investigation for evaluating tubal factors in her case?

A. Hysterosalpingo-contrast-ultrasonography (HyCoSy)
B. Hysteroscopy
C. Laparoscopy and dye test
D. Selective salpingography
E. X-ray Hysterosalpingography (HSG)

Answer [ ]

45 A primigravid woman has been in labour all day and on an oxytocin drip for the previous 8 hours. A decision is made for assisted vaginal delivery on account of delay in the second stage. There is no caput or moulding of the fetal head and the maternal condition is satisfactory.

Which of the following factors is essential before undertaking the delivery?

A. Arranging theatre as a difficult delivery is anticipated
B. Fetal head in the occipito-anterior position
C. Fully dilated cervix
D. Spinal analgesia
E. Normal fetal heart rate on the cardiotocograph

Answer [ ]

46 Regarding consent issues in contraceptive practice, which of these statements is correct?

A. Expressed (written or verbal) consent is needed for removal of subdermal implants

B. If a married woman is seeking sterilisation, her husband's consent should also be obtained

C. Implied or nonverbal consent is inadequate for practical procedures

D. Written consent and verbal consent are equally valid

E. Written consent is necessary for insertion or removal of IUDs

Answer [ ]

47 A woman who has suffered recurrent miscarriages has been found to have a normal karyotype, as has her partner. Which of the following management plans should be recommended for this couple to increase the chances of a successful term pregnancy?

A. Human chorionic gonadotrophin supplements until 12 weeks of gestation

B. Investigating the woman for diabetes

C. Prescribing progesterone during the first half of the pregnancy

D. Refer for preimplantation genetic diagnosis at the fertility clinic

E. Screening for antiphospholipid syndrome and prescribing aspirin and heparin if positive

Answer [ ]

48 In which of these situations is it advisable to perform an USS for a patient seeking termination of pregnancy?

A. The doctor is hoping to persuade her against termination

B. The patient is trying to choose between a medical or surgical method

C. The patient is undecided whether to continue with the pregnancy or not

D. The patient refuses vaginal examination

E. The uterus is larger than expected for the gestational age

Answer [ ]

49 A primigravid woman presents to labour ward at 32 weeks of gestation with vaginal bleeding. She is stable and the baby is well, but she is known to be rhesus negative. Her clinical notes confirm that she had her prophylactic anti-D injection at 28 weeks of gestation, administered by her midwife.

Select the most appropriate management option

A. Administer 250 IU anti-D and perform Kleihauer test

B. Administer 500 IU anti-D

C. Administer 500 IU anti-D and perform Kleihauer test

D. Ask the lab to check for residual anti-D from her prophylactic injection

E. No action necessary

Answer [ ]

50 A woman who has been on thyroxine 100 micrograms for 5 years attends surgery for antenatal booking at 8 weeks of gestation. The community midwife asks for your opinion.

Select the most appropriate management:

A. Leave the dose of thyroxine unchanged and refer to endocrine clinic
B. Leave the dose of thyroxine unchanged and refer to obstetric clinic
C. Leave the dose of thyroxine unchanged and refer to obstetric endocrine clinic
D. Increase the dose of thyroxine and refer to endocrine clinic
E. Increase the dose of thyroxine and refer to obstetric endocrine clinic

Answer [ ]

51 A woman attends the Early Pregnancy Unit for a scan at 8 weeks of gestation because she had a salpingectomy for a left-sided ectopic a year ago. She is asymptomatic but the scan shows an empty uterus with a mass in the right adnexa, thought to be another ectopic pregnancy. Methotrexate treatment is discussed to give her a chance of retaining her remaining fallopian tube.

Which factor would suggest surgical management is more appropriate than medical management of this second ectopic pregnancy?

A. Adnexal mass measuring 15 mm
B. hCG level of 500 IU/L
C. Previous ruptured ectopic pregnancy
D. No fetal heartbeat in the ectopic sac on scan
E. Patient has significant pain

Answer [ ]

52 A woman is admitted to hospital at 36 weeks of gestation because she has suspected H1N1 influenza. She is tachycardic, her temperature is 38°C, and she seems to be breathing very fast.

What is the upper threshold for the normal respiratory rate in pregnancy?

A. Ten breaths per minute
B. Fifteen breaths per minute
C. Twenty breaths per minute
D. Twenty-five breaths per minute
E. Thirty breaths per minute

Answer [ ]

53 A woman who is expecting her third child attends surgery at 36 weeks of gestation complaining of pain from symphysis pubis dysfunction.

Select the most appropriate management option:

A. Ask the obstetric team to arrange early induction of labour
B. Obstetric physiotherapy appointment
C. Prescribe nonsteroidal antiinflammatory drugs
D. Refer to an orthopaedic surgeon
E. Suggest elective caesarean delivery

Answer [ ]

54 Women with Turner syndrome sometimes have a mosaic karyotype where some cell lines have 45XO and some 46XX chromosomes.

Which of these statements is true about Turner mosaic patients?

A. They are all of short stature just like 45XO Turner women
B. They are at risk of osteoporosis at an early age
C. They cannot have children
D. They do not have any other Turner-associated congenital abnormalities such as renal tract
E. They do not usually have a uterus

Answer [ ]

55 Chorionic villus sampling can be used to detect sex-linked inherited conditions as well as trisomies. When counselling a woman choosing to have this test done, which of these statements is correct information to give her?

A. It can only be done in the first trimester of pregnancy
B. It carries a small risk of limb reduction defects in the fetus
C. The test is able to detect neural tube defects
D. The result is available in about a week
E. There is a miscarriage risk of 3 to 5 per cent

Answer [ ]

56 In women considering using POP that do not contain desogestrel for contraception, which of the following applies?

A. The bleeding pattern is likely to be amenorrhoea
B. The efficacy is reduced if the women weigh more than 75 kg
C. They should not be used in women with breast cancer (UKMEC4)
D. They are not suitable for women who are breast-feeding
E. They have a 12-hour window in which to take a pill they have missed

Answer [ ]

57 Regarding the duties of a doctor, which of these statements is correct?

A. A chaperone is needed for gynaecological pelvic examinations only if the doctor is male
B. Consent is not required for anomaly scans performed at 20 weeks of gestation
C. If you see a child with a proven sexually transmitted infection this must always be reported
D. When consenting a patient for a surgical procedure, only common complications need to be discussed
E. When treating a patient for a sexually transmitted infection, you always have a duty to inform the spouse regardless of the patient's consent

Answer [ ]

58 Which of these is a characteristic feature of physiological jaundice in the newborn?

A. Associated anaemia
B. Disappearance by the fourth day

C. Does not lead to kernicterus if not treated

D. Occurs more frequently in postdates infants

E. Onset after the first 24 hours of life

Answer [ ]

59 A 34-year-old woman has always attended for regular cervical screening and all her tests so far have been normal.

In which of the following circumstances would it be appropriate to take a smear from her?

A. She discovers a family history of cervical cancer

B. She is noted on examination to have a cervical erosion

C. She presents with a history of postcoital bleeding

D. She presents with a new diagnosis of genital warts

E. Three years after her previous cervical screen

Answer [ ]

60 NICE Guidelines suggest that low-dose aspirin (75 mg daily) is now recommended from 12 weeks of gestation to prevent pre-eclampsia in some pregnant women.

Which of these pregnant women should be taking low dose aspirin?

A. Chronic hypertension

B. Family history of pre-eclampsia

C. Maternal age more than 40 years

D. Multiple pregnancy

E. Pregnancy interval of greater than 10 years

Answer [ ]

Exam Paper 1

Answers

Extended Matching Questions

A	Anomaly scan at 20 weeks of gestation
B	Laparoscopy
C	Midstream urine specimen for culture
D	Repeat USS in 1 week
E	Repeat USS in 1 month
F	Routine booking scan
G	Serum βhCG assay
H	Serum lactate
I	Serum progesterone levels
J	Thyroid function test
K	Viability scan

These pregnant women have been admitted to hospital with excessive vomiting.
Select the most appropriate investigation for each patient.
Each option may be used once, more than once, or not at all.

1   A 39-year-old primigravid woman is admitted to hospital with vomiting at 8
    weeks of gestation. Her USS shows a 'snowstorm' appearance.

   G Serum βhCG assay

   *This ultrasound appearance is typical of hydatidiform mole that should be dealt
   with surgically. The baseline βhCG level helps the trophoblastic centre plan her
   subsequent follow-up and management.*

2   A primigravid woman is admitted to hospital with intractable vomiting for
    the first time at 16 weeks of gestation. She has seen her midwife a few
    times during the pregnancy already and everything seemed to be fine.

   C Midstream urine specimen for culture

   *It is unusual for hyperemesis to start in the second trimester so it is more likely
   that her symptoms are caused by urinary tract infection. She will already have
   had a booking scan that will have excluded molar pregnancy and twins.*

3 Having been treated for hyperemesis twice before, a primigravid woman is readmitted with further vomiting at 13 weeks of gestation. She is very dehydrated and her urine contains a great deal of ketones but nothing else. On her first admission at 8 weeks she had a scan that showed a twin pregnancy.

A Anomaly scan at 20 weeks of gestation

Although she has had recurrent admissions, this is not unusual with twin pregnancies and there is no need to worry about underlying causes such as UTI especially as her urine only shows ketones. Her next scan should be the anomaly scan at 20 weeks and she does not need another one before then.

A	Chorioamnionitis
B	Pelvic girdle pain
C	Placental abruption
D	Preterm labour
E	Pyelonephritis
F	Red degeneration of fibroid
G	Torsion of ovarian cyst
H	Urinary tract infection
I	Uterine rupture

The following clinical scenarios relate to women experiencing pain in pregnancy. For each case suggest the single most likely diagnosis.

Each option may be used once, more than once, or not at all.

4 A 35-year-old African woman presents at 34 weeks of gestation with severe continuous abdominal pain. There is no vaginal bleeding or history suggestive of ruptured membranes and fetal movements are normal. On examination the uterus is irregular, large for dates, and tender over the fundus. The CTG is reassuring.

F Red degeneration of fibroid

The salient feature here is her ethnic origin; fibroids are more common in African women, and the uterus is irregular. You will know from your revision that fibroids can undergo red degeneration in pregnancy even if you've never seen a case. Because the pain is continuous it makes the option of preterm labour unlikely even though it is a more common condition. The pain could be due to a concealed abruption but the whole uterus would be tender and abruption usually causes fetal distress.

5 A woman presents at 28 weeks of gestation feeling unwell with generalised abdominal pain for the last 12 hours. She gives a history of losing fluid per vaginam intermittently over the preceding 3 days. Fetal movements are present but reduced. On examination she is apyrexial and normotensive

but has a tachycardia of 120 bpm. On examination the uterus is tender and the symphysis-fundal height is 24 cm.

A Chorioamnionitis

The salient features in this case are the history suggestive of PROM and the significant tachycardia. PROM is a major risk factor for ascending infection, and in pregnant women a tachycardia usually precedes the pyrexia and is always a worrying sign. The pain is described as 'generalised' rather than intermittent (which might suggest option G – preterm labour). The small for dates uterus would fit with oligohydramnios due to ruptured membranes.

6   A 20-year-old woman in her first pregnancy presents to the labour ward complaining of a sudden onset of severe abdominal pain 6 hours ago. She hasn't felt any fetal movements since the pain started. There is no history of vaginal loss or bleeding. On examination her blood pressure is 170/110 mmHg, pulse 100 bpm, and she is apyrexial. Urinalysis shows protein++++. On abdominal palpation the uterus is hard and tender and the fetal heart cannot be detected.

C Placental abruption

The salient features in this case are the severe hypertension and proteinuria suggesting pre-eclampsia, the lack of fetal movements, and absent fetal heart suggesting an intrauterine death and the hard uterus suggesting the Couvelaire uterus of a large abruption. From your revision you know that abruption is a complication of pre-eclampsia and don't be distracted by the absence of vaginal bleeding as even large abruptions can be concealed.

A	Await result of fetal anomaly scan at 20 weeks of gestation
B	Inform the woman that Down syndrome is confirmed
C	Inform the woman that Down syndrome is excluded
D	Inform the woman that the risk for this pregnancy is low
E	Nuchal translucency scan at 11–13 weeks of gestation
F	Offer amniocentesis
G	Offer chorionic villus sampling
H	Offer Cordocentesis
I	Serum screening at 15–17 weeks of gestation

These clinical scenarios relate to women seeking prenatal testing for Down syndrome. For each woman select the most appropriate option.

Each option may be used once, more than once, or not at all.

7   A 38-year-old woman has a nuchal translucency test at 11 weeks of gestation and the risk of Down syndrome is calculated at 1 in 80. She requests a diagnostic test to be done as soon as possible.

G Offer chorionic villus sampling

The patient is keen on a diagnostic test that narrows the selection down to A, B, or C. The quickest result would be obtained by chorionic villus sampling because active placental cells will be dividing quickly enough to obtain a karyotype within 24–48 hours. Cordocentesis is reserved for later in pregnancy to investigate serious and rare conditions like fetal anaemia.

8 A primigravid 40-year-old woman is 10 weeks pregnant after many years of fertility investigations and she consults an obstetrician in private practice for antenatal care. She is concerned about the risk of having a baby affected by Down syndrome and wishes to have a diagnostic test with lowest possible risk of miscarriage.

F Offer amniocentesis

The patient wants a diagnostic test and the one with lowest risk of pregnancy loss is amniocentesis.

9 A 36-year-old woman presents late for antenatal care at 15 weeks' gestation in her first pregnancy because she was unaware that she was pregnant on account of irregular cycles. She has serum screening only done for Down syndrome and the result shows a 1 in 5,000 risk of the pregnancy being affected.

D Inform the woman that the risk for this pregnancy is low

Screening tests do not exclude Down syndrome but this low risk result is reassuring.

A	Delivery by caesarean section at 37 weeks of gestation is recommended
B	Elective caesarean section carries less fetal risks than vaginal birth
C	Emergency caesarean section in labour is as safe as elective section
D	Induction of labour is contraindicated
E	Induction of labour is recommended at 40 weeks of gestation
F	Pregnancy could continue to await spontaneous labour
G	The risk of scar rupture/dehiscence in labour is 10 per cent
H	Vaginal delivery is contraindicated for maternal reasons
I	Vaginal delivery is only possible if expected fetal weight is <4000 g

Each of these pregnant women is seeking advice about the management of her delivery. Select the most appropriate advice in each case.
Each option may be used once, more than once, or not at all.

10 A 22-year-old woman attends antenatal clinic at 36 weeks of gestation in her second pregnancy worried about her mode of delivery. Her current

pregnancy is uncomplicated and she previously had an elective caesarean section for placenta praevia.

F Pregnancy could continue to await spontaneous labour

The reason for her previous section is nonrecurrent so she should be able to have a vaginal birth this time. We would normally have a full discussion about the risks and benefits of VBAC and go through them again in the third trimester. Spontaneous labour is preferable to induced labour in this situation because the drugs we use to induce labour – prostaglandin and oxytocin – increase the risk of scar rupture. Induction is not completely contraindicated, just less safe but you could induce if there were good maternal reasons, for example, pre-eclampsia.

11 A 25-year-old woman attends your clinic at 37 weeks of gestation in her first pregnancy to discuss mode of delivery. She is anxious because scan confirms a breech presentation and she refuses to consider external cephalic version.

B Elective caesarean section carries less fetal risks than vaginal birth

The best option is external cephalic version because it reduces the incidence of breech presentation at term. If she won't accept this, then the 'Term Breech Trial' showed that section is safer for the breech baby than vaginal delivery.

12 A 34-year-old primigravid woman with a singleton uncomplicated pregnancy attends your clinic wishing to discuss mode of delivery. She is 38 weeks pregnant, having conceived following her third cycle of IVF. She has no complications and the baby is well grown.

F Pregnancy could continue to await spontaneous labour

Although this woman has had difficulty getting pregnant, she should now be treated like any other mother. There is no indication to interfere.

A	Anorexia nervosa
B	Anovulatory cycles
C	Asherman's syndrome
D	Haematocolpos
E	Juvenile type Granulosa cell tumour of the ovary
F	Kallman's syndrome
G	Munchausen's syndrome by proxy
H	Polycystic ovarian syndrome
I	Pregnancy
J	Sheehan's syndrome

These teenagers are referred by their GPs to gynaecology outpatients with amenorrhoea. Select the most likely diagnosis based on the clinical information given. Each option may be used once, more than once, or not at all.

13 Six months of secondary amenorrhoea in a 19-year-old professional model whose periods started at 12 years of age. She has a BMI of 16. Examination of the abdomen and pelvis is normal.

A Anorexia nervosa

The distracter is pregnancy, which is the most common cause of secondary amenorrhoea in teenagers, but the normal examination makes this less likely. Her BMI is extremely low and she is probably not ovulating. Disappearance of periods is an indication that anorexia is becoming very serious.

14 Secondary amenorrhoea of 4 months' duration followed by a week of intermittent light vaginal bleeding in a shy 18-year-old shop worker who weighs 68 kg. She has a mass palpable in the suprapubic region arising from the pelvis.

I Pregnancy

The mass could be an ovarian cyst but a granulosa cell tumour of the ovary is more likely to cause irregular bleeding than amenorrhoea and in any case they are extremely rare. Haematocolpos can also present with a lower abdominal mass, but the patient would have primary amenorrhoea, not secondary. Pregnancy is the most likely option.

15 A 15-year-old girl who has not yet started menstruating complains of lower abdominal pain for 3 days. You note that she has been admitted to hospital twice already during the previous 3 months with pain and suspect that she is avoiding school as exams are imminent. Her younger sister also has frequent episodes of pain but attained menarche recently at the age of 14 years.

D Haematocolpos

Imperforate hymen can cause cyclical pain as the haematocolpos gets bigger and it is not unusual to find a couple of hospital admissions have occurred before the diagnosis is reached. Many teenagers have anovulatory cycles but this causes irregular periods and menorrhagia rather than primary amenorrhoea.

A	Admission to isolation ward
B	Admission to maternity ward
C	Advise termination of pregnancy
D	Prescribe antibiotics
E	Prescribe acyclovir
F	Reassurance that no action necessary
G	Send blood for varicella zoster IgG levels
H	Varicella zoster immune globulin (VZIG)
I	Varicella zoster vaccination

These clinical scenarios relate to chickenpox in pregnancy.

Select the most appropriate management option for each pregnant woman. Each option may be used once, more than once, or not at all.

16   A woman whose first pregnancy is 28 weeks advanced is in the surgery for a routine check with the midwife. She sees a poster about chickenpox in pregnancy on the surgery wall and realises that she was exposed to a toddler with chickenpox 6 weeks ago at a birthday party. She had chickenpox herself as a child and is currently well.

F   Reassurance that no action necessary

The incubation period for varicella is 1 to 3 weeks so she would have developed it herself by now. As VZIG is only effective if given within 10 days of exposure, it is too late to consider that for this woman anyway. A personal history of chickenpox is 99 per cent predictive of the presence of serum varicella antibodies, so this woman does not even need testing for zoster IgG levels.

17   A newly qualified teacher is exposed to chickenpox at 20 weeks of gestation when a child in her class is sent home from school unwell with a fever and a rash. She did have some routine screening tests when she started her job 6 months ago but was not given any results. She visits her GP that afternoon, who contacts occupational health and discovers that the teacher is not immune to varicella zoster.

H   VZIG

There was a window of opportunity to vaccinate this woman against varicella before she got pregnant but now the only option is to give her VZIG to try and prevent her getting chickenpox (if that is what is wrong with the child in her class). It is still not recommended as part of a national screening programme to check antibody status and vaccinate all women in the United Kingdom like we do for rubella, but some occupational health departments do undertake this in high-risk groups such as teachers. If a woman contracts varicella in pregnancy she can become very ill with serious problems such as pneumonia and, of course, we worry about fetal varicella syndrome and infection of the newborn.

18   A woman whose current pregnancy is 15 weeks advanced takes her 3-year-old daughter to the GP because the child is unwell with a maculo-papular rash. The GP diagnoses chickenpox.

G   Send blood for varicella zoster IgG levels

If the woman had had chickenpox herself, she is likely to be immune so it is reasonable to check her antibody levels rather than prescribing VZIG. VZIG is manufactured from the plasma of blood donors and is a limited and expensive resource. If her antibodies are negative, there is still an opportunity to give VZIG up to 10 days.

Source: RCOG Green-top Guideline, No. 13, 'Chickenpox in Pregnancy'. Published 2015.

A	Computed Tomography (CT) scan of the pelvis
B	Barium enema
C	Diagnostic laparoscopy
D	Erythrocyte sedimentation rate

E	Faecal occult blood test
F	Laparoscopy and dye test
G	MRI scan of the pelvis
H	Serum estradiol levels
I	Transvaginal ultrasound scan
J	Triple swabs

Each of these clinical scenarios describes a woman presenting in primary care with pain that is likely to be gynaecological in origin. For each patient pick the most appropriate investigation given the clinical information provided.

Each option may be used once, more than once, or not at all.

19 An 18-year-old woman presents to her GP with cyclical pain for the previous 9 months. She is not yet sexually active and her mother had similar problems before starting a family.

C Diagnostic laparoscopy

If she is not sexually active she will not have pelvic inflammatory disease so the most likely diagnosis here is endometriosis, especially as it can run in families. Laparoscopy is the gold standard investigation as scan will not show up small deposits of endometriosis. MRI is sometimes used to investigate endometriosis, but only looking for deep deposits in sites such as the recto-vaginal septum in a patient where you already know the diagnosis.

20 An 18-year-old biology student presents to the University Student Health Centre for contraceptive advice. She mentions that she has experienced severe deep dyspareunia for several weeks and wishes to stop using Depo-Provera® as she has read that it can cause low estrogen levels, which she thinks is responsible for her problem.

J Triple swabs

It is more likely that she is suffering from pelvic inflammatory disease as a cause of her symptoms rather than vaginal atrophy so triple swabs would be the first investigation, especially as speculum examination would allow you to reassure her about the state of her vaginal skin at the same time. She does not need scan or laparoscopy unless her pain becomes chronic and a definite diagnosis is necessary.

21 When she attends the surgery for a routine smear a 51-year-old woman mentions to the practice nurse that she has had lower abdominal pain for several months associated with bloating and episodes of diarrhoea. Her symptoms have not responded to mebeverine, which one of your colleagues has prescribed recently. The nurse arranges for her to have a CA125 blood test and the result is 66 U/l.

I Transvaginal ultrasound scan

GPs are urged to do CA125 blood tests on women presenting with new onset of symptoms similar to irritable bowel after the age of 50 years and this result is raised. The next step is ultrasound, although there are many other conditions apart from ovarian cancer that can cause raised CA125. A thorough history and examination is recommended to avoid missing other pathology such as inflammatory bowel disease. The distracters in this question are the bowel investigation modalities, such as barium enema, and CT scan, which is more expensive than ultrasound and involves a dose of ionising radiation.

A	Cervical biopsy
B	Cervical smear at 3 months' postpartum
C	Colposcopy within 4 weeks
D	Counselling regarding increased risk of preterm labour
E	High vaginal swab
F	LLETZ
G	Repeat cervical smear in 12 months
H	Routine colposcopy
I	Routine smear for liquid-based cytology
J	Urgent smear for liquid-based cytology
K	Urine or endocervical swab for chlamydia trachomatis screen

These scenarios relate to women who have presented for cervical screening.

Select the most appropriate management plan for each woman based on the clinical information given.

Each option may be used once, more than once, or not at all.

22 A 26-year-old nulliparous woman recently had her first cervical smear, which is reported as showing severe dyskaryosis. She tells you she is delighted to have discovered that she is about 8 weeks pregnant.

C. Colposcopy within 4 weeks

Although this woman will have to wait until after she has delivered for treatment, someone must look at her cervix urgently to make sure that she is not one of the women with severe dyskaryosis who has cervical cancer already. Biopsy is possible in pregnancy if it is necessary.

23 A 26-year-old nulliparous woman complains of postcoital bleeding for the last 3 weeks. She has been recently assessed at the colposcopy clinic because of her second smear showed mild dyskaryosis.

K. Urine or endocervical swab for chlamydia trachomatis screen

One of the most common causes of postcoital bleeding in young women is chlamydia. As her cervix has recently been inspected at colposcopy, the smear history is irrelevant.

24 A 26-year-old nulliparous woman attends for contraceptive advice. She has never had a cervical smear but as the whole family attend your GP

practice you are aware that her sister had a hysterectomy for cervical cancer at the age of 28 years.

I. Routine smear for liquid-based cytology

The family history is not relevant as cervical cancer is not genetic. However, this woman has reached the age at which she should be enrolled on the screening programme and this seems like a good opportunity. Ethically the GP cannot mention the sister's medical history whilst trying to persuade her because of the confidentiality issue.

A	Abdominal x-ray (KUB) to look for calculus
B	Creatinine clearance
C	Flexible cystoscopy
D	FSH and LH levels
E	IVU
F	Micturating cystogram
G	Renal perfusion study
H	Serum urea and electrolytes
I	Three early-morning urine specimens for culture
J	Urodynamics (bladder pressure study)

Each of these clinical scenarios describes a woman presenting in primary care with urinary symptoms.

Select the most appropriate investigation based on the clinical information given.

Each option may be used once, more than once, or not at all.

25 A perimenopausal woman who is seeing you for HRT complains of urge and stress incontinence that is beginning to affect her social life as she cannot leave home without a pad.

J Urodynamics

The diagnosis is likely to be either detrusor instability or genuine stress incontinence and urodynamics will help you differentiate between them.

26 Since arriving in the country 3 months ago, a 47-year-old immigrant agricultural worker has experienced urinary frequency and urgency. She is at risk of losing her job as she cannot continue to work in the fields on account of her symptoms. She is still menstruating regularly but wonders if she is menopausal because she has night sweats. Pelvic examination reveals a minor cystocoele and a tender bladder.

I Three early-morning urine specimens for culture

Tuberculosis (TB) of the urinary tract is uncommon in the United Kingdom but possibly not in the country she has come from. It will not be picked up on routine

MSU – you need to send the whole of a morning void to the lab and specify TB testing.

27   The nurse running your smoking cessation programme sends a 61-year-old woman to see you on account of long-standing urinary incontinence that is made worse by her chronic cough. On testing her urine, you find microscopic haematuria.

C Flexible cystoscopy

Smoking is a risk factor for transitional cell carcinoma of the bladder, which should be excluded first before the incontinence is addressed, especially in view of the haematuria.

A	Arrange to see the woman on her own to ask her about domestic abuse
B	Arrange an independent translator and ask about domestic abuse
C	Ask the relatives if she is experiencing domestic abuse
D	Ask the community midwife to visit her at home
E	Contact the adult safeguarding team
F	Contact the police
G	Discuss child protection issues with the on-call social work team
H	Encourage the woman to confide in a close relative if she is being abused
I	Give the woman a card with contact numbers of agencies and refuges
J	Offer immediate admission to hospital

You are concerned about the possibility of domestic violence in each of these women who are attending the hospital for antenatal care.

Select the best course of action in each case.

Each option may be used once, more than once, or not at all.

28   Whilst performing an anomaly scan at 20 weeks of gestation, the ultra-sonographer notices several bruises of different colours on the abdomen of a timid 17-year-old primigravid woman. Her 25-year-old boyfriend is also present to watch the scan and when she is asked questions (such as her address and date of birth) he supplies the answers.

A Arrange to see the woman on her own to ask her about domestic violence

29   At 02.30 hours in the morning a 19-year-old primigravid woman presents to labour ward with postcoital bleeding. Her pregnancy is 32 weeks of gestation and she is unaccompanied.

On examination you notice that she has a 'black eye' and some circular bruises on her arms. Speculum examination reveals a tear in the posterior vaginal fornix which is not actively bleeding and the cervix is healthy. The baby is moving well, the uterus is not tender, and the CTG is normal.

J Offer immediate admission to hospital

30 A 26-year-old immigrant woman attends antenatal clinic at 34 weeks with her sister-in-law who translates for her, as she speaks no English at all. This is her first pregnancy and she is having growth scans on account of recurrent ante-partum haemorrhage. The growth of the baby is fine, but when you are auscultating the fetal heart you notice some circular lesions on the maternal abdomen that look like cigarette burns.

B Arrange an independent translator and ask about domestic abuse

Domestic violence is a common problem that crosses social boundaries and sometimes results in extreme outcomes, that is, the death of the woman. In some areas of the country up to a quarter of women booking for antenatal care will have experienced some sort of domestic abuse that can take many forms: violence, sexual abuse, psychological abuse, control of her finances, and so forth.

Obstetricians and GPs should have some knowledge of this issue as they are well placed to identify the problem in the first place. Clinicians should be aware of the existence of agencies and facilities able to help protect the woman and be able to discuss the subject with a patient at short notice.

Women should be asked about the possibility of domestic abuse at some stage in their antenatal care without any other family members or acquaintances being present, in case they are part of the problem. If necessary translators paid by the NHS such as 'language-line' should be used.

If a woman discloses that she is being subjected to violence, you may need to arrange admission to a place of safety such as hospital. There could be child protection issues if he is harming the children as well so if there are children in the equation, don't forget their needs.

A	Advise against flying
B	Advise against travel after 32 weeks of gestation
C	Advise against travel after 36 weeks of gestation
D	Aspirin 75 mg for duration of flight and several days afterwards
E	Avoid flying in first trimester
F	Graduated compression stockings
G	Hydration and mobilization during flight
H	Low molecular weight heparin for duration of flight
I	Low molecular weight heparin for flight and several days afterwards

J	Reassurance/no special measures needed
K	Take out travel insurance that covers pregnancy complications

Select the most appropriate advice for a woman wishing to go on a commercial flight during pregnancy, given the clinical information provided.

Each option may be used once, more than once, or not at all.

31 A primigravid woman with an uncomplicated 22-week pregnancy and a BMI of 25 wishes to fly to New Zealand to attend a wedding. She fractured her tibia and fibula 2 days ago and is wearing a plaster on her leg but the airline has assured her that a wheelchair will be available for her use at the airport. She is concerned about the risks of air travel in pregnancy and seeks your advice.

A Advise against flying

The recent fracture with plaster is hazardous because significant swelling can occur in flight, which might compromise the circulation to the limb.

32 A 25-year-old primigravid woman with a singleton pregnancy wishes to fly from London to Paris for a fashion show and shopping trip at 34 weeks of gestation. She seeks your advice because she is concerned about the risk of thromboembolism and is wondering about catching a train instead.

J Reassurance/no special measures needed

For short-haul flights no specific measures are likely to be required.

33 A primigravid woman who is pregnant with twins wishes to visit her mother in South Africa and seeks advice about when she should plan to fly.

B Advise against travel after 32 weeks of gestation

The main worry is the risk of going into labour in flight and delivering without appropriate medical aid, which is clearly more of a risk with twins rather than a singleton pregnancy.

If the pregnancy were singleton, you would advise against travelling after 37 weeks although some airlines insist on 36 weeks as a cutoff.

34 A primigravid woman who has been referred to antenatal clinic at 31 weeks of gestation for management of severe anaemia with a haemoglobin of 70 gm/L, asks if she can take a short-haul flight to Italy to go on holiday the day after tomorrow.

A Advise against flying

Although airline cabins are pressurized, the barometric pressure is significantly lower than at sea level. Severe anaemia with a haemoglobin <75 gm/L is a contraindication to air travel because of the potential reduction in blood oxygen saturation of 10 per cent due to reduced pO_2 at altitude.

Source: Scientific Impact Paper, No. 1, 'Air Travel and Pregnancy' (May 2013);

www.rcog.org.uk.

A	Audit
B	Case-based discussion
C	Case presentation in a practice meeting
D	Lecture with PowerPoint presentation
E	Mini clinical evaluation exercise
F	Observation of the technique
G	Practical session using a patient
H	Practical simulation session using a manikin (dummy)
I	Reflective practice
J	Show a video of the technique
K	'Skills drills' session
L	Small group tutorial

Each of these scenarios describe a teaching situation that you may encounter during your training. Select the most appropriate method for delivering the required learning objective.

Each option can be used once, more than once, or not at all.

35   A new medical student is starting in your GP practice who has never done gynaecology before. You are asked to ensure that they have been taught to do speculum examination by the end of their first week.

H Practical simulation session using a dummy

The best way to learn any practical technique is to see it demonstrated then to have a go at it yourself preferably with feedback. The only way to deliver that to a medical student having a go for the first time is to run a practical session using a dummy, before you let them loose on a patient.

36   Last week you taught a new trainee how to counsel a patient who wants to be sterilised. Now you want to check whether they have learnt the principles you taught them.

E Mini clinical evaluation exercise

Mini clinical evaluation exercise is ideal for watching a trainee interact with a patient and giving feedback to improve their performance.

A	Anaphylactic rash
B	Eczema
C	Erythema multiforme

D	Pemphigoid gestationis
E	Polymorphic eruption of pregnancy
F	Prurigo (atopic eruption) of pregnancy
G	Psoriasis
H	Striae gravidarum
I	Urticaria

These clinical scenarios relate to women seeking help with skin conditions they have developed in pregnancy. From the preceding list choose the most likely diagnosis given the examination findings.

Each option may be used once, more than once, or not at all.

37 A primigravid woman presents to her GP at 30 weeks of gestation with itching all over her abdomen. On examination she has pink linear wrinkles, and she has clearly been scratching them.

H Striae gravidarum

She could have any itching skin condition but the description of linear wrinkles means that these are likely to be striae.

38 A primigravid woman has slightly raised papules and plaques across her gravid abdomen, thighs, and buttocks. There are no lesions around the umbilicus.

E Polymorphic eruption of pregnancy

Sparing of the umbilicus suggests this diagnosis

A	Amlodipine
B	Bendroflumethazide
C	Hydralazine
D	Labetalol
E	Magnesium Sulphate
F	Methyldopa
G	Nifedipine
H	Ramipril

These clinical scenarios relate to pregnant women presenting with hypertensive problems. In each case choose the most appropriate drug to treat the patient.

Each option may be used once, more than once, or not at all.

39 A 25-year-old primigravida is referred to the obstetric unit because her blood pressure is 150/100 mmHg on a routine check at 38 weeks of gestation. On admission her blood pressure is repeated twice and found to be 165/100 mgHg and 158/110 mmHg. Urinalysis reveals 2+ proteinuria.

D Labetalol

Although this woman clearly has pre-eclampsia and may need magnesium sulphate and delivery, you must stabilise her blood pressure first as she is at risk of intracerebral bleeding with a blood pressure this high.

40 A 32-year-old woman with gestational hypertension at 37 weeks of gestation has a blood pressure of 150/105 mmHg despite taking labetalol 200mg t.d.s. for several days. She is asymptomatic and has no proteinuria.

G Nifedipine

This woman has pregnancy induced hypertension and not pre-eclampsia. This drug would be the preferred second line.

Source: NICE Guideline on 'Hypertension in Pregnancy; Diagnosis and Management CG107. Published 2010, updated 2011.

www.nice.org.uk

Exam Paper 2

Answers

Single Best Answers

1   A woman who has three children has unfortunately conceived whilst using a copper coil for contraception. She attends surgery after a positive pregnancy test and thinks that she is probably 7 weeks pregnant. Having talked to her husband, she is not too upset and is intending to keep the pregnancy. She feels well and has no vaginal discharge, pain, or bleeding.

Select the most appropriate course of action:

A.   Perform a full STI screen as infection is likely to cause miscarriage

B.   Prescribe a course of antibiotics prophylactically

C.   Remind the midwife that the coil needs removing at her postnatal appointment

D.   Send her for a routine booking scan mentioning the coil on the scan request form

E.   *Take the coil out as there is a risk of septic miscarriage

Although removing the coil may cause miscarriage, leaving it in the uterus is more likely to result in pregnancy loss. Not only that, miscarriage is more likely to be complicated by infection if the coil is still present, so the advice is to remove it.

There is a risk of ectopic pregnancy when a woman conceives with a coil in situ so an earlier scan than 12 weeks is indicated.

2   As she is completing the hospital discharge paperwork for a recently delivered mother on the maternity ward one of the midwives accidentally puts her copy of the list containing details of women currently on the ward into the handheld notes, so that the patient takes the list home with her.

Which of these options is the most appropriate course of action for the midwife in charge of the ward to take?

A.   Ask the woman's community midwife to visit and retrieve the list

B.   *Complete an incident form and inform the Information Governance Lead

C.   Send the police to retrieve the list from the patient's house

D.   Telephone the woman and ask her to shred the list

E.   Write to the woman and ask her to return the list

This is a serious breach of confidentiality and the person responsible for information governance will have to be informed. The action to be taken is their decision.

3 A 26-year-old primigravid woman has a routine appointment with her community midwife at 32 weeks of gestation. Her ankles and feet are so swollen that she has had to wear sandals instead of shoes and can no longer wear her rings. Her BP at booking was 120/70 mmHg and it is now 130/80 mmHg. Urinalysis is negative.

On examination she does have bilateral varicose veins and both ankles are mildly oedematous but there is no redness or tenderness in either leg.

Which is the most appropriate management option?

A. *Advise the use of compression stockings
B. Arrange lower-limb venous Doppler studies
C. Commence low-dose aspirin
D. Refer to an obstetrician
E. Request serum U&E and urate testing

This patient does not have pre-eclampsia although it would be prudent to recheck her BP earlier than normal. Her oedema is likely to be physiological related to pregnancy and is not a problem (apart from the discomfort) unless she does develop pre-eclampsia. As she has varicose veins too, some of her discomfort may be alleviated by compression stockings.

4 A 20-year-old woman is admitted to the gynaecology ward over a bank holiday weekend with lower abdominal pain, deep dyspareunia, vaginal discharge, and a fever of 38°C. She has no gastrointestinal symptoms, is using the pill for contraception, and is halfway through a packet. On examination there is suprapubic tenderness and bimanual pelvic examination elicits cervical motion tenderness. Urinalysis is negative as is her pregnancy test.

Which of the following is the most appropriate management plan?

A. Take triple swabs and prescribe appropriate antibiotics according to sensitivities
B. Prescribe doxycycline 100 mg twice daily for 14 days
C. Prescribe metronidazole 400 mg and cephalexin 500 mg t.d.s. for 14 days
D. *Prescribe metronidazole and ofloxacin 400 mg b.d. for 14 days
E. Administer azithromycin 1 g intramuscular injection and refer to the GUM clinic

Broad spectrum antibiotics that will cover chlamydia infections and possibly gonorrhoea as well as anaerobes are needed. You should not wait for the culture results as the sequelae of not treating acute PID are serious (pelvic abscess, tubal damage, infertility, and ectopic).

If the culture reveals gonorrhoea you might need to change the ofloxacin because of increasing resistance to quinolones in the United Kingdom.

Source: British Association for Sexual Health and HIV (BASHH) Clinical Effectiveness Group 'UK National Guideline for the Management of Pelvic Inflammatory Disease' (2011).

5 Obstetric units utilise a 'maternity dashboard' that describes items such as the caesarean section rate, the percentage of forceps deliveries, the number of home births, the number of inductions of labour, and the number of third-degree tears per month, and so forth.

The purpose of this 'dashboard' is to:

A. Check on the performance of individual obstetricians for revalidation
B. ***Compare the outcomes of their maternity services with other units**
C. Keep track of the costs incurred on labour ward
D. Present the data to the CNST inspectors
E. Reduce the risk of litigation in relation to labour

Maternity dashboards were introduced a few years ago to give the obstetricians and midwives working in a hospital some idea of how their services were performing in relation to neighbouring hospitals. Obviously the demographics of the local population will have some effect on the outcomes, but sometimes problems are flagged up that can be solved by changing protocols and guidelines, for example, reducing the induction rate will produce a fall in the caesarean section rate.

6 Following the realisation that suicide was the leading cause of maternal death in the 2000–2002 triennium, GPs are expected to be aware of issues concerning the mental health of pregnant women.

Which one of the following statements is true with regard to psychiatric problems in pregnant women?

A. A previous history of puerperal psychosis carries a recurrence risk of 5 per cent
B. A woman with a history of depression should be always be referred for a formal psychiatric opinion during pregnancy
C. The risk of suicide increases during pregnancy
D. ***New mothers who commit suicide are more likely to die by violent means rather than overdose**
E. The Edinburgh depression scale may be used to screen for the risk of a psychotic depressive illness occurring

The Edinburgh scale is used to screen for postnatal depression symptoms and is of no use in predicting serious psychotic illness that, in relation to pregnancy, is usually a serious delusional state with a rapid onset 'out of the blue' and swift deterioration.

The risk of a psychotic illness recurring after the next pregnancy is frighteningly high and these women should be offered prenatal counselling so that they are aware of the risk. These issues were highlighted by the 2000–2002 Confidential Enquiries.

The recurrence risk for a major depressive illness, for example, bipolar disorder, is similarly high at about 50 per cent and there should be a plan of care written in conjunction with a psychiatrist that is available in all the woman's clinical notes.

The actual risk of suicide is lower in pregnancy but there is a massive increase following delivery and maternal suicide features as a leading cause of death in the triennial maternal mortality reports.

Because suicide is often associated with psychotic illness the attempt is much more likely to be serious and irretrievable, that is, death by hanging, stabbing, or jumping rather than the usual 'female' method of overdose.

7 Following a ward round with the registrar on labour ward you are left with a list of tasks to do. Which job takes priority over the rest?

A. Clerking a new patient admitted with raised blood pressure at 39 weeks of gestation

B. Discharging a patient recovering after a severe postpartum haemorrhage to the postnatal ward

C. Inserting an IV line for a patient in labour with a previous caesarean scar

D. Obtaining consent for postmortem from a mother who is waiting to be discharged having delivered her stillborn baby 6 hours ago

E. ***Performing a fetal blood sample on account of late decelerations on the CTG at 5 cm dilatation**

Checking for fetal distress in the abnormal CTG situation is the most pressing item on this list. The hypertensive new patient may actually have pre-eclampsia and be at risk of fitting so this would be the next priority. The IV access for the patient undergoing vaginal birth after caesarean is on account of the risk of scar rupture and not that urgent.

8 Six days after a difficult hysterectomy and bilateral salpingo-oophorectomy operation for endometriosis, a woman presents to the surgery with right loin pain. She reports that she did have some pain and 'felt shivery' when she was discharged from hospital 3 days before. She now looks very unwell with a temperature of 38°C. There is no vaginal bleeding or discharge. On examination she is tender in the right renal angle and right hypochondrium. You take a midstream urine specimen and can see that she needs readmission for antibiotic treatment.

Which of the following investigations would be the most appropriate to check for an underlying cause when she gets to hospital?

A. ***CT urogram**

B. Laparoscopy

C. Serum amylase

D. Three swab test with methylene blue in the bladder

E. USS of the gallbladder and liver

The suspicion is that she has ureteric damage, although a similar picture could occur with UTI or an abscess. The three swab test is to look for vesico-vaginal fistula.

9 You are clerking a new patient in gynaecology clinic with pelvic pain and trying to sort out a differential diagnosis. As well as the pelvic pain, which one of the following is a recognised symptom of endometriosis?

A. Abdominal bloating

B. ***Dyschezia**

C. Postcoital bleeding

D. Primary dysmenorrhoea

E. Superficial dyspareunia

Dyschezia refers to pain on defaecation and means that there is endometriosis in the Pouch of Douglas or in the recto-vaginal septum. Endometriosis patients get secondary dysmenorrhoea, not primary dysmenorrhoea. There is no reason for the cervix to bleed so postcoital bleeding is not usually caused by endometriosis. If they do get dyspareunia, it is deep dyspareunia rather than superficial (as superficial means that there is something wrong in the vagina or vulva).

10 Two years after her last menstrual period a woman aged 51 presents with severe dyspareunia that is so bad that she can no longer tolerate

intercourse. She was glad to see the end of her periods because they were becoming increasingly troublesome and has not experienced any vasomotor symptoms. On speculum examination the vulva and vagina look very atrophic and opening the speculum causes a small amount of bleeding by splitting the skin at the introitus.

What is the most appropriate treatment in her case?

A. Fenton's operation to enlarge the vaginal introitus
B. Dilators
C. Psychosexual counselling
D. Transdermal estradiol and progestogen patches
E. *Vaginal estradiol pessaries

As her symptoms are confined to the genital tract she only needs local treatment, not systemic HRT. Sequential therapy would bring a return of her bleeding, which she would not be keen on, having been glad to get rid of her periods. There is no point in doing a Fenton's operation to enlarge the introitus or attempting dilation before restoring the vaginal skin as without estrogen the skin would just continue to split.

11 A postmenopausal woman presents to gynaecology clinic with an advanced utero-vaginal prolapse. Which of the following clinical problems is not likely to be attributable to the prolapse?

A. Constipation
B. Digitation
C. Recurrent cystitis
D. Ulceration of the vaginal walls
E. *Vaginal bleeding

Digitation means having to reduce the prolapse with a finger to facilitate defaecation. Women with procidentia often have pressure sores on the vaginal walls because of trauma. Although bleeding may be coming from ulceration of the vaginal walls, it would be prudent to exclude more sinister causes such as endometrial cancer.

12 Following a normal delivery a baby is unexpectedly in poor condition and you are the first person on the scene. His heart rate is 80 bpm and his extremities are blue. His body has some muscle tone and he grimaces when pinched but is not yet making any respiratory effort.

What Apgar score would you give him at one minute?

A. 2
B. *4
C. 6
D. 8
E. 10

He scores 1 for heart rate <100; 1 for blue extremities; 1 for some muscle tone; 1 for grimacing; and 0 for respiratory effort.

13 The main purpose of organising a bladder pressure (urodynamic) study for a woman whose presenting symptoms are a mixed picture of stress and urge incontinence with nocturia is:

A. Check for urinary fistula
B. Diagnose problems with bladder emptying

C. ***Differentiate detrusor instability from genuine stress incontinence**

D. Find out whether her symptoms are due to utero-vaginal prolapse

E. Prevent subsequent medico-legal problems if she does not respond to treatment

Some women develop 'de novo' bladder instability following operations for stress incontinence (which increase the pressure at the bladder neck). Requesting a bladder pressure study prior to a stress incontinence operation may be advisable to protect the gynaecologist against the accusation that they got the initial diagnosis wrong; but the main reason is to sort out the patients with unstable bladder in the first place who need anticholinergics and bladder drill, not surgery.

14 You are counselling a woman about having an evacuation of uterus to deal with her first trimester miscarriage. With regard to the surgical management of miscarriage, which of these statements is correct?

A. Avoiding surgery is advisable if the uterus is septic

B. Histological proof that the uterus contained trophoblastic tissue will always exclude ectopic pregnancy

C. Medical management is associated with an increased incidence of pelvic infection

D. Perforation of the uterus during surgical evacuation is more likely in incomplete rather than missed miscarriage

E. *** Women having a surgical evacuation should be screened for Chlamydia trachomatis**

There is a reduction in clinical pelvic infection after medical evacuation compared with surgical (7.1 per cent vs. 13.2 per cent; p < 0.001). The risk of a patient developing an infection after surgical evacuation with subsequent fertility problems can be reduced if screening for Chlamydia is undertaken routinely. If the uterus contains infected tissue, surgical evacuation is the best management. Ectopic cannot be completely excluded by finding trophoblastic tissue in the uterus as there are rare patients with a heterotopic pregnancy (one pregnancy in the uterus and another in the fallopian tube). In missed miscarriage the cervix is often tightly closed and difficult to dilate, making perforation of the uterus much more likely during surgical evacuation. Having said that, surgical evacuation is more effective than medical management in this group of patients.

15 A woman with preexisting type 2 diabetes that was previously treated with metformin and glibenclamide switched to insulin during pregnancy to improve her blood glucose control. The insulin was stopped after delivery and she is breast-feeding her baby.

Select the most appropriate management advice during the time she is breast-feeding:

A. Avoid any oral blood glucose lowering medication whilst breast-feeding

B. ***Both metformin and glibenclamide can be taken whilst breast-feeding**

C. Metformin should be avoided until she ceases breast-feeding

D. She should have a snack before breast-feeding

E. There is an increased risk of hypoglycaemia during breast-feeding

The hypoglycaemia issue only applies to women who are on insulin and breast-feeding.

Source: NICE Guideline, No. NG3, 'Diabetes in Pregnancy; Management from Preconception to the Postnatal Period' (2015).

16 A 25-year-old woman presents to the Early Pregnancy Unit with brown vaginal discharge. She is unsure of her last menstrual period but thinks the gestational age might be about 7 weeks. The USS has shown a small sac in the uterus with no contents. On vaginal examination you find no pelvic tenderness.

What is the most suitable management plan?

A. Booking scan at 12 weeks of gestation
B. Evacuate the uterus and send the contents for histological examination
C. Laparoscopy
D. ***Repeat USS in 1 week**
E. Serial urine βhCG assays with the next test 48 hours later

As she is unsure of the gestation, there is still a chance that she has an intrauterine pregnancy (of lesser gestation than she estimates from her unsure last menstrual period). A decidual ring in the uterus can look like a gestation sac on scan, however, so you still have not ruled out ectopic pregnancy. Serial hCG titres every 48 hours will help, but it is serum, not urine.

17 A 47-year-old woman presents with a 6-month history of regular heavy menstrual bleeding. She has had normal smears in the past and pelvic examination is unremarkable. Histology on a 'pipelle' sample of the endometrium and USS are reported as normal. She had a DVT following a long-haul flight in the past but is otherwise healthy.

Which of the following is the most appropriate treatment option for her menorrhagia?

A. COC
B. Hysterectomy
C. ***Levonorgestrel releasing IUS (Mirena®)**
D. Norethisterone 15 mg daily from day 5–26 of menstrual cycle
E. Tranexamic acid

She cannot use either tranexamic acid or the combined pill because of the DVT risk and she is too old for the pill anyway. Hysterectomy is not first line management and cyclical Norethisterone is no longer recommended for dysfunctional uterine bleeding.

18 A 14-year-old schoolgirl attends the Teenage Family Planning Clinic requesting emergency contraception after a mid-cycle condom breakage.

Her parents are unaware of her sexual activity and do not approve of the relationship with her 22-year-old partner because he has another girlfriend who is currently pregnant.

She is clearly Fraser-competent.

Select the most appropriate action in this situation:

A. Referral to police because of underage sexual activity
B. Referral to social services to investigate her sexual relationship with an adult
C. Referral to GUM clinic for full sexually transmitted disease screening

D. Refuse to supply contraception until parents give consent

E. ***Supply contraception and arrange follow-up appointment**

There is a duty of care to this teenager to help her prevent an unwanted pregnancy that is reasonable as you have decided that she understands the issues and is competent to make a decision for herself. You should be concerned about the age discrepancy between the teenager and her partner, and there are overtones of possible child abuse or exploitation that need addressing on a separate occasion. The best course of action regarding that would be to discuss her case with your local child protection agency but we have not given you this option. Involving her parents is a good idea and you should encourage her to do so, but you cannot do this yourself without her consent because of confidentiality. Informing the police, whilst legally correct, is not an appropriate first response to this situation as her contraceptive needs outweigh all other considerations.

19 A 16-year-old woman presents to the surgery with primary amenorrhoea and a pelvic USS requested by one of your GP colleagues suggests that the uterus is absent. She has normal breast and pubic hair development and is 166 cm tall with a BMI of 23.

Which of these conditions is likely to be responsible for her amenorrhoea?

A. XYY syndrome

B. Gonadal dysgenesis

C. ***Mullerian agenesis**

D. Kleinfelter syndrome

E. Turner syndrome

Causes of primary amenorrhoea, in descending order of frequency, are gonadal dysgenesis, Mullerian agenesis, and testicular feminization.

Because this patient has other signs of pubertal development that are sex steroid-dependent, we can conclude that some ovarian function is present. This excludes such conditions as gonadal dysgenesis as a possible cause of her primary amenorrhoea.

Turner syndrome women are usually of short stature and have a uterus.

Mullerian defects are the only plausible cause, and the diagnostic evaluation in this patient would be directed toward both confirmation of this diagnosis and establishment of the exact nature of the Mullerian defect.

Mullerian agenesis, also known as Mayer-Rokitansky-Kuster-Hauser syndrome, presents as amenorrhoea possibly also with absence of a vagina as well as absent uterus. The incidence is approximately 1 in 10,000 female births and the karyotype is 46,XX. There is normal development of breasts, sexual hair, ovaries, tubes, and external genitalia. There are associated skeletal (12 per cent) and urinary tract (33 per cent) anomalies.

Ten per cent of cases of primary amenorrhoea have testicular feminization, or congenital androgen insensitivity syndrome, which is an X-lined recessive disorder with a karyotype of 46,XY. In these patients the amount of sexual hair is significantly decreased.

Patients with Kleinfelter syndrome typically have a karyotype of 47,XXY and a male phenotype. XYY syndrome and Turner syndrome often present with amenorrhoea, but these patients have a uterus.

20 Having presented at 34 weeks of gestation with an antepartum haemorrhage, a multigravid woman is found to have a major degree of placenta praevia. The bleeding settles and her haemoglobin the following day is 105 gm/L with normal parameters and ferritin levels. She has experienced trouble tolerating oral iron preparations in her previous pregnancies because of constipation.

Select the most appropriate management option:

A. *A blood sample should be obtained once a week for 'group and save'
B. Autologous blood deposit should be arranged
C. Prescribe parenteral iron
D. She should alter her diet to increase iron intake
E. She should have a blood transfusion to increase her haemoglobin level above 12 gm/L

She is not technically anaemic yet (in the second and third trimester anaemia is defined as Hb <105 gm/L), but she is at risk of haemorrhage because of the placenta praevia. In women at high risk of transfusion and with no clinically significant alloantibodies, group and screen samples should be sent once a week to exclude any new antibody formation and keep blood available if necessary.

Source: RCOG Green-top Guideline, No. 47, 'Blood Transfusion in Obstetrics' (2015).

21 One of the pregnant women in your practice has just been found to be HIV positive. She has just had a swab taken at the hospital as part of a routine screen and the result showing bacterial vaginosis has been faxed to the surgery. She is asymptomatic.

Select the most appropriate course of action:

A. *Prescribe oral metronidazole 400 mg b.d. for 5 days
B. Repeat the swab
C. Reassure her that it will not affect the pregnancy
D. Treat her only if she develops a discharge
E. Treat with high-dose 2 g oral metronidazole

BV is known to be associated with preterm delivery.

However, in asymptomatic pregnant women, NICE does not recommend routine screening for BV because there is no evidence that identifying and treating it makes any difference to the preterm birth rates. In HIV-positive pregnant women, bacterial vaginosis increases the risk of mother-to-child transmission of HIV.

Oral metronidazole is the treatment of choice but not the single high-dose regimen.

Sources: British Association for Sexual health and HIV (BASHH) 'Guideline on Bacterial Vaginosis' (2012) www.bashh.org; NICE Clinical Knowledge Summary on bacterial vaginosis (2014) www.nice.org.uk

22 Vaginal birth after caesarean (VBAC) used to be known as 'trial of scar'. Which of the following signs or symptoms would prompt concern that a previous caesarean scar is dehiscing during labour in a woman having a VBAC?

A. Contractions become more painful
B. Leakage of liquor per vaginam

C. Maternal bradycardia

D. Slow progress of labour

E. ***Uterine contractions cease**

The main symptom of dehiscence is continuous pain (in between contractions) that will not be masked by an epidural. Signs include fresh vaginal bleeding, fetal distress, and cessation of contractions.

23 A primigravid woman who is 16 weeks pregnant asks for advice because she has been exposed to a case of chickenpox 5 days ago. She cannot remember having chickenpox as a child and there is nothing about that in her records at the surgery so a serum test was taken just after exposure which was negative for IgG antibodies. Select the most appropriate management option:

A. Administer oral acyclovir for 7 days

B. ***Give varicella zoster immune globulin (VZIG) as soon as possible**

C. Intravenous acyclovir

D. Order sputum culture and chest x-ray

E. Prescribe a course of zanamivir or oseltamivir

All nonimmune pregnant women exposed to varicella should be given VZIG as soon as possible after exposure. It is effective up to 10 days after contact and can be delayed until serology results are known.

Source: RCOG Green-top Guideline, No. 13, 'Chickenpox in Pregnancy' (2015).

24 A woman has chosen to deliver her third baby at home and has gone into labour at 38 weeks of gestation. The community midwife has only just left the labour ward on her way to the house, having collected a cylinder of Entonox. The woman's husband telephones the surgery to say that her waters have just gone and he can see the cord hanging out of the vagina.

Select the most appropriate instruction to give him on the telephone:

A. Encourage his wife to start pushing

B. Push the cord back in to her vagina

C. ***Put her into the knee-chest position**

D. Take her straight to hospital in the car

E. Wrap the cord in a warm towel

The most important thing is to get the presenting part off the cord so it does not compress it. Replacing the cord in the vagina or wrapping it in a towel is not advised as handling of the cord should be kept to a minimum.

Source: RCOG Green-top Guideline, No. 50 on 'Umbilical Cord Prolapse' (2014).

25 A nulliparous woman whose partner is HIV positive wishes to get pregnant whilst minimising her risk of HIV infection through unprotected intercourse with her partner. He is compliant with his HAART and is clinically well.

What advice should be given?

A. Avoid sexual intercourse until he has a plasma viral load of less than 5,000 copies/ml

B. HIV transmission can be eliminated by sperm washing and intrauterine insemination

C. Prescribe broad spectrum antibiotics to cover intercourse

D. She should be prescribed HAART as well

E. ***Unprotected intercourse should be limited to the time of ovulation**

Sperm washing reduces, but does not eliminate, the risk of HIV transmission.

She should be screened for other infections but you would not offer routine prophylaxis.

There is nothing to be gained by the female partner taking HAART.

He should have a viral load of less than 50 copies per ml in the 6 months before attempting conception.

Source: NICE guideline CG156 `Fertility problems: assessment and treatment' clinical guideline on Fertility (updated 2016).

26 An USS was performed to locate a 45-year-old woman's intrauterine copper device because the strings were not visible when she attended the surgery to have it changed. The abdominal USS report confirmed that the IUD was in the uterine cavity but also found a 5 cm complex ovarian cyst with no free fluid in the pelvis. She has no symptoms at all, so this is an incidental finding.

Select the best management option:

A. Another scan in a few weeks to see if the cyst has gone

B. Change the IUD and ignore the cyst as it is <7 cm

C. Refer for diagnostic laparoscopy

D. Send blood for all the tumour markers including AFP and hCG

E. ***Serum CA125 level**

The cyst is complex so cannot be ignored.

CA125 is needed to work out the 'risk of malignancy index' (RMI) although the details on the scan are a little sparse and a repeat TV scan may be indicated.

Diagnostic laparoscopy is not usually helpful as we make management decisions on the RMI.

She does not need all the tumour markers as she is more than 40 years old so this is not likely to be an embryonic tumour.

Source: RCOG Green-top Guideline, No. 62, 'Management of Suspected Ovarian Masses in Premenopausal Women'. RCOG/BSGE Joint Guideline (2011).

27 You see a woman in clinic with urinary frequency and urgency who you suspect might have overactive bladder (detrusor instability) and counsel her about it.

Which of these statements is correct with regard to detrusor instability?

A. Bladder drill (retraining) is ineffective

B. It can be confidently diagnosed from the history without further investigation

C. ***It may be a symptom of multiple sclerosis**

D. It will respond to oral duloxetine

E. Pelvic floor physiotherapy is not indicated

It can be difficult to tell from her symptoms whether the diagnosis is unstable bladder or genuine stress incontinence. The bladder is an unreliable witness. For example, in patients with instability, a cough will provoke a detrusor contraction that results in urinary leakage. if the woman has mixed symptoms, a bladder pressure study is usually indicated to sort out the diagnosis.

Pelvic floor physiotherapy helps both genuine stress incontinence and instability.

28   Women with a BMI > 30 at booking are at increased risk of vitamin D deficiency and are advised to supplement their diet with 10 micrograms of vitamin D daily during pregnancy and breast-feeding.

The main reason for taking vitamin D is:

A.   To prevent haemorrhagic disease of the newborn

B.   To prevent intrauterine growth restriction

C.   To prevent neural tube defects

D.   To prevent pre-eclampsia

E.   ***To prevent rickets in the neonate**

Prepregnancy BMI is inversely associated with serum vitamin D concentrations and obese pregnant women are at increased risk. A quarter of women in the United Kingdom aged 19 to 24 are at risk of vitamin D deficiency, probably because we do not get enough exposure to sunlight.

Source: CMACE/RCOG Joint Guideline, 'Management of Women with Obesity in Pregnancy' (2010).

29   In the 2014 MBRRACE report on maternal deaths there was a decrease in the maternal mortality rate to 10.12 maternal deaths. What is the denominator for the maternal mortality rate?

A.   The number of maternal deaths per hundred deliveries

B.   ***The number of maternal deaths per hundred thousand maternities**

C.   The number of maternal deaths per million maternities

D.   The number of maternal deaths per thousand maternities

E.   The number of maternal deaths per thousand pregnancies

30   A 45-year-old woman presenting with urinary incontinence is diagnosed with overactive bladder and starts treatment with immediate-release oxybutynin tablets. She reads on the leaflet that constipation can be a side effect.

Which of these statements is appropriate advice to give her regarding this side effect of oxybutynin?

A.   ***Adverse effects such as constipation indicate that the treatment is starting to work**

B.   Constipation side effects should prompt cessation of treatment

C.   Laxatives will not work if she continues to take the oxybutynin

D.   Every patient should routinely take laxatives whilst they are taking oxybutynin

E.   The chance of the tablets causing constipation is less than 1 per cent

Constipation is very common and should be treated as in any other patient, rather than stopping the anticholinergics.

Source: NICE Guideline, No. CG171, 'Urinary Incontinence in Women'. Published 2013, updated 2015.

31 A 23-year-old woman presents to the surgery complaining of intermenstrual and postcoital bleeding. She is not using any contraception as she is trying to get pregnant.

Select the most likely diagnosis:

A. Cervical polyp
B. ***Chlamydia infection**
C. Endometrial polyp
D. Nabothian follicle on the cervix
E. Squamous cancer of the cervix

In a woman of this age, chlamydia is relatively common and cervical/endometrial polyps are not. Nabothian follicles are mucous retention cysts on the cervix and are covered with normal epithelium, so they don't bleed. Squamous cancer of the cervix, whilst it does occur in women under 25 years, is rare.

32 Obstetric units often audit the decision-to-delivery interval for caesarean section as a marker of their performance. According to the 2011 NICE guideline, what should the interval be for a category 2 caesarean section where there is maternal or fetal compromise that is not immediately life threatening?

A. 30 minutes
B. 45 minutes
C. 60 minutes
D. ***75 minutes**
E. No time limit for this category

The urgency of a caesarean is standardised to ensure clear communication between staff, but NICE only suggests a time limit for the first two categories – 30 minutes for category 1 (immediate threat) and 75 minutes for category 2.

Source: NICE Guideline, No. CG132

'Caesarean section'. Published 2011, updated 2012.

33 An immigrant woman presents late for antenatal care at 39 weeks of gestation having just arrived in the country from Latvia. The baby is presenting by the breech and external cephalic version is indicated but she cannot sign the consent form as she has no English at all.

Select the best course of action with regard to consent for the procedure:

A. Ask her husband to sign the consent form
B. ***Find a translator**
C. Get permission through a court order
D. Give her a leaflet in Latvian to read and then ask her to sign
E. Ignore as consent not needed because it is not an operation

Where a woman's capacity to consent is in doubt legal advice is obtained in accordance with the Mental Capacity Act 2005, but the main issue here is to find someone, preferably not a relative, to translate whilst consent is obtained. Most Trusts in the United Kingdom have access to facilities such as 'language line' although this is time consuming and difficult.

Relatives cannot consent on behalf of an adult patient.

34   A woman whose BMI is 42 books for antenatal care in her fourth pregnancy. She is 27 years old and her general health is good although she does smoke ten cigarettes daily. Her previous pregnancies and deliveries have been straightforward.

Select the most appropriate recommendation regarding low molecular weight heparin (LMWH) for thromboprophylaxis in her case?

A.   LMWH antenatally only if she develops two more risk factors

B.   ***LMWH for 1 week postnatally if she has a normal delivery**

C.   LMWH for 6 weeks postnatally regardless of the mode of delivery

D.   LMWH is not effective enough for morbidly obese women

E.   LMWH throughout pregnancy and for 6 weeks postpartum

All women with a BMI > 40 should be offered postnatal thromboprophylaxis regardless of their mode of delivery for a minimum of 1 week. If a woman with a BMI > 30 has two additional risk factors she should be offered LMWH antenatally – this woman has only one (smoking). If a woman has been given antenatal LMWH because she is high risk, then it should be continued for 6 weeks postpartum.

Source: CMACE/RCOG Joint Guideline, 'Management of Women with Obesity in Pregnancy' (2010) and RCOG Green-top Guideline, No. 37a, 'Thrombosis and Embolism during Pregnancy and the Puerperium, Reducing the Risk' (2015).

35   A primigravid woman at 33 weeks of gestation is referred to the antenatal clinic because the uterine fundus is large for dates. USS reveals a very high amniotic fluid index, confirming the diagnosis of polyhydramnios.

Which is the most appropriate next investigation?

A.   Cardiotocograph

B.   ***Glucose tolerance test**

C.   Pass a nasogastric tube when the infant is delivered

D.   Serial growth scans

E.   Toxoplasmosis IgM titre

Fifty to sixty per cent of cases are idiopathic.

Maternal diabetes should be excluded as it would alter the antenatal care.

If there is a trachea-oesophageal fistula in association with an oesophageal atresia, you can still see a stomach bubble because the amniotic fluid passes down the trachea, so all babies with polyhydramnios need an nasogastric tube passing at delivery to check for patency.

You need to exclude parvovirus too, which is not part of a TORCH screen.

Source: The Obstetrician and Gynaecologist, 'Polyhydramnios in Singleton Pregnancies', 16 (3) (2014).

36   You are asked to review a woman who had a forceps delivery of her first baby 12 hours ago after a long labour because she is keen to go home. The midwives are unhappy to let her leave the hospital yet because she has not passed urine since delivery.

Which statement is correct with regard to the management of her bladder and urine output?

A.   Dehydration is the most likely cause

B.   Intermittent self-catheterisation is inadvisable straight after delivery

C.   Referral to urology is indicated

D.   ***She is at risk of long-term detrusor failure**

E.   Voiding problems are likely to be related to damage to her bladder from the forceps

Retention of urine postpartum may go unrecognised unless midwifery staff are vigilant. Overdistension of the bladder can result in detrusor failure and long-term voiding problems, which could result in the woman having to self-catheterise. Midwives will normally catheterise a woman who has not passed urine by 6 hours postpartum to prevent this happening. There is no need to involve urology at this stage.

37   The following women leave the pre-op clinic without having their full blood count (FBC) taken and the nurse asks you if they need to be called back to the clinic.

   In which case does it not matter, that is, which of them does not really need to have it done before the operation?

A.   27-year-old woman having an ovarian cystectomy

B.   ***30-year-old woman being sterilised laparoscopically**

C.   40-year-old woman having an endometrial ablation

D.   42-year-old woman having a hysteroscopy for menorrhagia

E.   50-year-old woman undergoing cystoscopy for recurrent infections

The woman being sterilised is not likely to be anaemic, neither is she likely to bleed during the operation.

38   A woman books with a community midwife in her first pregnancy and gives a history of having being treated for manic episodes whilst at university. She has been well since and is not currently under the care of a psychiatrist or taking any medication.

   Which information is correct in terms of the effect of her mental health history on the pregnancy?

A.   ***Bipolar disorder is a strong predictor for postpartum psychosis**

B.   Her risk of developing puerperal psychosis is 2 per 1,000

C.   She is more likely to become mentally ill during pregnancy than postpartum

D.   She is unlikely to commit suicide once the baby is born

E.   The history of bipolar disorder will not affect the pregnancy at all

The incidence in the general population is 2 per 1,000 births, but women with a previous history of bipolar disorder are much more at risk and the chance of developing psychosis is as high as 30 to 50 per cent in some studies. The incidence increases rapidly after delivery – 50 per cent present within the first week after birth, 75 per cent within the first 6 weeks, and 90 per cent within 90 days.

Suicide is an important preventable cause of maternal death in the United Kingdom and the mode of suicide in puerperal psychosis is often violent, unlike the way in which women 'normally' kill themselves, that is, overdose. Unfortunately, these mothers commit suicide in such a way that they cannot be rescued. In the 2006–2008 CEMACE Report, 31 per cent of suicide deaths were due to hanging, another 31 per cent due to jumping from a height, whereas only 10 per cent were associated with taking an overdose.

Source: 'Review of Postnatal Affective Disorders,' The Obstetrician and Gynaecologist 10 (3) (2008) MBRRACE-UK report `Saving lives, improving mothers' care' – latest version December 2016; www.npeu.ox.ac.uk NICE Guideline, `Antenatal and Postnatal Mental Health: clinical management and service guidance' (updated 2015).

39 A 24-year-old primigravid primary school teacher is in the early third trimester when one of her pupils develops German measles. On review of the woman's previous blood tests during pregnancy, there are no rubella IgG antibodies detected.

Select the most appropriate course of action:

A. ***Defer rubella vaccine until postnatal period**
B. Give rubella vaccine to her immediately
C. Prescribe rubella immunoglobulin to reduce the chance of infection
D. Reassure that no further action necessary at any stage
E. Refer to hospital for a scan

If she does not have IgG antibodies then she is not immune, but the pregnancy is third trimester so it is less worrying in terms of fetal effects, even if she gets rubella during pregnancy. You cannot vaccinate during pregnancy as it is a live attenuated virus vaccine. There is no immunoglobulin that will prevent her getting rubella. There is nothing to be gained by scanning the fetus (although middle cerebral artery Doppler looking for fetal anaemia is done following parvovirus infection).

40 A 39-year-old woman with a BMI of 39 requests referral to gynaecology clinic for laparoscopic sterilisation. She has four children all delivered by caesarean section and currently uses barrier contraception. She has recently been diagnosed with type 2 diabetes and gives a history of heavy intermenstrual bleeding for 6 months.

Which is the most appropriate initial management option?

A. Arrange vasectomy instead
B. Opportunistic cervical smear
C. Pelvic USS
D. ***Refer for endometrial biopsy**
E. Suggest Mirena® IUS insertion

This woman is at risk of endometrial pathology such as hyperplasia or cancer because she is diabetic and overweight, in spite of being under the age of 40. Planning her contraception takes second place to diagnosing her irregular bleeding.

41 A pregnant woman in the first trimester has just been in contact with a patient with swine flu (H1N1) and seeks advice having seen posters about the condition in your surgery. She has asthma but no other medical problems and is currently well with no respiratory symptoms at all

Which of the following is correct advice to give in this situation?

A. Asthma is a contraindication to vaccination against swine flu
B. She should have antiviral therapy instead of the vaccine
C. The safety of H1N1 vaccines in the first trimester is well documented

D.   *The vaccination should be offered immediately

E.   Vaccination is contraindicated in pregnancy

Asthma is associated with an increase in respiratory complications and pregnant women are more likely to have serious complications requiring hospital admission. Although the safety of H1N1 vaccines in the first trimester is unknown, closely related vaccines have been shown to be safe with no increased risk of miscarriage or fetal abnormality.

The vaccination should be given but may not be effective at this stage because the patient may already have contracted swine flu, and be in the incubation phase. In any case vaccination is not fully effective for 3 weeks and is not wholly protective (75 per cent effective).

The patient needs to be advised to look out for early signs of infection to allow early treatment with antiviral therapy but it is not used as prevention.

RCOG/RCM Joint statement on Swine flu (2009) www.rcog.org.uk; MMBRACE-UK 2014 report covering the swine flu epidemic in 2011.

42   Following a course of supervised physiotherapy for stress incontinence, a 48-year-old woman still experiences frequent episodes of incontinence of urine. She is about to go to Australia for 2 months and is seeking further help with her symptoms so that her holiday is not spoiled by incontinence.

Select the most appropriate advice:

A.   *Duloxetine tablets

B.   Electrical stimulation to levator ani muscle

C.   Oxybutynin tablets

D.   Transvaginal tape procedure

E.   Wear a pad

This woman is seeking immediate help and surgery is not appropriate just before embarking on a long-haul flight. If she has already had a course of supervised physiotherapy it is not likely that electrical stimulation will make a difference quickly enough and the only pharmacological treatment on the list for stress incontinence is duloxetine.

43   A Jehovah's Witness is being seen in the pre-operative clinic. She is having a hysterectomy for menorrhagia and her haemoglobin is 90 gm/L.

Select the most appropriate management option:

A.   Arrange a 'cell saver' for the operation

B.   Cancel the operation as it is too dangerous

C.   *Postpone the operation and prescribe iron

D.   Prescribe erythropoietin

E.   Sign a Jehovah's Witness 'advance directive'

Transfusion of whole blood, including pre-operative autologous donation, and blood components is unacceptable to Jehovah's Witnesses but they don't usually object to cell-saver use or factors that stimulate erythropoiesis. They usually carry an Advance Decision Document listing which blood products and procedures are acceptable to them.

For this patient, all of the options are possible, but her procedure is not urgent and there is time to optimise her haemoglobin if the operation is postponed.

44 A woman attends surgery asking for fertility investigations as she stopped taking the pill 3 years ago and is not yet pregnant. She has a past history of an episode of pelvic inflammatory disease following a surgical termination of pregnancy as a teenager. Her partner's semen analysis is normal. Pelvic examination reveals a retroverted uterus that is slightly tender.

Which is the most suitable investigation for evaluating tubal factors in her case?

A. Hysterosalpingo-contrast-ultrasonography (HyCoSy)
B. Hysteroscopy
C. *Laparoscopy and dye test
D. Selective salpingography
E. X-ray Hysterosalpingography (HSG)

Women who are not known to have co morbidities (such as pelvic inflammatory disease, previous ectopic pregnancy, or endometriosis) should be offered HSG because this is a reliable test for ruling out tubal occlusion, and it is less invasive and makes more efficient use of resources than laparoscopy. Women who are thought to have comorbidities should be offered laparoscopy and dye so that tubal and other pelvic pathology can be assessed at the same time.

Source: NICE clinical guideline CG156 'Fertility problems: assessment and treatment'. Published 2013, updated 2016.

45 A primigravid woman has been in labour all day and on an oxytocin drip for the previous 8 hours. A decision is made for assisted vaginal delivery on account of delay in the second stage. There is no caput or moulding of the fetal head and the maternal condition is satisfactory.

Which of the following factors is essential before undertaking the delivery?

A. Arranging theatre as a difficult delivery is anticipated
B. Fetal head in the OA position
C. *Fully dilated cervix
D. Spinal analgesia
E. Normal fetal heart rate on the CTG

This should be an easy delivery as the baby's head is well engaged and there is no sign of cephalo-pelvic disproportion. We would only plan to do an assisted delivery in theatre if we thought there was a good chance of having to proceed to caesarean section. There should be adequate analgesia but a pudendal block may be sufficient. The factors that must be in place for a successful assisted delivery are that the fetal head is not palpable abdominally, the bladder and bowel are empty, the cervix is fully dilated, and the position of the head is known. The 'normal CTG' is unnecessary as often we perform assisted delivery because we are worried about the baby's condition and want to bring the second stage to an end quickly.

46 Regarding consent issues in contraceptive practice, which of these statements is correct?

A. Expressed (written or verbal) consent is needed for removal of subdermal implants
B. If a married woman is seeking sterilisation, her husband's consent should also be obtained

C.   Implied or nonverbal consent is inadequate for practical procedures
D.   ***Written consent and verbal consent are equally valid**
E.   Written consent is necessary for insertion or removal of IUDs

> *If a woman attends a clinic seeking contraceptive advice and chooses the IUD or implant methods, submitting herself to the insertion procedure implies consent. Most clinics seek verbal or written consent.*

47   A woman who has suffered recurrent miscarriages has been found to have a normal karyotype, as has her partner. Which of the following management plans should be recommended for this couple to increase the chances of a successful term pregnancy?

A.   Human chorionic gonadotrophin supplements until 12 weeks of gestation
B.   Investigating the woman for diabetes
C.   Prescribing progesterone during the first half of the pregnancy
D.   Refer for preimplantation genetic diagnosis at the fertility clinic
E.   ***Screening for antiphospholipid syndrome and prescribing aspirin and heparin if positive**

> *This is a difficult situation for couples to face and they are usually desperate to pursue any form of treatment that might increase their chances of a successful pregnancy. However, the only manoeuvres that have been proved to work are the identification and treatment of antiphospholipid syndrome and regular reassurance scans during the first trimester (can't explain why this should work).*

> *Source: RCOG Green-top Guideline, No. 17, 'The Investigation and Treatment of Couples with Recurrent First-Trimester and Second-Trimester Miscarriage'. Published 2011.*

48   In which of these situations is it advisable to perform an USS for a patient seeking termination of pregnancy?

A.   The doctor is hoping to persuade her against termination
B.   The patient is trying to choose between a medical or surgical method
C.   The patient is undecided whether to continue with the pregnancy or not
D.   The patient refuses vaginal examination
E.   ***The uterus is larger than expected for the gestational age**

> *If the uterus is large for dates she may have a multiple pregnancy, a molar pregnancy, or the dates may be wrong. Ultrasound does not usually aid the choice of method and should definitely not be used to upset the patient or pressurise her not to go ahead with termination, which must be her decision having weighed up the pros and cons. Counselling should be nonjudgemental.*

> *If she refuses vaginal examination you will not be sure of the gestation (and also lose the opportunity for STI screening).*

49   A primigravid woman presents to labour ward at 32 weeks of gestation with vaginal bleeding. She is stable and the baby is well, but she is known to be rhesus negative. Her clinical notes confirm that she had her prophylactic anti-D injection at 28 weeks of gestation, administered by her midwife.

Select the most appropriate management option

A.   Administer 250 IU anti-D and perform Kleihauer test
B.   Administer 500 IU anti-D

C. ***Administer 500 IU anti-D and perform Kleihauer test**
D. Ask the lab to check for residual anti-D from her prophylactic injection
E. No action necessary

She still needs anti-D in view of the recent bleed because the prophylactic dose will not cover this new event. There will be residual anti-D in her circulation, so you need to let the lab know about her prophylactic dose. She gets 500 IU because the gestation is more than 20 weeks. The Kleihauer test is necessary because you have to make sure that the dose is enough to cover the amount of feto-maternal haemorrhage that has occurred.

50 A woman who has been on thyroxine 100 micrograms for 5 years attends surgery for antenatal booking at 8 weeks of gestation. The community midwife asks for your opinion.

Select the most appropriate management:

A. Leave the dose of thyroxine unchanged and refer to endocrine clinic
B. Leave the dose of thyroxine unchanged and refer to obstetric clinic
C. Leave the dose of thyroxine unchanged and refer to obstetric endocrine clinic
D. Increase the dose of thyroxine and refer to endocrine clinic
E. ***Increase the dose of thyroxine and refer to obstetric endocrine clinic**

The requirement for thyroxine is increased in pregnancy by 30 to 50 per cent above the preconception dosage. In addition, the absorption of thyroxine may be reduced, so it is important to increase the dose early in pregnancy. There is evidence of a higher miscarriage rate and psychomotor and IQ deficits in infants born to mothers with undiagnosed or inadequately treated hypothyroidism (including subclinical hypothyroidism).

Source: NICE Clinical Knowledge Summary 'Hypothyroidism' (2016) www.cks .nice.org.uk.

51 A woman attends the Early Pregnancy Unit for a scan at 8 weeks of gestation because she had a salpingectomy for a left-sided ectopic a year ago. She is asymptomatic but the scan shows an empty uterus with a mass in the right adnexa, thought to be another ectopic pregnancy. Methotrexate treatment is discussed to give her a chance of retaining her remaining fallopian tube.

Which factor would suggest surgical management is more appropriate than medical management of this second ectopic pregnancy?

A. Adnexal mass measuring 15 mm
B. hCG level of 500 IU/L
C. Previous ruptured ectopic pregnancy
D. No fetal heartbeat in the ectopic sac on scan
E. ***Patient has significant pain**

NICE Guideline 154 on ectopic pregnancy and miscarriage states that surgery should be offered if:

- The patient has significant pain
- There is an adnexal mass of 35 mm or larger
- There is a fetal heartbeat visible on scan in the ectopic sac
- Serum hCG is 50,000 IU/L or more

52 A woman is admitted to hospital at 36 weeks of gestation because she has suspected H1N1 influenza. She is tachycardic, her temperature is 38°C, and she seems to be breathing very fast.

What is the upper threshold for the normal respiratory rate in pregnancy?

A. 10 breaths per minute
B. 15 breaths per minute
C. ***20 breaths per minute**
D. 25 breaths per minute
E. 30 breaths per minute

53 A woman who is expecting her third child attends surgery at 36 weeks of gestation complaining of pain from symphysis pubis dysfunction.

Select the most appropriate management option:

A. Ask the obstetric team to arrange early induction of labour
B. ***Obstetric physiotherapy appointment**
C. Prescribe nonsteroidal antiinflammatory drugs
D. Refer to an orthopaedic surgeon
E. Suggest elective caesarean delivery

Neither induction of labour nor caesarean delivery are recommended in this condition although the patients put their clinicians under severe pressure to arrange this. Spontaneous onset of labour and normal delivery offer the best prospects of recovering quickly after birth. Nonsteroidals are contraindicated because of the theoretical risk of causing premature closure of the ductus. Physiotherapy and analgesia are the mainstays of treatment.

54 Women with Turner syndrome sometimes have a mosaic karyotype where some cell lines have 45XO and some 46XX chromosomes.

Which of these statements is true about Turner mosaic patients?

A. They are all of short stature just like 45XO Turner women
B. ***They are at risk of osteoporosis at an early age**
C. They cannot have children
D. They do not have any other Turner-associated congenital abnormalities such as renal tract
E. They do not usually have a uterus

Women with karyotype 45XO are usually of short stature, but women with a mosaic karyotype can be of normal height. They have small ovaries but normal pelvic organs otherwise. They usually present with secondary amenorrhoea as teenagers but can have children using donated eggs as long as they have received enough estrogen to grow the uterus to normal proportions at puberty.

They are at risk of osteoporosis because of low estrogen levels and need HRT until normal menopausal age.

55 Chorionic villus sampling can be used to detect sex-linked inherited conditions as well as trisomies. When counselling a woman choosing to have this test done, which of these statements is correct information to give her?

A. It can only be done in the first trimester of pregnancy
B. ***It carries a small risk of limb reduction defects in the fetus**

C. The test is able to detect neural tube defects
D. The result is available in about a week
E. There is a miscarriage risk of 3 to 5 per cent

CVS refers to taking a biopsy of the placenta and can be done at any gestation but tends to be called placental biopsy when performed later in pregnancy. The idea is that women can get a diagnosis early enough in pregnancy to allow surgical termination but the earlier it is done, the more chance of harm to the fetus. The risk of limb reduction defects is the main reason that it is deferred until 11 weeks rather than being done earlier in pregnancy.

56 **In women considering using POP that do not contain desogestrel for contraception, which of the following applies?**

A. The bleeding pattern is likely to be amenorrhoea
B. The efficacy is reduced if the women weigh more than 75 kg
C. ***They should not be used in women with breast cancer (UKMEC4)**
D. They are not suitable for women who are breast-feeding
E. They have a 12-hour window in which to take a pill they have missed

POPs are well known for producing an unpredictable bleeding pattern: 20 per cent amenorrhoea, 40 per cent irregular, and 40 per cent of women with a normal pattern. This leads to discontinuation of the method in between 10 and 25 per cent of users within the first year of use.

There is no evidence that the efficacy of POPs is reduced in women with a high BMI although many practitioners prescribe double doses for them.

Cerazette®, which contains desogestrel, has a 12-hour window; the others only have 3 hours.

57 **Regarding the duties of a doctor, which of these statements is correct?**

A. A chaperone is needed for gynaecological pelvic examinations only if the doctor is male
B. Consent is not required for anomaly scans performed at 20 weeks of gestation
C. ***If you see a child with a proven sexually transmitted infection this must always be reported**
D. When consenting a patient for a surgical procedure, only common complications need to be discussed
E. When treating a patient for a sexually transmitted infection, you always have a duty to inform the spouse regardless of the patient's consent

It is good practice to offer a chaperone for consultations whatever the sex of the doctor. Anomaly scans do require consent although this can be verbal or written.

If you diagnose a child with a sexually transmitted infection the child protection services must be informed as the age of consent is 16 years in England and Wales, under the Sexual Offences Act 2003.

Complications that are rare but of important consequence to the patient must be discussed when obtaining consent.

Confidentiality prevents you from informing a spouse about a sexually transmitted infection without consent although it is your duty to try and persuade them to allow disclosure. However, if the benefit to the spouse's health outweighs the patient's confidentiality, such as with HIV infection, the situation may be different. You would be well advised to discuss with your defence/protection society.

58 Which of these is a characteristic feature of physiological jaundice in the newborn?

A. Associated anaemia

B. Disappearance by the fourth day

C. Does not lead to kernicterus if not treated

D. Occurs more frequently in postdates infants

E. *Onset after the first 24 hours of life*

Physiological jaundice usually peaks at 2 to 4 days of life and resolves within 2 weeks. If the baby is also anaemic there could be a more sinister cause associated with haemolysis and further investigation is warranted. Phototherapy is very effective at reducing bilirubin levels so kernicterus is possible but a rare event.

59 A 34-year-old woman has always attended for regular cervical screening and all her tests so far have been normal.

In which of the following circumstances would it be appropriate to take a smear from her?

A. She discovers a family history of cervical cancer

B. She is noted on examination to have a cervical erosion

C. She presents with a history of postcoital bleeding

D. She presents with a new diagnosis of genital warts

E. *Three years after her previous cervical screen*

Genital warts are a different virus from CIN so this would not be an indication for an opportunistic smear; neither is there a genetic component. Postcoital bleeding could be due to cervical cancer but she needs a speculum examination not a smear. Cervical erosions are irrelevant. At the age of 34, she will be on a three-yearly screening programme.

60 NICE Guidelines suggest that low-dose aspirin (75 mg daily) is now recommended from 12 weeks of gestation to prevent pre-eclampsia in some pregnant women.

Which of these pregnant women should be taking low-dose aspirin?

A. *Chronic hypertension*

B. Family history of pre-eclampsia

C. Maternal age more than 40 years

D. Multiple pregnancy

E. Pregnancy interval of greater than 10 years

If a woman has one high-risk factor (previous hypertensive disease in pregnancy, chronic kidney disease, autoimmune disease such as SLE, antiphospholipid syndrome, diabetes mellitus, or chronic hypertension) or two moderate-risk factors (first pregnancy, age 40 or over, pregnancy interval > 10 years, BMI >35, family history, or multiple pregnancy) she should take aspirin from 12 weeks of gestation until term.

Source: NICE Guideline, No. CG107 'Hypertension in Pregnancy: diagnosis and management' Published 2010, updated 2011.

www.nice.org.uk.

Useful Web Addresses

www.rcog.org.uk for Green-Top Guidelines/advice on consent/patient information leaflets

www.gmc-uk.org for 'Duties of a Doctor', ethical issues and consent

www.fsrh.org for Faculty of Reproductive and Sexual Health clinical guidance/ UK Medical Eligibilty Criteria for contraceptive use

www.bashh.org for genito-urinary medicine guidance (British Association for Sexual Health and HIV)

www.nice.org.uk for NICE guidance and clinical knowledge summaries on many women's health topics

www.cancerscreening.nhs.uk for information on cervical screening and human papilloma virus vaccination

www.fpa.org.uk for contraception and abortion information

www.fetalanomaly.screening.nhs.uk for details of the NHS Fetal Anomaly Screening Programme (FASP)

www.bhiva.org for clinical guidance about HIV

Index

abdominal bloating, diagnosis and management of, 87, 206
abdominal mass, assessment of, 84
abdominal pain, in non-pregnant women, 205–6
  copper coil IUD and, 98
  diagnosis of, 85–86, 205–6, 233–34, 241, 263–65
  ovarian torsion, 112
  pelvic inflammatory disease, 205
abdominal pain, in pregnancy
  diagnosis of, 84, 229, 258–59
  early pregnancy, 87
  ectopic pregnancy diagnosis, 107–8
  emergency care procedures, 41–42, 148–49
  group B streptococcus and, 60
  infectious disease and, 46
  pre-eclampsia and, 149
  vaginal bleeding and, 45
abdominal x-ray, intrauterine insertion complications, 129–30
abortion. *See* termination of pregnancy
acne, in adolescent patients, contraception for management of, 82, 201
actinomycosis, copper coil IUD and, 216
adenomyosis, 108, 206
adnexae tenderness
  diagnosis of, 85
  dysmenorrhoea, pelvic pain and dyspareunia, 85
  ectopic pregnancy and, 87
  pelvic inflammatory disease, 205
  in vitro fertilisation and, 13–14
adolescent patients
  abortion procedures in, 29, 132
  amenorrhoea in, 76, 231–32, 245, 261–62, 280
  cervical smears for, 210
  contraceptive counseling for, 82, 89–91, 95, 210, 211–12, 218

emergency contraception in, 98, 245, 279–80
human papilloma virus vaccine for, 12, 109
infectious disease and pregnancy in, 46
labour and delivery for, 58
menstrual bleeding in, 78, 195–96
postcoital bleeding in pregnancy and, 154
postpartum contraceptive counseling for, 67
pregnancy in, 39, 145
adult respiratory distress syndrome, pulmonary oedema and, 162
advance directives, 66, 182
advanced maternal age
  miscarriage and, 108
  oral contraception and, 183
  prenatal screening and, 147, 148
airway management
  anaesthesia in asthmatic patient and, 127
  placental delivery complications and, 167
amenorrhoea
  in adolescent patients, 76, 231–32, 245, 261–62, 280
  iliac fossa pain with, 84
  pregnancy diagnosis and, 19, 85, 262
  primary *vs.* secondary, 7, 103
  secondary sexual characteristics and, 76, 194
amnihook, 172
amniocentesis, Down syndrome screening, 148, 259–60
amniotic fluid volume, 250
  diabetic pregnancy patients, 37
amniotomy
  indications for, 165
  vaginal bleeding following, 59
anaemic patients, hysterectomy complications in, 28

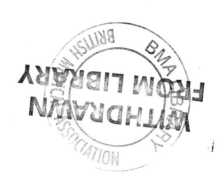